# THE FIGHT OF OUR LIVES

# DAVID LEVITHAN AND GABRIEL DUCKELS

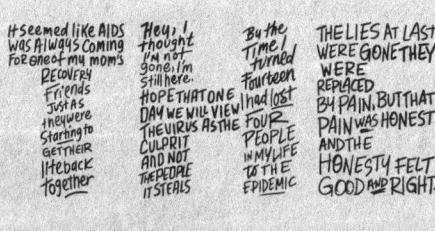

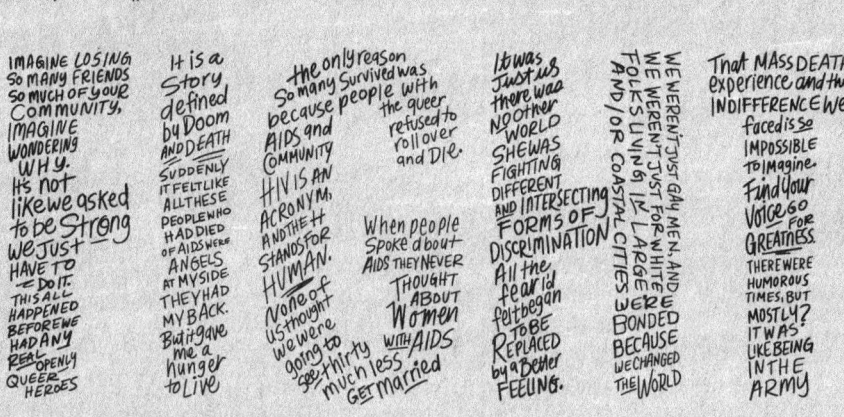

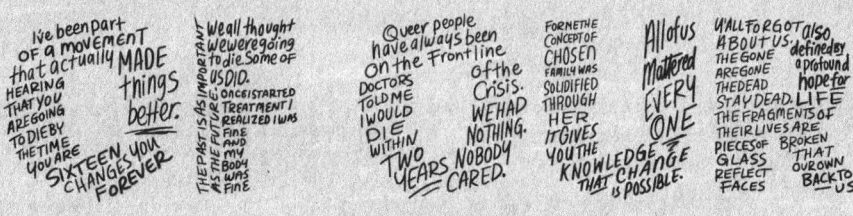

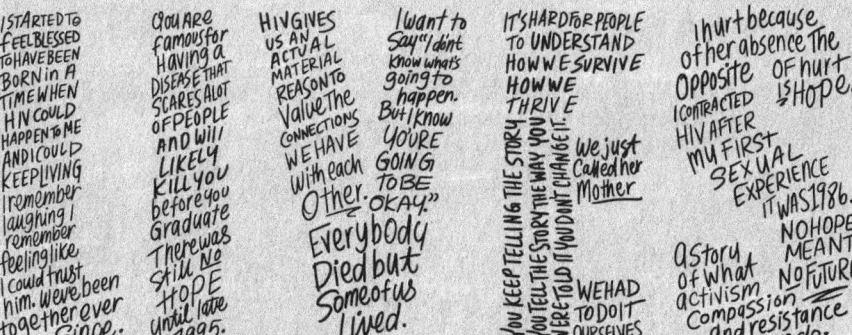

# AIDS IN AMERICA

ALFRED A. KNOPF • NEW YORK

A Borzoi Book published by Alfred A. Knopf
An imprint of Random House Children's Books
A division of Penguin Random House LLC
1745 Broadway, New York, NY 10019
penguinrandomhouse.com
getunderlined.com

Text copyright © 2026 by David Levithan and Gabriel Duckels
Interior illustrations (pages 330–341) copyright © 2026 by Brian Selznick

Penguin Random House values and supports copyright. Copyright fuels creativity, encourages diverse voices, promotes free speech, and creates a vibrant culture. Thank you for buying an authorized edition of this book and for complying with copyright laws by not reproducing, scanning, or distributing any part of it in any form without permission. You are supporting writers and allowing Penguin Random House to continue to publish books for every reader. Please note that no part of this book may be used or reproduced in any manner for the purpose of training artificial intelligence technologies or systems.

Knopf, Borzoi Books, and the colophon are registered trademarks of Penguin Random House LLC.

For permissions, see "Notes and Sources" on pages 439–453.

Library of Congress Cataloging-in-Publication Data is available upon request.
ISBN 978-0-593-71092-0 (trade)—ISBN 978-0-593-71093-7 (lib. bdg.)—
ISBN 978-0-593-71094-4 (ebook)

Book design by Cathy Bobak
The text of this book is set in 11-point Warnock Pro.
Title lettering by Alix Northrup

Manufactured in the United States of America
1st Printing

The authorized representative in the EU for product safety and compliance is Penguin Random House Ireland, Morrison Chambers, 32 Nassau Street, Dublin D02 YH68, Ireland, https://eu-contact.penguin.ie.

Random House Children's Books supports the First Amendment and celebrates the right to read.

*For all the people in this book, and everybody affected by HIV and AIDS, then and now.*

# CONTENTS

Prelude . . . . . . . . . . . . . . . . . . . . . . . . . . . . . . . . . . . . . . . . . . . . . . . . . . . . 1

A Note About This Book . . . . . . . . . . . . . . . . . . . . . . . . . . . . . . . . . . . . . 5

Some Terms Used in This Book . . . . . . . . . . . . . . . . . . . . . . . . . . . . . . 7

A Brief Overview of the AIDS Epidemic, in Facts
and Figures . . . . . . . . . . . . . . . . . . . . . . . . . . . . . . . . . . . . . . . . . . . . . . . 9

A Brief Overview of the AIDS Epidemic, Through the Story
of My Uncle, Robert Levithan . . . . . . . . . . . . . . . . . . . . . . . . . . . . . . 15

A Boy, Lost in History: Robert Rayford . . . . . . . . . . . . . . . . . . . . . . . 22

HIV and AIDS: The Basics . . . . . . . . . . . . . . . . . . . . . . . . . . . . . . . . . . 27

Timeline: 1978–1982 . . . . . . . . . . . . . . . . . . . . . . . . . . . . . . . . . . . . . . 31

The Accidental, Deliberate Poster Boy: Ryan White . . . . . . . . . . . . . 44

Complications . . . . . . . . . . . . . . . . . . . . . . . . . . . . . . . . . . . . . . . . . . . 59

"Health Care" by M.L. . . . . . . . . . . . . . . . . . . . . . . . . . . . . . . . . . . . . . 71

"June 25" by Essex Hemphill . . . . . . . . . . . . . . . . . . . . . . . . . . . . . . . 73

Testimony: Robert Levithan . . . . . . . . . . . . . . . . . . . . . . . . . . . . . . . . 75

Luna Luis Ortiz . . . . . . . . . . . . . . . . . . . . . . . . . . . . . . . . . . . . . . . . . . 79

Derinthia Williams . . . . . . . . . . . . . . . . . . . . . . . . . . . . . . . . . . . . . . . 92

Kalee Garland . . . . . . . . . . . . . . . . . . . . . . . . . . . . . . . . . . . . . . . . . . . 97

Timeline: 1983–1986 . . . . . . . . . . . . . . . . . . . . . . . . . . . . . . . . . . . . . 103

Young People Schoolin' Other Young People: Zines, Raps,
Comics, and Beyond . . . . . . . . . . . . . . . . . . . . . . . . . . . . . . . . . . . . . 124

*How to Have Sex in an Epidemic* and the Denver Principles . . . . . . . . . . 136

How to ACT UP When SILENCE=DEATH . . . . . . . . . . . . . . . . . . . . . . . 141

Peggy Sue . . . . . . . . . . . . . . . . . . . . . . . . . . . . . . . . . . . . . . . . . . . . . 156

"Stop the Church" .................................................. 171

Milo Miller ........................................................... 183

Fighting Words: Larry Kramer vs. Anthony Fauci ..................... 188

Addressing the Need: Needle Exchange and HIV/AIDS. ............... 201

Tina Valentin Aguirre. ............................................. 208

HIV Is Not a Deadly Weapon. ...................................... 223

Timeline: 1987–1991 ............................................... 228

As the World Watched: Rock Hudson and Magic Johnson ............ 245

"A Little Magic and a Lot of Faith" by Patricia Eldridge ............. 252

Pedro Zamora and the New Reality ................................ 256

What We Lost ..................................................... 262

Deaths in the Neighborhood. ...................................... 268

Ed Wolf. ........................................................... 276

Floyd Sklaver. ..................................................... 282

Blood Sisters. ..................................................... 286

John D'Amico ..................................................... 289

"Parachute" by Tim Dlugos ........................................ 295

Testimony: Robert Levithan ........................................ 299

"Tiara" by Mark Doty .............................................. 301

"What the Living Do" by Marie Howe ............................... 304

Elizabeth Coleman ................................................ 306

Todd Theringer. ................................................... 310

"Letter to Roger" by Deryl K. Deese ................................ 317

Ricky Tucker. ..................................................... 320

"Thousands of Angels" by Anna Forbes. ............................ 324

The Names ....................................................... 326

"Aunt Ida pieces a quilt" by Melvin Dixon ........................... 342

CONTENTS | ix

Refuge in Their Final Days . . . . . . . . . . . . . . . . . . . . . . . . . . . . . . . 346

Timeline: 1992–1996 . . . . . . . . . . . . . . . . . . . . . . . . . . . . . . . . . . . . 350

Testimony: Robert Levithan. . . . . . . . . . . . . . . . . . . . . . . . . . . . . . 366

"Non, Je Ne Regrette Rien" by David Warren Frechette . . . . . . . . . . . . . . . . 372

"Litany" by Christopher Gorman. . . . . . . . . . . . . . . . . . . . . . . . . 375

Timeline: 1997–Present . . . . . . . . . . . . . . . . . . . . . . . . . . . . . . . . . 379

Mallery Jenna Robinson. . . . . . . . . . . . . . . . . . . . . . . . . . . . . . . . . 395

Q . . . . . . . . . . . . . . . . . . . . . . . . . . . . . . . . . . . . . . . . . . . . . . . . . . . 401

Justin Smith. . . . . . . . . . . . . . . . . . . . . . . . . . . . . . . . . . . . . . . . . . . 404

Kay Poyer. . . . . . . . . . . . . . . . . . . . . . . . . . . . . . . . . . . . . . . . . . . . . 409

Antonio Boone . . . . . . . . . . . . . . . . . . . . . . . . . . . . . . . . . . . . . . . . 416

Sarah Schulman . . . . . . . . . . . . . . . . . . . . . . . . . . . . . . . . . . . . . . . 419

"Remembrance" by Kenneth McCreary . . . . . . . . . . . . . . . . . . . . 426

"Happy Anniversary" by Robert Vazquez-Pacheco . . . . . . . . . . . . . . . . . . . 427

"Little Prayer" by Danez Smith . . . . . . . . . . . . . . . . . . . . . . . . . . . . 429

Excerpt from "Committing to Memory" by Paul Monette . . . . . . . . . . . . . 430

Excerpt from "The Tomb of Sorrow" by Essex Hemphill. . . . . . . . . . . . . . . 432

Testimony: Robert Levithan . . . . . . . . . . . . . . . . . . . . . . . . . . . . . 434

Notes and Sources. . . . . . . . . . . . . . . . . . . . . . . . . . . . . . . . . . . . . 439

Bibliography . . . . . . . . . . . . . . . . . . . . . . . . . . . . . . . . . . . . . . . . . . 455

Suggested Reading on the Global AIDS Crisis . . . . . . . . . . . . . . . . . . . . . 459

Acknowledgments. . . . . . . . . . . . . . . . . . . . . . . . . . . . . . . . . . . . . 461

Resources . . . . . . . . . . . . . . . . . . . . . . . . . . . . . . . . . . . . . . . . . . . 465

# Prelude

This is a story of what fear, ignorance, and prejudice can do.
It is also a story of what activism, compassion, and resistance can do.
It is a story defined by doom and death.
It is also defined by a profound hope for life.

Imagine ten of your friends.
Now imagine that six or seven of them have an incurable, deadly disease.
You rage against the indifferent government that won't stop what's killing them. You sit at their bedsides, keep vigil as they struggle, diminish, and grasp. You attend their funerals, except when their parents say you are not welcome, covering the truth with their own versions. You try to keep track of the friends and acquaintances you have lost. Eventually, there are so many, you lose count.
Death is everywhere, and there isn't a thing you can do to stop it—except pressure the people who *can* do something to stop it. The federal government. Local governments. Drug companies. The general public. You want to scream at people in the supermarket to make them listen to you. You want to shake any news reporter who isn't paying attention. You want to overpower the self-righteous bystanders who say that people like you had it coming, that you deserve to die.
It is a seemingly endless fight. And as friend after friend keeps dying, you wonder if you will be next.

You cannot do much alone. But there is strength as a community. The enemies wanted people with AIDS to give up, give in, go quietly.

They did not.

But as in any war, many died along the way.

The AIDS crisis refers to a distinct period between the early 1980s and the mid-1990s, when hundreds of thousands of people in the United States faced a deadly new disease that had no treatment and no cure. It is hard for us now to imagine the devastation, the grief, the injustice that the generations before us went through. Diagnosis as a near-certain death sentence. Being given a year, maybe two, to live. And even now, nearly thirty years since the first successful treatments were found, people still become HIV+ and people still die from AIDS-related illness. Because HIV/AIDS continues to be aided and abetted by forces of bigotry, indifference, and shame.

We are going to ask you to start here:
  Imagine losing so many friends, so much of your community.
  Imagine wondering why.
  Imagine finding a way to fight back.

By the start of the twenty-first century, combination therapy meant that HIV no longer had to be a death sentence for people with access to health care. But by that time, almost *half a million* Americans had died. As we finish this book, just over a million people in the United States are living with HIV. Combination therapy means that many of these people are able to live healthy, fulfilling lives, in which being HIV+ doesn't have to be any different from having any other chronic condition. These are the two inextricably connected pieces of HIV history: the terrible legacy of the AIDS crisis in the United States in the 1980s and 1990s and the unresolved but vastly improved circumstances for HIV+ people today.

We tell this story because it is dangerous to forget it. We tell this story because as much as it is a story of negligence and suffering, it is also a story of activism and fighting back. It's as much about life as it is about death. It is a story of protest—on both individual and community levels. It is a story of doing everything you can to sound the alarm until those in power find the alarm more unbearable than the silence.

There are so many voices who were lost. We gather some of them here, even as we acknowledge the many who died without leaving written traces. For some, there wasn't enough time to get their stories down in the suddenness of their dying. For others, there was a record left behind . . . but then it fell into the hands of the family members who wanted to deny how they'd lived. Insult on top of injury; invisibility on top of death. It only made the rest of us more defiant, more determined to never be erased.

We honor all those who survived. We are grateful to a number of them for talking to us so you can read their stories here in their own words. There are now generations of queer people who weren't alive in the 1980s and 1990s, who can't possibly remember what it was like unless we tell them. Ours has always been an oral history, often told in whispers and code. But now it can be a matter of public record, and we can bring the past back to life.

The story of HIV/AIDS in America is a complicated one, with hundreds of thousands of characters and just as many subplots. But at heart, the story is disturbingly simple: At a time when LGBTQ+ people in America were starting to make progress in our fight for equality, we were hit with a horrific disease, and many people were willing to let us die, along with so many others, whether in the United States or around the world.

At the start, HIV/AIDS had plenty of accomplices. Like bigotry. Like indifference. Like racism. And shame. AIDS did not just decimate the gay community; in America, almost half of all people with hemophilia died because of a tainted blood supply. As with so many plagues in America, poor people and people of color were disproportionately affected. Babies were born HIV+ because the virus was in their mothers' blood. People who were addicted to intravenous drugs were especially vulnerable, as were people living or working on the street, in no small part because society saw them as marginal, dispensable.

The only reason it wasn't worse, the only reason so many survived, was that people with AIDS and the queer community refused to roll over and die. We would not go quietly. We would not allow the government and the corporations to ignore us. With medical activism that was unprecedented in American history, people with AIDS and their allies fought back. Ultimately, far too late, treatments were found.

This is not a happy ending. There is no ending yet. There is still no cure. There are treatment and prevention options, but those treatment and prevention options cost money, creating a financial divide for medical health. And the bigotry, the indifference, the racism, the shame, and the homophobia sadly remain. As we write this, there are renewed existential threats on funding to fight HIV/AIDS, both in America and globally, from a hostile administration that seems willing to let people die in order to achieve its political aims.

This is why we are vigilant. We learned vigilance the hard way.

There are many lessons carried through these pages. At heart, there is this:

We, the generations after, must remember.

Many of us died.

Those of us who didn't must carry on in their names.

In order to do this, we need to know what happened. And why.

## A Note About This Book

This book is a mix of narrative nonfiction, interviews, reprinted works from the 1980s and 1990s, and a few creative approaches to tell the story of what happened during the AIDS epidemic. It is not a strictly chronological telling—rather than try to present things in a rigidly linear way, we will weave in and out of times and topics, hoping that in the assemblage we can tell as much of the story as possible within the number of pages we have.

The earliest and hardest decision we made was to limit our narrative to the United States. The AIDS epidemic is a massive global epidemic, and we cannot tell the worldwide story here with the depth we believe it deserves. For people who want to read more about the global experience of AIDS, we have listed other works in our suggested reading at the end.

Even keeping the scope to the United States, we know there is no way that we can convey all the stories from that time. We have done our best to create a representative sampling here, drawn from all the different genders, races, communities, and identities that were affected by HIV/AIDS. And at the same time, we are acutely aware that there will inevitably be important voices missing. Our hope is that this is just the start of our project, and not an end in itself.

If, as you are reading this book, it sometimes feels as if different pieces are crashing together, that is deliberately meant to echo (in some small way) the dissonance of living during the height of the AIDS crisis, before a treatment was discovered, and the reality of living with HIV now, when treatment is available. The tension between the past tense and the present tense is irresolvable: We ask you to stay with that tension. At the height of the crisis, people with HIV/AIDS had so much to navigate at once—health and politics and family and friends and activism and art and despair and getting through the day. The book will try to navigate many of these at the same time as well.

The chapters marked "Source Material" have not been altered from their original publication in the 1980s or 1990s. It is important to ground these sections in the times in which they were written, when the umbrella terms "LGBTQ+" and "queer" were not used like they are today. As a result, "gay" is often used as an umbrella term or the focus is given to gay men within the excerpts from the past, even though a number of other people (queer and nonqueer) were also devastated by the disease.

At certain junctures of the book, we present "Timeline" sections—these are meant to fill in the blanks of the overall history. But, again, we caution you that these timelines exist separately from the chapters surrounding them and are not meant to give the book a chronological structure.

There's also the matter of narration. Since the two of us wrote this book together, we may use an authorial "we" from time to time. When it slips into a first-person "I," we signpost who's speaking by putting one of our names in brackets.

We'll start with the definitions of a few terms we use a lot in the book, followed by two overviews, to give you a sense of the larger picture before we go into the specific stories.

## Some Terms Used in This Book

While these phrases and acronyms are defined within context throughout the book, we want to give you a brief primer here, for your reference as you read.

**ACT UP:** Stands for the AIDS Coalition to Unleash Power. Founded in 1987, this activist group was responsible for many of the most effective, audacious protests during the AIDS crisis, and it remains active today.

**AIDS:** Acquired Immune Deficiency Syndrome. It is diagnosed when HIV's infiltration of the body has reached the point where the immune system is seriously compromised.

**AIDS-related complications:** Because AIDS weakens a body's immune system, allowing germs (such as bacteria, viruses, and fungi) and toxins to do lethal damage, people do not die of AIDS itself, but instead die of the diseases that AIDS prevents the body from fighting off; these are often referred to as "AIDS-related complications."

**CDC:** The Centers for Disease Control and Prevention, the US government agency tasked with combating epidemics.

**FDA:** The Food and Drug Administration, responsible for the approval of all drugs for medical use.

**GRID:** Before doctors knew what AIDS was, they briefly (erroneously) called it this, for Gay-Related Immune Deficiency.

**HAART:** Highly Active Antiretroviral Therapy. In the 1990s, it was discovered that this combination of drugs could prevent HIV from replicating itself.

**HIV:** Human Immunodeficiency Virus—a virus that attacks and weakens a person's immune system.

**HIV+/HIV−:** Pronounced "HIV positive" and "HIV negative." If you are the former, you have HIV in your body, and if you are the latter, you do not.

**Kaposi's sarcoma (KS):** A rare form of cancer that can attack people with AIDS. People with Kaposi's sarcoma often get lesions—purple, brown, red, or pink marks that blotch across the body as the cancer progresses. These became strongly associated in the public's mind with what a person with AIDS looked like.

**PrEP:** Pre-exposure prophylaxis, a drug approved in 2012 to prevent HIV transmission.

**PWA:** Person With AIDS or People With AIDS. In the Denver Principles in 1983, activists insisted that these terms, and not "AIDS victim" or "AIDS victims," were the proper terms for those with AIDS, empowering them and not defining them by their disease.

**T-cells (or CD4 cells):** White blood cells that fight off infections. HIV attacks these cells and renders them useless. An HIV+ person's health is measured by the number of T-cells (or CD4 cells) they have per milliliter of blood. If someone's T-cell count drops below a dangerously low count of 200, they are diagnosed with AIDS.

**U=U:** Undetectable = Untransmittable. A development from the late 1990s. Once HIV is treated with the right medication, it will not show up on standard blood tests anymore, and cannot be passed from one person to another.

# A Brief Overview of the AIDS Epidemic, in Facts and Figures

When we talk about the AIDS crisis, we are most often describing a distinct period between the early 1980s and the mid-1990s when there was no treatment and AIDS spread unchecked around the world. First, there are the staggering numbers, the census of the sick and the dead. The figures below are from the Centers for Disease Control's *HIV/AIDS Surveillance Report* from 1980 through December 2001, the most accurate figures for the United States. Please keep in mind that because of the stigma involved, many AIDS cases went unreported and many AIDS deaths were said to have other causes—so these numbers are likely far lower than the real numbers. But even if they underrepresent, they still give a clear, painful view of the virus's deadly trajectory.

(Sources for all facts and figures in this book can be found in the Notes and Sources section at the end.)

## Before 1981: 100 new cases, 31 deaths

There is no single date when we can say the AIDS epidemic began. Because the virus can be present in the body for up to a decade before symptoms occur, it is impossible to pinpoint its emergence. As you will see in the case of Robert Rayford, there may have been isolated cases that went unnoticed by doctors before the 1980s. It is only when a few cases happen in a localized area that doctors begin to see a pattern.

## 1981: 339 new cases, 130 deaths

The first reports of a "gay pneumonia" or "gay cancer" appear in medical journals and local newspapers as clusters of young gay men in urban areas come down with unusual infections and/or a rare cancer called Kaposi's sarcoma. Similar conditions are also found in infants in New York City who contracted it from their mothers, pointing to the fact that the disease is not, in fact, unique to gay men.

## 1982: 1,201 new cases, 466 deaths

The Centers for Disease Control (CDC) uses the term AIDS (acquired immune deficiency syndrome) for the first time, replacing GRID (gay-related immune deficiency). The source of the disease and how it spreads are still unknown, nor is there any way to test for it. Cases are discovered in hemophiliacs, who have become infected through blood transfusions.

## 1983: 3,153 new cases, 1,511 deaths

AIDS wards begin to appear in hospitals in major cities. The CDC adds female partners of men with AIDS as an "at-risk" group, and also warns blood banks of a possible problem with the US blood supply. Activists raise the alarm about a lack of funding to fight the disease while also cautioning the gay population in particular to be aware. French scientists discover the retrovirus—HIV (human immunodeficiency virus)—that causes AIDS.

## 1984: 6,368 new cases, 3,526 deaths

American scientists confirm the connection between HIV and AIDS.

## 1985: 12,044 new cases, 6,996 deaths

The first blood test is released to diagnose HIV/AIDS. And when famous actor Rock Hudson reveals he has AIDS, the world takes notice in a way it hasn't before. President Reagan mentions AIDS for the first time in a speech. Meanwhile, a *Los Angeles Times* poll finds that a majority of Americans favor quarantining people with AIDS. Patients are often subject to isolation, stigma, and ridicule—as shown in the treatment of hemophiliac teenager Ryan White, who is HIV+ and prevented from going to his school.

There are 89 percent more new cases in 1985 than in 1984. Of those who have been diagnosed with AIDS, 51 percent of all adults and 59 percent of all children have died.

## 1986: 19,404 new cases, 12,183 deaths

Defying conservatives, the surgeon general issues a report encouraging the use of condoms, sex education, and voluntary testing to prevent the spread of AIDS. Meanwhile, the CDC reports that Black and Latine people are disproportionately affected by AIDS.

## 1987: 29,105 new cases, 16,488 deaths

ACT UP (AIDS Coalition to Unleash Power) is formed to protest governmental and corporate malfeasance in helping people with AIDS. AZT is the first drug approved by the FDA (Food and Drug Administration) to fight AIDS; it is highly (and often prohibitively) expensive and has many potentially toxic side effects.

## 1988: 36,126 new cases, 21,244 deaths

Grassroots needle-exchange programs begin to help prevent intravenous drug users from infecting themselves through dirty needles.

### 1989: 43,499 new cases, 28,054 deaths

The National Commission on AIDS, formed by Congress, first meets. The number of new cases continues to grow, as AZT does not prove to be the cure that many hoped it would be.

### 1990: 49,546 new cases, 31,836 deaths

ACT UP protestors at the NIH (National Institutes of Health) demand more treatments, fast-track approvals of AIDS drugs, and a clinical trial system that is more inclusive, particularly of women and people of color.

### 1991: 60,573 new cases, 37,106 deaths

The red ribbon becomes the symbol of AIDS awareness. But even if people are talking about it, there is still no cure, and the infection rate is only rising.

### 1992: 79,657 new cases, 41,849 deaths

AIDS becomes the leading cause of death for US men ages twenty-five to forty-four.

### 1993: 79,879 new cases, 45,733 deaths

The CDC expands its list of clinical indicators of AIDS to include pulmonary tuberculosis, recurrent pneumonia, and invasive cervical cancer, which leads to more accurate diagnoses in women and drug users.

### 1994: 73,086 new cases, 50,657 deaths

AIDS is now the leading cause of death for all Americans ages twenty-five to forty-four.

### 1995: 69,984 new cases, 51,414 deaths

The number of cases of AIDS in the US passes 500,000. The first protease inhibitor is approved for use in fighting AIDS. HAART (highly active antiretroviral therapy) becomes the newest treatment for people with AIDS.

### 1996: 61,124 new cases, 38,074 deaths

The HAART combination therapy proves to be effective, and the numbers of new cases and deaths decline for the first time in the epidemic. While AIDS is no longer the leading cause of death for all Americans ages twenty-five to forty-four, it is still the leading cause of death for Black Americans in that age range, highlighting the disparity of care.

### 1997: 49,379 new cases, 21,846 deaths

UNAIDS (the Joint United Nations Programme on HIV/AIDS) estimates 30 million people worldwide have HIV. Meanwhile, the use of HAART in America leads to a 48 percent decline in deaths from AIDS.

### 1998: 41,829 new cases, 18,148 deaths

The CDC reports that Black Americans account for 49 percent of AIDS-related deaths in America. The AIDS-related mortality rate for Black people is ten times higher than the rate for white people and three times higher than the rate for Latine people.

### 1999: 38,811 new cases, 16,762 deaths

According to the World Health Organization (WHO), AIDS has become the fourth-biggest cause of death in the world and the biggest cause of death in Africa. It is estimated that 33 million people are living with AIDS and 14 million have died worldwide.

## 2000: 36,087 new cases, 14,499 deaths

President Clinton announces the Millennium Initiative to find vaccines for HIV/AIDS and other diseases. (Twenty-five years after the millennium, there is still no HIV vaccine.)

## 2001: 24,855 new cases, 8,998 deaths

In the twenty years between 1981 and 2001, including cases where the year of death couldn't be determined, there are 816,149 new cases and 467,910 deaths in the United States alone. To put that in perspective, 418,500 Americans died in all of World War II.

## 2002 to 2025:

Throughout the 2000s, 2010s, and 2020s, the number of infections decreases overall within the United States but is still substantial. Transmission rates among gay men remain significant (especially in underserved communities, in terms of race and income), and there is an uptick when the opioid crisis creates a new generation of intravenous drug users. The "cocktail" of medications introduced with HAART continues to be an effective way to manage HIV, with treatment enabling people with HIV to maintain levels of the virus that are not transmittable or detectable. (The science of HIV/AIDS will be explained further in a later part of this book.)

CDC data for 2022 (the latest year for which we have data at the time of this book's completion) says that 37,981 people ages thirteen and up were diagnosed with HIV in this year. Of these, 76 percent received care for HIV and 65 percent were virally suppressed, meaning they were undetectable and untransmittable. It is estimated there are 1.2 million people living with HIV in America by the end of 2022. In 2025, deep cuts to governmental funding for HIV/AIDS care and research have led to urgent concern that HIV rates and AIDS-related deaths will rise again in the United States and abroad.

# A Brief Overview of the AIDS Epidemic, Through the Story of My Uncle, Robert Levithan

I [David] now want to rewind the overview and share it with you again, mapping it out against the life of my uncle Bobby, who you'll be hearing from throughout this book. At the risk of giving away the ending, I will tell you that Bobby lived with HIV for over thirty years, and that my closest knowledge of AIDS comes from him. I share the overview of his story below with two caveats: First, I don't mean to claim that Bobby—a white gay man from a supportive (emotionally and financially) family—is in any way emblematic of all people with AIDS. In fact, one of the biggest misstatements you can make in talking about AIDS is to imply that *anyone* is emblematic of the very wide, very diverse population of people with AIDS. I'm sharing this one story to tell you one story, not to tell you anything more than that. Which leads to the second caveat: There was much more to my uncle than his HIV status, although as you'll see later, he very proudly took on the mantle of AIDS counselor and AIDS elder. I want to introduce him here, in this way, to show you what these numbers mean against one man's experience, before we use his own words to tell you more.

## Before 1981: 100 new cases, 31 deaths

Robert grew up the youngest of three brothers. (The oldest was my dad, the middle my uncle Jack.) His childhood was very suburban and very straight... although he sensed early on that he might be more into boys than girls. It wasn't until he hit college in the 1970s that he found his crowd... and once he did, he plunged right into the dynamic, subversive wave of gay culture that moved through New York City after the Stonewall Riot. He was (among other things) an actor, a taxi driver, a waiter, an off-off-Broadway theatrical producer, a sound engineer, and a muse. He traveled through Italy with his lover, the photographer Peter Hujar, and was also photographed by contemporaries like Robert Mapplethorpe and Duane Michals. He danced in the movie version of *Hair.* He went to the bars and had many boyfriends. He never settled down, even though there was a part of him that wanted to find someone worthy of the settling.

Because HIV can live in your body for over a decade before making itself known, and because so many of his lovers (including Peter) would later die because of AIDS, Robert always assumed he contracted HIV sometime in the 1970s. (He would often pinpoint it to the summer of 1975.) He had no idea what the risk was then. No one did.

### 1981: 339 new cases, 130 deaths

He will always remember where he was sitting—at a round metal table in Park Avenue Plaza in Manhattan—when an acquaintance asks him if he's heard about this gay cancer going around. Thirty years old, this is the first time he learns about it: not from the news, not from the government or a doctor, but from the gay whisper network.

### 1983: 3,153 new cases, 1,511 deaths

Robert becomes a crisis counselor at the newly formed Gay Men's Health Crisis (GMHC). He is devasted when Jeffrey, the first person he works with, dies.

Scientists trying to figure out how AIDS works put out a call to gay men, asking them to donate blood that can be analyzed as part of a larger study. Robert's blood is taken to audition the blood test that will become available the following year.

Robert participates in the test . . . but he asks not to be notified of the results. He knows it is likely that he's been infected . . . but because there isn't any treatment, he doesn't see the point of knowing whether or not he's positive. If he gets really sick, then he'll know he's really sick.

## 1987: 29,105 new cases, 16,488 deaths

Friends die. Former lovers die. Acquaintances die.

Robert immerses himself in the work of caring for those who are ill.

Later, he writes, "I remember in 1987, realizing that in the midst of my work in the AIDS community, I had become the person I always wanted to be."

## 1988: 36,126 new cases, 21,244 deaths

"AIDS made a lot of us veterans of grief. I left New York City in the Fall of 1988 for Southern California and eventually Santa Fe, New Mexico, because it started to feel like there were ghosts on every corner. But geography couldn't solve that problem. Eventually, Santa Fe was just as ghost-filled."

## 1990: 49,546 new cases, 31,836 deaths

"I clearly remember waking up on January 1, 1990 and feeling a sense of despair as I looked at the decade leading up to 2000. I was expecting to lose most of my friends and most of my colleagues in the AIDS community. How would I live through it?"

Robert's doctor dies. Robert goes to his office to get his medical records—and it is in the lobby of this dead doctor's building that he opens his file and discovers that his earlier blood sample tested positive. He has HIV.

## 1991: 60,573 new cases, 37,106 deaths

Robert's friend Cynthia O'Neal and the movie director Mike Nichols start an AIDS support organization called Friends in Deed. A few years later, Friends in Deed will become Robert's base as he runs workshops there. A family friend named Jonathan Larson will attend these workshops and will use them as the basis for the AIDS support group in his musical *Rent*. In that musical, people with AIDS ask, "Will I lose my dignity? Will someone care?" It is Robert's job to say no to the first question, yes to the second question, and then to explain the how and the why.

### 1992: 79,657 new cases, 41,849 deaths

AIDS becomes the leading cause of death for US men ages twenty-five to forty-four.

### 1994: 73,086 new cases, 50,657 deaths

"I was aware of breath, and oxygen and IVs. . . ."

In May, opportunistic infections nearly kill Robert. He hangs on to life at St. Vincent Hospital in Santa Fe, barely able to breathe.

After ten days in the hospital, he is released . . . but it takes him months to recover his stamina and strength. He feels he is living on borrowed time, so he decides to take off to Europe for one last farewell tour, using up most of his savings and much of his energy.

### 1995: 69,984 new cases, 51,414 deaths

So many of his close friends have died. People he's counseled have died. Peter and Mathew have died. Johnny has died. Dick and Rick have died. Horatio and Louis. Bob. Aswan. Jeffrey. Carole. Felicity. Others, like Michael, are very sick.

Robert manages to finish graduate school and becomes a psychotherapist. He lets his hair grow, works out at the gym, and has weekly acupuncture. He continues his daily doses of vitamins and herbs and adds sometimes harsh, sometimes helpful prescription drugs and vitamin C drips, as well as wildly expensive (not covered by insurance) gamma globulin IVs. He prays to God, to the Great Mother, to the sky and the earth. He despairs each time he thinks he might be sickening or losing ground, and cheers when he feels progress or his blood work improves.

Still, the trajectory isn't good. According to the doctors, if his T-cell count drops below 200, he is considered to have AIDS.

Robert's count drops to 20. His immune system is wrecked, an open door to any infection that wants to attack.

Then something miraculous occurs.

As a direct result of lobbying by AIDS activists, the FDA holds a lottery for early access to the first successful protease inhibitor, Crixivan. Doctors for people in the trial will receive the drug from its manufacturer, Merck, before full FDA approval. In a break from medical tradition, there will be no "placebo control"—meaning that everyone in the trial will get the medication instead of only half the participants.

Robert literally wins the lottery, his number chosen to allow him access to the drug. After an excruciating two-month waiting period, he is given the medication by his doctor.

His T-cell count doubles in the first three weeks. Four months later, it rises above 200. He is still HIV+, but he no longer has AIDS.

Up to this point, doctors had no idea if an immune system could rebuild itself. Robert's does.

## 1996: 61,124 new cases, 38,074 deaths

A year after starting the medication, Robert's T-cell count is up to a healthy 360.

Friends who do not have access to the cocktail (the slang name for the combination of medications in the HAART protocol) continue to die.

## 1997: 49,379 new cases, 21,846 deaths

Robert dives into his role as an AIDS counselor. His focus is on people like him, who were certain they were going to die . . . and then didn't. Many ran through their savings or burned bridges in their relationships, thinking there wouldn't be any future for them. And then there was.

## 1998–2016:

Over the next eighteen years, Robert writes and lectures on "Outliving Myself" for a range of audiences. Like many people with AIDS, he feels his status has made him understand life more and has guided him into caring a lot less what other people think. He dies in 2016 of a cancer completely unrelated to HIV . . . but his spirit and words can be found throughout this book.

There is no formal start to the AIDS epidemic, no definitive first case. For years, many thought there was a specific "patient zero"—one of the first humans with HIV who then spread it to many other people ... who then spread it to more people ... and so on. But that has proven to be a myth, and the earliest cases of HIV/AIDS can only give us a vastly incomplete picture.

Take, for instance, the strange, sad case of Robert Rayford. . . .

> *The autopsy poses fresh questions, withholding rather than providing answers. What killed Robert?*

## A Boy, Lost in History: Robert Rayford

Robert Rayford is fifteen years old and he's in trouble.

It's early 1968. He's sick, scared, and alone.

He takes himself to the hospital.

Just south of downtown St. Louis, City Hospital is an imposing building with six floors and a tower. The building was constructed in 1846 but destroyed by a fire ten years later. It was then rebuilt. Fifty years later, it was destroyed a second time by a vast tornado that tore apart swaths of the city. In 1907, the building was rebuilt one final time. The site remained in use as a hospital until it fell into disrepair in the late 1980s, twenty years after Robert arrived at its door.

We don't know much about Robert, but what we do know is important: He's a Black boy from Old North, a historically Black district in the city. His family lives below the poverty line in an underserved neighborhood. It's him, his mother, and his brother. He first feels sick in 1966 but only checks himself into City Hospital early in 1968. He arrives at the hospital unaccompanied.

The medical professionals who examine Robert find him to be quiet, distrusting. They speculate that he has a learning disability. There is no doubt he has some kind of serious ailment. He has swelling around his body: swollen genitals, swollen hemorrhoids. There is evidence of advanced chlamydia infection at multiple sites on his body and—unusual—in his bloodstream. Pushed for further information, Robert discloses that he's been intimate with a girl from his neighborhood, but the doctors dismiss this as insubstantial.

Robert stays in the hospital.

His condition gets worse.

The doctors hypothesize that he might have been sleeping with men, or has been subjected to sexual abuse. It's possible he's been an underage sex worker. The swelling around his anus implies that he has received anal sex. The doctors speculate whether he's somehow contracted some strange illness from a faraway place—but Robert has never left the Midwest, let alone the country.

He is a medical mystery that refuses to be solved.

Months go by, and then a year. Robert's condition deteriorates.

Doctors operate on him. He bends forward like an old man when he walks or stands. He is in pain, and none of the doctors can pinpoint why.

Later, one of his doctors, Memory Elvin-Lewis, will say, "He was not communicative. He barely said boo. He never told us what he was doing." She will also say, "He was the typical fifteen-year-old who is not going to talk to adults, especially when I'm white and he's Black."

He turns sixteen on the third of February 1969.

By the middle of May, he is dead. His cause of death is listed as lymphedema, or generalized body swelling.

The story could end here.

It doesn't.

Soon after Robert's death, Robert's mother gives permission for an autopsy. Under the sterile light of the autopsy room, the doctors find scars that imply, as they earlier suspected, that he received anal sex, perhaps had been raped. Less expectedly, the doctors discover lesions on his body—purple marks that indicate Kaposi's sarcoma, a rare skin cancer associated with elderly Italian men, not teenage Black boys. The autopsy poses fresh questions, withholding rather than providing answers. What killed Robert?

At the time of his death, doctors have no idea.

In the early 1970s, a report is published that examines his case and raises a possible connection between his chronic case of chlamydia and the swollen, engorged skin around his penis, scrotum, and thighs. Robert is described as exhibiting "moderate mental retardation"—the harsh language of his autopsy refers to him as a "wasted Negro boy" who died in part due to inanition (exhaustion from malnourishment).

The pieces of the puzzle of Robert's short life and death don't come together for another fifteen years, when HIV/AIDS enters the medical community's consciousness. If Robert were still alive, he would be in his early thirties, still young.

He is gone, but traces of him remain.

Elvin-Lewis had samples from the autopsy put into storage. For years he is an unexplained mystery in a laboratory archive, a ghost on ice. Reading the reports about the unfolding AIDS crisis, Elvin-Lewis orders the retrieval of the samples from the freezer and transports them to a testing center.

Her hunch proves correct.

Robert's tissue tests positive for HIV.

The mystery of Robert's death seems to be solved. Suddenly, it all makes sense: the onslaught of infections that antibiotics wouldn't shift; the way his body grew skeletal before the doctors' eyes, no matter what they threw at it. The most likely scenario is that this young Black boy from St. Louis is the first person in America known to have died because of AIDS.

In 1968.

Thirteen years before 1981, when the "gay cancer" is "discovered."

History is a story we tell ourselves to understand where we've come from, where we're going, and who "we" are. That's why the histories that get taught in schools and universities are never neutral but formed around certain ideals of what it means to be American. The past bleeds into the present. We look at the past and expect it to be neatly organized. As though history can be a straight river of cold fact that rushes us without stopping from "back then" to "right now." But the past is a place that we can return to as visitors, and sometimes we have to be detectives.

No photographs can be found of Robert Rayford. No letters in which we might see his handwriting. No record of any words he said, feelings he felt. His brother died in 2007, his mother in 2011. There is no one left to ask. The cells from his body were stored in a laboratory in New Orleans and destroyed in Hurricane Katrina in 2005.
All we have are records of his illness.
The rest is uncertainty.

There is uncertainty, too, in why we talk about him here.
The news about Robert rewrote the conventional narrative that HIV/AIDS appeared in the early 1980s in New York and California. His case challenges the accepted history of an epidemic that continues to disproportionately affect young Black boys and men.
Robert likely *wasn't* the first case of HIV/AIDS in the United States.
He just happened to be the one whose doctor kept a trace.

The gone are gone; the dead stay dead. The fragments of their lives are pieces of broken glass that reflect our own faces back at us.

The limited information we have about Robert comes through the perspective of his doctors: white people he didn't trust or connect with. Our memory of Robert is burdened by the bias of these doctors, the tragedy of his circumstances, and the intervention he represents in the accepted history of the epidemic. Thinking about his short life and premature death means recognizing the limits of what we know. It means feeling the frustration of those limits and looking for his humanity anyway. This task requires—demands—that we rewind to that first moment again: A fifteen-year-old boy in great pain shows up alone at the door of a hospital he hopes will help him. His face may have fallen into shadow, but we can still sense what it is like for him to take those hard steps.

He feels his own daunting uncertainty, asks one of the scariest questions we can ask ourselves: What is happening to me?

In this moment, he is not the first of anything.

In this moment, he is just like us.

# HIV and AIDS: The Basics

One of the scariest parts of the HIV/AIDS epidemic was that for years doctors didn't know what the disease was or how it worked. Now, decades later, we have a better (but still not perfect) way of defining HIV and AIDS and understanding how HIV works within our bodies.

## How Do HIV and AIDS Work?

The immune system is the body's defense mechanism against infections and disease. There are two parts of the immune system: the innate immune system and the acquired immune system. The innate immune system is the body's rapid-response system, made of barriers like skin and mucous membranes that prevent outside germs and toxins from entering too deeply. The acquired immune system makes proteins called antibodies to defend us against specific germs (such as bacteria, viruses, and fungi) and toxins. These antibodies zero in on the invaders and get rid of them. Then, after the acquired immune system fights off the infection, it ideally remembers the microbes it defeated so it can defend the body more effectively against that specific kind of attack if it occurs again. Our bodies do this all the time, since we come into contact with tens of thousands of germs every single day.

HIV stands for human immunodeficiency virus—meaning that HIV is a virus that attacks and weakens a person's acquired immune system. The immune system uses many kinds of white blood cells to fight infections. One kind of white blood cell is the CD4 cell, or T-cell—and CD4 cells are the ones that HIV attacks. HIV bombards a CD4 cell and gets inside it. Once it's broken through, it uses the inner machinery of the CD4 cell to replicate itself. Eventually, the virus takes over, killing the CD4 cell. Then the new copies of HIV attack other CD4 cells, slowly compromising the immune system and rendering it much less effective in fighting new infections. The immune system will try to fix this by making even more CD4 cells, but ultimately it can't keep up with the attacking virus, so it can't protect the body from other infections. That's when people with HIV get sick. The HIV itself is not what makes them sick—instead, it weakens the body's defenses so bacteria, viruses, and other agents of disease can beat the immune system and sicken the body.

AIDS stands for acquired immune deficiency syndrome. It is diagnosed when HIV's infiltration of the body has reached the point where the immune system is seriously compromised and the viral load (the quantity of virus in a given volume of fluid, like blood) has reached a dangerous level, with the CD4 count dropping below 200 cells per milliliter of blood. People with AIDS are particularly vulnerable to opportunistic infections and other serious illnesses.

It is important to note that today many people can live with HIV and treat it so it doesn't become AIDS. If you contract HIV today and it is diagnosed, you go on medication pretty much immediately; you can't pass on the virus, and your life carries on as normal. That's the miracle of science. But in the 1980s and much of the 1990s, this was not the case, and there was no way for doctors to prevent HIV from eventually leading to AIDS. For that reason, in this period living with HIV was all too often a fatal condition.

## How Does HIV Spread?

The only way for untreated HIV to spread to your body is for someone else's HIV-infected blood, semen, vaginal fluid, rectal fluid, or breast milk to enter your bloodstream. One way for this to happen is during vaginal or anal sex with a penis. Another way is if you use a needle that has HIV-infected blood on it. Mothers whose blood is HIV infected can pass it to their babies during pregnancy. And in America, it wasn't until 1985 that blood and blood products used in hospitals for transfusions were screened for HIV, so people receiving transfusions, particularly hemophiliacs, were vulnerable.

People with HIV do not necessarily show signs of illness immediately, although it's common to have a sudden, brief flu-like illness a few weeks after you have contracted HIV. It's often the case that people with HIV live with it for many years before it is diagnosed, which is why getting tested for HIV is so important. Prior to the first blood test for HIV/AIDS in 1985, it was nearly impossible to know for sure whether you were HIV+ (HIV positive) or HIV– (HIV negative), especially if you weren't showing symptoms.

Because doctors at first couldn't pinpoint the cause of HIV, there was fear that it was transmitted through coughing, sneezing, kissing, physical contact, shared utensils, or contact with body fluids other than blood, semen, vaginal/rectal fluids, or breast milk (like saliva, mucus, tears, and urine). These fears are the cause of a lot of the hatred and bigotry that has been directed toward queer people and/or people with HIV/AIDS since the epidemic began. None of these fears proved true; HIV cannot be transmitted in any of these ways.

**How Are HIV and AIDS Treated?**

There is no single drug that can treat AIDS. But in the 1990s, it was discovered that combinations of drugs known as ART (antiretroviral therapy) or HAART (highly active antiretroviral therapy) could treat HIV. This medicine prevents HIV from replicating itself. And without new HIV being generated, it is easier for the immune system to recover from it and reduce the viral load within the blood. The earlier someone living with HIV begins treatment, the more effective it can be. These days, most people living with HIV need to take only one pill a day, with minimal side effects. Their day-to-day lives are just like anybody else's; their life expectancy is the same as anyone else's. But being HIV+ does mean they need consistent access to quality health care to maintain treatment.

## Is There a Cure for HIV or AIDS?

Once HIV is in your body, it will stay there. There is still no "cure" that will erase it from your blood entirely—not yet. However, for more than ten years, it's been proven that treatment helps the viral load in most HIV+ people stay undetectable. "Undetectable" means that the amount of HIV in your blood is so low that you cannot transmit it and you are not likely, with continued treatment, to get sick from it. HIV is called "undetectable" at this stage because it will not show up on standard blood tests anymore, although it can still be tracked with more advanced tests.

There are also ways now to massively decrease your likelihood of getting HIV from contact with someone who has it. There is no vaccine, like for diseases such as polio or smallpox, but there are medications that greatly reduce the risk of transmission. In 2012, the FDA approved PrEP (pre-exposure prophylaxis) treatment as a means for people to prevent HIV transmission. PrEP builds "walls" around a person's CD4 cells so HIV cannot infiltrate them; when HIV cannot get into CD4 cells and replicate, it has no way of staying in the body. Most people who are on PrEP take it every day, but new, longer-acting forms of PrEP (such as a bimonthly injection) bring this drug closer and closer to resembling a vaccine. There is also in some circumstances PEP (post-exposure prophylaxis), approved in 2005, which is medication that can be taken within seventy-two hours of potential exposure in order to prevent infection.

Treatments like ART and PrEP are among the developments that activists in the 1980s and 1990s were fighting for. But access to these drugs is easiest for those who have the health insurance to afford it. Making sure that everyone has access to ART and PrEP is an ongoing challenge that inspires further activism to this day.

## TIMELINE

# 1978–1982

## 1978

In the 1970s, New York City is the heroin capital of America. People who develop serious problems with heroin are often unhoused and prone to being incarcerated—a loop of problems that leads straight back to using heroin. By 1978, health professionals in New York begin to notice a surge in deaths among heroin users in the city . . . but it isn't exactly cause for widespread alarm, because these people are already susceptible to health problems associated with premature death.

Among themselves, some practitioners call this ailment "Rikers Island adenopathy" ("adenopathy" means the enlargement of lymph nodes). Since 1932, Rikers has housed one of the country's largest correctional and rehabilitative institutions—picture a set of ugly concrete buildings in the shape of crosses, stamped across a tiny island only a handful of miles from Manhattan, one of the wealthiest but most unequal parts of the United States. There are prison riots throughout the 1970s to protest overcrowding; the name of the prison evokes images of squalid, harsh conditions.

In the late 1970s, Sheldon Landesman is at the start of his career at a medical center in Brooklyn as an assistant professor. Landesman becomes familiar with "Rikers Island adenopathy" when his ward receives several patients sent over from Rikers. The patients exhibit "persistent fever, wasting, weight loss, and large lymph nodes."

At the same time, many people working with vulnerable adults in the city begin to refer to "junkie pneumonia" or "the dwindles" as a cause of death. Bodies found on the sidewalk; skinny people getting skinnier, wasting away. But these rumors receive little attention.

> **I actually believe that AIDS kind of existed among this group of people first, because if you look back, there was something called junkie pneumonia, there was something called the dwindles that addicts got, and I think this was another early AIDS population way too helpless to ever do anything for themselves on their own behalf.**
> **—Activist Betty Williams**

## June 1981

After the Stonewall Riot in 1969, queer people were increasingly visible as a population in major American cities. Queer people lived in "gayborhoods" or "gay ghettos"—in the postwar decades, new communities slowly formed as queer people migrated to run-down areas to find escape from intolerance. By the late 1970s, gay men in particular were becoming recognized as a demographic with increasing power. In 1977, Harvey Milk was the first openly gay man elected to San Francisco's board of supervisors—a symbol of change. His assassination only eleven months after his election raised tensions across the nation and emphasized to many queer people their need to organize and be visible as a community.

In June 1981, the Centers for Disease Control publishes a report on five cases of *Pneumocystis carinii* pneumonia (PCP, or just pneumocystis pneumonia) in gay men in Los Angeles. It's the same kind of rare pneumonia that is killing some of the heroin users, but these crucial connections aren't being made yet, nor is any connection being made to the incidences of Kaposi's sarcoma that will come to be seen as the "gay cancer." These five men had other infections too, the kinds of infections that a body should be able to fight off on its own—the first indication that this strange, shared sickness might point to an immune disorder. The men are all short of breath, sick in a way that nobody can understand or predict. The regular treatment options don't work as expected; the problems don't go away. Three of the five men studied in the report are dead by the time it's published. Not enough people are paying attention—not yet—but the implication of these cases begins to send shock waves among those who are.

In July, the LGBTQ+ newspaper the *Bay Area Reporter* refers to "Gay men's pneumonia" in one of the first examples of press coverage of the disease. Buried in the back pages, the feature is part of a short article that urges gay men with breathing problems to consult their clinician in the hope that they may avoid the same fate as the five men in the CDC report. The article implies that the cause of these cases of pneumonia might be amyl nitrate, or "poppers"—a legal party drug since proven to have had no role in the spread of HIV.

> Symptoms include fever, a cough that is dry or only minimally productive of sputum, and progressive shortness of breath. The **progressive shortness of breath** is considered the most specific symptom. Therefore, any Gay man who is **really** sick and has the above-mentioned symptoms, **including progressive shortness of breath**, is advised to see his physician.

## August 1981

On August 11, writer Larry Kramer hosts a meeting at his apartment that over eighty gay men attend. The guest of honor is Dr. Alvin Friedman-Kien, a dermatologist and virologist at New York University's Medical Center, who earlier in the year had been shocked to see two new cases of the rare Kaposi's sarcoma in a two-week period. He contacted colleagues and Physicians for Human Rights, a newly formed group of gay doctors who treated gay men, and within four weeks found out about twenty other cases in New York City and six in California. He alerted the CDC to these findings in June—but no funding for further study has been given to him by either governmental or private sources.

Activist Andy Humm would later recall, "We listened intently, respectfully, and full of dread as the soft-spoken Dr. Friedman-Kien described the devastation he was seeing in his practice and hearing from other physicians treating gay men. You could have heard a pin drop."

Humm remembers that Kramer passed a hat at the event . . . and later stood on the dock at the gay vacation spot Fire Island with a tin can to collect money. (He made sixty dollars.)

Dr. Larry Mass, who later founded Gay Men's Health Crisis with Kramer, Paul Popham, Edmund White, and Paul Rapoport, thought that they needed to raise the alarm—but also needed to be mindful of the public's reaction:

> As a medical doctor, I wanted us to be careful about what we said, so that we weren't giving out misinformation or starting a panic. I was also worried about civil rights issues, since we had no such protections in place. Homophobia was pervasive, a powder keg ready to explode.

Overall, $6,635 is raised at this meeting—the only significant amount donated to any such research in 1981.

## December 1981

Arye Rubinstein is a doctor at the Albert Einstein College of Medicine in the Bronx. He studied in Switzerland with a specialty in pediatric health: His vocation is to help children with severe allergies and immune disorders. In 1979 he starts to see children who are experiencing recurring infections, and by 1981 he is getting seriously concerned. He treats (or tries to treat) five different children who all have unusual recurring symptoms—some kind of immune disorder he hasn't seen before. Like the gay men in Los Angeles and heroin users in other parts of New York City, the children have PCP, a rare form of pneumonia. The kids are Black and come from underserved and impoverished homes in the city.

The children's symptoms remind Rubinstein of the recent studies about a mysterious immune disorder among gay men. Their glands are swollen. They are susceptible to recurring viral and bacterial infections, none of which the usual treatments can budge.

After further investigation, Rubinstein's team learns that several of the mothers of these children were or are drug users. Several of the women report that they relied on or still rely on sex work for their income. Rubinstein queries if these sick young children could be experiencing the same enigmatic condition that has been reported about gay men: the drip-drip of infections and a failing immune system.

His colleagues dismiss his hypothesis.

## December 1981

"I'm Bobbi Campbell, and I have 'gay cancer.'"

With these words, written in an article on the front page of the *San Francisco Sentinel*, Bobbi Campbell, a twenty-nine-year-old registered nurse from San Francisco, becomes the first person with HIV/AIDS to publicly disclose his status.

The title of the article?

"I WILL SURVIVE!"

Campbell's openness comes as no surprise. Six weeks earlier, he became only the sixteenth young person to be diagnosed with Kaposi's sarcoma. Rather than hide his condition, he took photos of his lesions and posted them, along with an explanation of his illness, in the window of the Star Pharmacy in the Castro, San Francisco's gay neighborhood—the first-ever AIDS awareness poster (even if Campbell wasn't aware of the ultimate name of his illness yet).

In his *Sentinel* article, Campbell embraces his role, jokingly referring to himself as a "Kaposi's Sarcoma Poster Boy." But, he figured, "The purpose of a poster child is to raise interest and money in a particular cause, and I do have aspirations of doing that regarding 'gay cancer.' . . . I'm writing because I have a determination to *live*. You do, too—don't you?"

## January 1982

Gay Men's Health Crisis in New York City becomes the first community-based service provider for people with HIV/AIDS in the country. Founded by a mix of writers, doctors, and activists, it hits the ground running. It holds its first fundraiser ("Showers") at the Paradise Garage in April, raising $50,000. And in May, a GMHC volunteer named Rodger McFarlane sets up the world's first information and counseling hotline for people concerned about HIV/AIDS. He uses his home phone and gets over a hundred calls on the first night.

## April 1982

US Representative Henry Waxman of Los Angeles convenes a congressional hearing about HIV/AIDS . . . not in Washington but at the Los Angeles Gay and Lesbian Community Services Center. In his opening statement, Waxman declares:

> I also want to look at the larger questions of the depth of Federal commitment to the continuation of research on these illnesses. In 1982, the overall funding of the Centers for Disease Control was effectively cut by 20 percent.
>
> The administration's 1983 budget does not even keep pace with inflation and will mean a further effective cut of 7 percent. The study of these relatively rare and poorly understood diseases will surely suffer.
>
> Biomedical research funding has been treated in a similar fashion. In 1983, Mr. Reagan proposes to allow 1,000 fewer new research grants than in 1981.
>
> With such shortsighted Federal policies of disease control and research, we can only expect slower cures and larger epidemics. Public health officials are confronted with impossible choices: Research can be done on cancer only if it is not done on infectious diseases. Herpes surveillance may be done only if syphilis is uncontrolled.

Last year's budget cuts have limited our ability to deal with familiar diseases and syndromes that we understand. There is little margin for new problems. If a new Kaposi's or Legionnaire's disease occurs next year, we might not be able to respond.

This pennywise and pound-foolish approach to prevention and research is a cause of concern for everyone.

CDC and NIH have begun important work on this new syndrome. The implications for immunology and for cancer research in general are tremendous. We must not allow that start to be undermined. As a nation, we cannot afford to slow down our efforts to understand, control, and cure such disease.

I want to be especially blunt about the political aspects of Kaposi's Sarcoma. This horrible disease afflicts members of one of the Nation's most stigmatized and discriminated-against minorities. The victims are not typical, Main Street Americans. They are gays, mainly from New York, Los Angeles, and San Francisco.

There is no doubt in my mind that if the same disease had appeared among Americans of Norwegian descent, or among tennis players, rather than among gay males, the responses of both the Government and the medical community would have been different....

We can't talk about the gay cancer. There is a cancer which seems predominantly to affect gay men, but it is a cancer and a public health concern for all Americans. Above all, I intend to fight any effort by anyone at any level to make public health policy regarding Kaposi's Sarcoma or any other disease on the basis of his or her personal prejudices regarding other people's sexual preferences or lifestyles.

## May 1982

The mainstream media won't pay attention to HIV/AIDS until May 1982, when a notorious headline makes its way onto the front page of *The New York Times* . . . science section: "New Homosexual Disorder Worries Health Officials." The article describes the spread of a mysterious immune disorder afflicting and killing a growing number of gay men in gay areas of major cities. It reports that 335 people have been diagnosed and 136 have already died. Even though it notes cases among heterosexuals, the *Times* quotes researchers calling the alarming condition GRID, for gay-related immunodeficiency. The term's use in the *Times* sends it into the mainstream—with the effect that people start to think there is a new "gay plague" caused by being gay.

The article strikes a warning note that will prove to be all too true:

> According to both the Centers for Disease Control and the National Cancer Institute in Bethesda, Md., GRID has reached epidemic proportions and the current totals probably represent "just the tip of the iceberg."

Hearsay about "the gay cancer" spreads. These rumors establish a shadowy connection between gay men and a mysterious form of killer pneumonia. People speculate about immune system failure in this population—and question what this might imply about the sexual lives of gay men in the busiest gayborhoods. These rumors will thicken like smoke in the years ahead. And gay men and other queer people will continue to be disproportionately affected by the spread of HIV/AIDS, often having their needs (and deaths) ignored by a society that remains prejudiced against difference.

> We had heard stuff about, you know, people being sick. I remember in 1980 we had started to hear stuff. Of course, in New York it was like, "Oh, those sluts in San Francisco are getting some disease." So that's what we had heard. So, there were vague stories about it, and no one really knew anything.
>
> —Activist Robert Vazquez-Pacheco

## July 1982

The identities and behaviors first associated with AIDS were shrouded in stigma. Using heroin. Being gay. Having sex with men. Having sex for money.

But hemophilia is a less stigmatized condition that the average person seldom thinks about unless they know someone directly affected by it. People living with hemophilia undergo regular blood transfusions to maintain their health, because if they cut themselves, their blood doesn't clot properly and they risk bleeding to death. In July 1982, a report announces the appearance of—you guessed it—a rare type of pneumonia in this small and mostly unseen population. The appearance of PCP among hemophiliacs raises alarm bells, because it suggests that the national blood supply could be contaminated. If this is true (and it *is* true), the national blood supply is transmitting the same random infection that has begun to sicken and kill gay men, other queer people, sex workers, and some of the nation's drug-using population.

By the time the report on PCP among hemophiliacs comes out, the majority of the patients it describes have already died. The blood supply in the United States isn't screened for HIV until 1985. Of the 10,000 hemophiliacs living in the US in the 1980s, more than 4,000 will die due to AIDS.

## September 1982

As scientists around the country compare notes and assemble information about this new condition, a number of names are used to describe it. At first, the CDC calls it "4H" to gather together the first groups of people deemed to be vulnerable: homosexuals, Haitians (who saw a disproportionately high spread of the disease in their community), heroin users, and hemophiliacs. The name is oversimplistic to the point of being offensive, although it demonstrates the diverse and marginal range of human beings who are associated with the crisis in these first months and years.

Early on, a representative of the National Cancer Institute describes 4H, or GRID, as posing a possible threat to all Americans, but too many stories in this era of HIV/AIDS suggest that it is directly connected to gay people and gay identity. As though no one else has to question their own vulnerability; as though *not being gay* is protection enough. Likewise, "4H" draws attention to the vulnerability of certain behaviors and certain identities, without acknowledging the societal structures that make some people more at risk than others. As "GRID" and "4H" become fixed into the language of the public, they take on dramatic proportions, setting up a number of associations that become foundational to how Americans think about HIV/AIDS.

In September 1982, the term "acquired immune deficiency syndrome," shortened to "AIDS," is used for the first time in a Centers for Disease Control report. The CDC's definition is "a disease at least moderately predictive of a defect in cell-mediated immunity, occurring in a person with no known cause for diminished resistance to that disease." This painfully neutral language tries to acknowledge the diversity of possible cases—picture the sickly children on Rubinstein's ward in the Bronx, the drug users seeking a fix on Rikers Island, the disparate hemophiliacs in the American population, or the queer people in gayborhoods like Greenwich Village in Manhattan or the Castro in San Francisco. The exact cause of AIDS—why is everyone suddenly getting sick?—remains unknown.

HIV/AIDS weaves through communities of people who were already unseen, marginalized, sometimes barely surviving. Politicians and journalists and educators don't want to talk about people who use drugs or men who have sex with men. They don't want to talk about dying babies in underfunded hospitals in predominantly Black parts of New York City. From the beginning of the crisis, many of the people most affected by HIV/AIDS are poor, Black, Latine, underserved, gay, trans—people whose stories have been conveniently disregarded or even discarded by mainstream society.

## October 1982

On October 15, conservative journalist Lester Kinsolving becomes the first reporter to ask a question about the new epidemic at a White House briefing. Instead of somberly mourning the hundreds of people who have died at this point, Larry Speakes, the acting press secretary for President Reagan, makes gay jokes, egged on by the laughter of the other reporters (almost entirely straight men) in the room.

This is a transcript from that briefing.

```
KINSOLVING: Larry, does the President have any
reaction to the announcement by the Centers for
Disease Control in Atlanta, that A-I-D-S is now an
epidemic and have over 600 cases?

SPEAKES: A-I-D-S? I haven't got anything on it.

KINSOLVING: Over a third of them have died.
It's known as "gay plague." (Laughter.) No,
it is. I mean it's a pretty serious thing that
one in every three people that get this have
died. And I wondered if the President is aware
of it?

SPEAKES: I don't have it. Are you . . . Do you?
(Laughter.)

KINSOLVING: You don't have it. Well, I'm relieved
to hear that, Larry! (Laughter.)

SPEAKES: Do you?

KINSOLVING: No, I don't.

SPEAKES: You didn't answer my question. How do you
know? (Laughter.)

KINSOLVING: In other words, the White House looks
on this as a great joke?
```

SPEAKES: No, I don't know anything about it, Lester.

KINSOLVING: Does the President, does anybody in the White House know about this epidemic, Larry?

SPEAKES: I don't think so. I don't think there's been any—

KINSOLVING: Nobody knows?

SPEAKES: There has been no personal experience here, Lester.

KINSOLVING: No, I mean, I thought you were keeping—

SPEAKES: I checked thoroughly with Dr. Ruge [the president's physician] this morning and he's had no—(laughter)—no patients suffering from A-I-D-S or whatever it is.

KINSOLVING: The President doesn't have gay plague. Is that what you're saying or what?

SPEAKES: No, I didn't say that.

KINSOLVING: Didn't say that?

SPEAKES: I thought I heard you on the State Department over there. Why didn't you stay there? (Laughter.)

KINSOLVING: Because I love you, Larry, that's why. (Laughter.)

SPEAKES: Oh, I see. Just don't put it in those terms, Lester. (Laughter.)

KINSOLVING: Oh, I retract that.

SPEAKES: I hope so.

Empathy should transcend the fear of "the other," but in America that doesn't occur often enough. When AIDS was primarily seen as affecting gay men, drug users, and Black immigrants, it was easy for the population at large (including the media, including the government) to turn a blind eye.

But when it strikes the Boy Next Door?

That's something completely different.

*Did portraying him as an "innocent victim" implicate those who became HIV+ through sex or drug use as being somehow guilty of their own sickness?*

# The Accidental, Deliberate Poster Boy: Ryan White

There are many notable celebrities who died because of AIDS. Most were famous before they had AIDS. There are far fewer who became famous *because* they had AIDS.

Ryan White was the most famous of them all.

In America in the late 1980s, most people knew who Ryan White was: an ordinary boy in extraordinary circumstances, a young fighter who was exposed to HIV/AIDS because he was a hemophiliac. He had famous friends like Elton John and Michael Jackson. He went on talk shows and was on the covers of magazines. He was straight, but he was also the subject of merciless taunts—plenty of "Ryan White jokes" were disseminated over the airwaves of shock-jock radio and in schoolyards across the nation. Most people knew his plight was no laughing matter. After one school kicked him out, another welcomed him with open arms. He lived much longer than anyone expected, but he still died far too young, a month before his high school graduation, at age eighteen.

Ryan White didn't ask to be a celebrity, nor did he ask to become the face of AIDS in America. But for a while, that's exactly what he was. And the fact that a straight white teen boy from the heartland was the face of AIDS raises a lot of interesting questions about queer erasure and media attention in the fight against AIDS. Because even if Ryan White was not representative of the majority of people with AIDS, he was a deeply effective symbol, conveying the toll of AIDS to an otherwise indifferent country.

* * *

Ryan was born on December 6, 1971, in Kokomo, Indiana. His family immediately discovered that he had severe hemophilia—which means that his blood wouldn't clot as quickly as it was supposed to. Without clotting, a hemophiliac will keep bleeding and bleeding, leaving the constant risk that a cut or injury will become very serious very fast. In order to prevent this, Ryan was given blood products drawn from other people's plasma to help his own blood clot. Before April 1985, donated blood wasn't screened for HIV. So sometime before the fall of 1984, Ryan received transfusions that contained HIV. By Christmas that year, he was in the hospital and diagnosed with AIDS.

He was told he probably had six months to live.

One of Ryan's doctors, Howard Markel, later wrote:

> Although there is no cure for hemophilia, doctors treat the bleeding episodes with injections of factor 8 to help the clotting process along. But in the years before the threat of HIV/AIDS became widely understood, this substance was pooled and isolated from thousands of anonymous and untested blood donations. What no one knew back then was that every time a pediatrician administered this seemingly lifesaving elixir (and I was one of those pediatricians), there was a real risk of administering an HIV-contaminated dose. Hence, we doctors were unknowingly infecting our hemophiliac patients with the human immunodeficiency virus. Virtually every hemophiliac I treated in the mid-1980s has since died from AIDS. This was the way Ryan White became infected with HIV sometime in the late 1970s or early 1980s.

A thirteen-year-old with AIDS would have already been a significant story. As of July 1985, the CDC didn't have any guidelines for dealing with young people with AIDS. CDC spokesperson Betty Hooper said, "We know of 148 cases of pediatric AIDS. We are beginning to get cases in children around the country."

It is within the context of this unpreparedness and uncertainty that Ryan White made the news. His school, Western Middle School in Russiaville, Indiana, refused to let him return to class after his diagnosis. The administrators and many parents were scared—even though they were told HIV/AIDS wasn't transmitted by airborne activity, how could they know for sure?

> With all the things we do and don't know about AIDS, I just decided not to do it.
> —School Superintendent James Smith

> I'm pretty upset about it. I'll miss my friends mostly.
> —Ryan White
> (both quoted in the *Los Angeles Times,* July 31, 1985)

Reporters descended on the White household. "I understand why the school is scared," Ryan said, "but they should just listen to the facts." Many parents didn't want to listen to the facts; they were afraid that Ryan would endanger their children by breathing or coughing or bleeding on them. Ryan and his mother sued the school for him to be let back in; in response, over a hundred other parents threatened to sue the school if Ryan returned to class. These parents raised money through bake sales, going door to door, and holding an auction in the school gymnasium to pay for the lawyers arguing to keep Ryan out.

The judge ruled in Ryan's favor. Ryan went back to school . . . and some parents pulled their children from classes and set up an alternate school in an American Legion hall. Although some students were supportive, others were hostile, writing "FAG" on Ryan's locker, saying he had threatened to spit on them so they'd die, and taunting him in the halls with the jokes that were making the rounds.

> What kind of bread do fags eat?
> Ryan White bread.

The town was divided. Since there wasn't any social media in the mid-1980s, people took to the local paper to write letters defending Ryan or, more often, criticizing him and his mother. Some of Ryan's friends were told they couldn't play with Ryan anymore, that they had to stay away from his house. Stores that were once welcoming were now cold when Ryan's mother came in.

Then someone shot a bullet through a window of the Whites' house.

The message was clear: They were not welcome in the place they'd lived for years.

As he went in and out of the hospital, Ryan's fame grew. Most of the stories about him had the same way of describing him, emphasizing how normal, how average, what an everyboy he was.

> Despite the fact that AIDS is laying waste to Ryan's 60-lb. body, he has all the cravings of a normal teenager.
>
> —*People*

> His fresh-faced innocence provided a different perspective—an eye-opening realization that anyone could fall victim to the disease, and a call for the world to help, rather than shun, those afflicted with AIDS.
>
> —*The Indianapolis Star*

Other accounts talked about how he was an honor student, a good friend, a good son, the boy next door. At under five feet two and weighing less than a hundred pounds, he was hardly a threatening figure. He used humor and talk of faith to disarm the people who were afraid of him and of AIDS. "Why were they so scared?" White asked at one point. "Maybe it was because I wasn't that different from everyone else. I wasn't gay; I wasn't into drugs. I was just another kid from Kokomo. . . . Maybe that made me even more of a goblin."

People, both famous and not famous, reacted strongly to this, and

Ryan White became a very important symbol. To put it bluntly, many Americans who didn't care when AIDS was killing gay men in their twenties or Black women in their thirties or IV drug users in their forties suddenly cared a lot about AIDS when it was killing a straight white teen boy in Indiana. He was so "normal," he could have been their son, or grandson, or neighbor. He was so "normal" that if it could happen to him, it could happen to anyone. You couldn't argue that he had brought it upon himself. He was an innocent. And most people could unite against a disease that was killing innocent children.

This was not the story that Ryan White told; it was the story the media told *about* Ryan White. It raises a host of disturbing questions: If Ryan hadn't been so "normal" (i.e., straight, white), would he have still been seen as deserving sympathy on such a grand scale? Did portraying him as an "innocent victim" implicate those who became HIV+ through sex or drug use as being somehow guilty of their own sickness?

Ryan appeared on the cover of *People* three times. Tellingly, all the other famous-for-having-AIDS people who made the cover of *People* (as opposed to famous-and-then-having-AIDS) were also straight and white. There was Alison Gertz, whose date with a bisexual man led to her becoming infected. There was Kim Bergalis, whose dentist had infected her. There was Elizabeth Glaser, the wife of actor Paul Michael Glaser; like Ryan, she'd become HIV+ through a blood transfusion.

> Her date came with champagne, roses . . . and AIDS. Eight years later, Ali Gertz, 24, is fighting for her life and warning women that, yes, it *can* happen to you.
>
> —*People* cover, July 30, 1990

> Two years after routine dental surgery, college student Kim Bergalis developed AIDS. Now her dentist is dead of the disease, and she charges that he infected her.
>
> —*People* cover, October 22, 1990

> Ten years ago, Elizabeth Glaser was infected with the AIDS virus during a blood transfusion. Unaware, she passed it on to her two children; her daughter, Ariel, died at age 7. "My hope," she says, "is that others can learn from what I've been through."
> —*People* cover, February 4, 1991

All these people, and the coverage of their stories on TV shows and in magazines like *People*, did an effective job of getting the message across to America: *AIDS is not just a homosexual disease.* This helped much of America take HIV/AIDS more seriously. The media knew what it was doing in using these stories as sympathy lures. In its hard-hitting story "24 Hours in the Crisis That Is BREAKING AMERICA'S HEART," *People* opened the article on the cover itself, with a picture of an ill Ryan White in his jean jacket, being cradled in his mom's arms, alongside five paragraphs that start, "Ryan White is 15, and he is dying. 'Mom, I'm freezing,' he calls out." Then it goes on to say: "There are theologians who say that hell is cold—that ice, not fire, is the eternal torment. Ryan White has every reason to agree."

This is, in itself, heartbreaking and infuriating, confrontational and unsparing. What follows is even more interesting—the editors of *People* used this opening salvo to lead readers to not just Ryan's story but the story of a number of people dying with AIDS—sex workers and housewives, gay men in devoted relationships and gay men alone in hospices facing their unsparing last days. Also nurses and caregivers, parents who refused to be there for their suffering children, and parents who were willing to do anything to save them. The spotlight shines on the "normal child" to draw you in, then expands to show all the other people who are suffering and surviving.

Ryan White's misfortune was a rare misfortune—being born with hemophilia, then contracting HIV/AIDS. But what's remarkable about him is how he and his mother turned this rare misfortunate into an even more rare opportunity, leveraging it to build a bigger platform than a "normal" American teenager could ever expect to have. Like any queer kid his age, Ryan found his very existence made him an activist. Even as two diseases were ravaging his body, he did not shy away from speaking out. He pushed it as far as it could go.

During an episode of *The Phil Donahue Show,* a popular talk show at the time, Ryan appeared with his big celebrity crush, fifteen-year-old TV star Alyssa Milano. In front of the live studio audience, Alyssa kissed Ryan on the cheek, just to show that AIDS couldn't be spread by such casual contact. It was a groundbreaking moment, with a significant backlash—a backlash that turned Milano into an activist like White.

Ryan went to Washington in March 1988 and testified to the Commission on the HIV Epidemic:

> I came face to face with death at thirteen years old. I was diagnosed with AIDS: a killer. Doctors told me I'm not contagious. Given six months to live and being the fighter that I am, I set high goals for myself. It was my decision to live a normal life, go to school, be with my friends, and enjoying day to day activities. It was not going to be easy.
>
> The school I was going to said they had no guidelines for a person with AIDS. The school board, my teachers, and my principal voted to keep me out of the classroom even after the guidelines were set by the I.S.B.H. [Indiana State Board of Health], for fear of someone getting AIDS from me by casual contact. Rumors of sneezing, kissing, tears, sweat, and saliva spreading AIDS caused people to panic.
>
> We began a series of court battles for nine months, while I was attending classes by telephone. Eventually, I won the right to attend school, but the prejudice was still there. Listening to medical facts was not enough. People wanted one hundred percent guarantees. There are no one hundred percent guarantees in life, but concessions were made by Mom and me to help ease the fear. We decided to meet them halfway:
> - Separate restrooms
> - No gym

- Separate drinking fountains
- Disposable eating utensils and trays

Even though we knew AIDS was not spread through casual contact. Nevertheless, parents of twenty students started their own school. They were still not convinced. Because of the lack of education on AIDS, discrimination, fear, panic, and lies surrounded me:

- I became the target of Ryan White jokes
- Lies about me biting people, spitting on vegetables and cookies, urinating on bathroom walls
- Some restaurants threw away my dishes
- My school locker was vandalized inside and folders were marked FAG and other obscenities

I was labeled a troublemaker, my mom an unfit mother, and I was not welcome anywhere. People would get up and leave so they would not have to sit anywhere near me. Even at church, people would not shake my hand.

This brought on the news media, TV crews, interviews, and numerous public appearances. I became known as the AIDS boy. I received thousands of letters of support from all around the world, all because I wanted to go to school. Mayor Koch, of New York, was the first public figure to give me support. Entertainers, athletes, and stars started giving me support. I met some of the greatest like Elton John, Greg Louganis, Max Headroom, Alyssa Milano (my teen idol), Lyndon King (Los Angeles Raiders), and Charlie Sheen. All of these plus many more became my friends, but I had very few friends at school. How could these people in the public eye not be afraid of me, but my whole town was?

It was difficult, at times, to handle; but I tried to ignore the injustice, because I knew the people were wrong. My family and I held no hatred for those people because we realized they were victims of their own ignorance. We had great faith that with patience, understanding, and education, that my family and I could be helpful in changing their minds and attitudes around. Financial hardships were rough on us, even though Mom had a good job at G.M. The more I was sick, the more work she had to miss. Bills became impossible to pay. My sister, Andrea, was a championship roller skater who had to sacrifice too. There was no money for her lessons and travel. AIDS can destroy a family if you let it, but luckily for my sister and me, Mom taught us to keep going. Don't give up, be proud of who you are, and never feel sorry for yourself.

Having lived with a chronic illness since birth, Ryan was perhaps more able than others his age to understand his sickness. Certainly the love and support of his mother, sister, grandparents, and other family members, as well as friends, helped him accomplish what he accomplished. And his famous friends didn't hurt in spreading the word.

Other kids in similar situations had even harder reactions to face. Ricky, Robert, and Randy Ray were hemophiliac brothers who contracted AIDS from blood transfusions when they were all younger than eight. Their parents fought for them to attend school in Arcadia, Florida—and a week after the court ruled in their favor, their house was burned to the ground and they were forced to leave town. Channon Lee Phipps was in fifth grade when he was infected through tainted blood products. After his school in California barred him, he sued and won the right to return to class. But his family life wasn't as stable as Ryan's; his parents were teenage drug addicts who were out of the picture. Channon was raised by his aunt, whom he later sued for siphoning off money from the trust established in his name. When he got to junior high, he was not made to feel welcome. Classmates gave him a hard time. He was afraid of all the germs around him. He got sick more often. After the bullying was too much, he got into a fistfight. He decided he couldn't do it anymore and quit school when he was in seventh grade.

By the time he died of complications from AIDS and hemophilia at age twenty, he had been convicted of two drug offenses, telling a reporter that the drugs were his way of staving off depression.

Irene Emerson lost two of her hemophiliac sons, Steve and Richard, to AIDS in the 1980s. Steve had been one of Channon's best friends. As she left Channon's memorial service, Emerson told a reporter, "Most of the hemophiliacs are dead; almost all of them have died. When I heard Channon had died, I began thinking of who I should call to let them know. But there isn't anybody. They're all dead."

Things got better for Ryan White before his health got worse. Knowing that the divisions in their hometown weren't likely to be bridgeable, the Whites moved to Cicero, another town in Indiana, which was much more accepting of them. Ryan attended Hamilton Heights High School with little incident.

Imagine you are in high school, and you are famous for having a disease that scares a lot of people and is likely to kill you before you graduate. You have friends who support you, who you can confide in . . . but none of them are going through anything close to what you're going through. You still find bullies and passive-aggressive fear when you walk the halls—kids and adults who steer clear of you. While you try to make it to class, try to pass your exams and do your group projects, you are also out of school a lot. Sometimes it's to be flown to LA to hang out with Michael Jackson or to be onstage as Elton John sings a song to you. Other times—much more often—you're back in the hospital. You deal with relentless coughing, shingles, *Pneumocystis,* chills, fevers, exhaustion, and vomiting that never seems to stop. At the same time, you stress for weeks about who to ask to prom . . . but when prom comes along, you're in the hospital, barely able to move.

This was what Ryan's last year of life was like.

In March 1990, Ryan flew to Los Angeles to host an Oscars after-party with, among others, former President Ronald Reagan and former First Lady Nancy Reagan. There is steep irony here, because Reagan famously didn't mention AIDS until late in his fourth year in office, which was also the fourth year of public knowledge of the plague. In fact, in the press conference where he first addressed AIDS, he was asked about kids with AIDS being kept out of schools. Instead of taking Ryan's side and defending his right to be in school, Reagan took both sides and didn't answer a thing.

> Q: Mr. President, returning to something that Mike [Mike Putzel, Associated Press] said, if you had younger children, would you send them to a school with a child who had AIDS?
>
> PRESIDENT: I'm glad I'm not faced with that problem today. And I can well understand the plight of the parents and how they feel about it. I also have compassion, as I think we all do, for the child that has this and doesn't know and can't have it explained to him why somehow he is now an outcast and can no longer associate with his playmates and schoolmates. On the other hand, I can understand the problem with the parents. It is true that some medical sources had said that this cannot be communicated in any way other than the ones we already know and which would not involve a child being in the school. And yet medicine has not come forth unequivocally and said, "This we know for a fact, that it is safe." And until they do, I think we just have to do the best we can with this problem. I can understand both sides of it.

White's trip to Los Angeles had to be cut short because he was so ill. Back in Indiana, he was hospitalized for a respiratory infection and never left the hospital.

> **I was having so much trouble breathing I had to have an oxygen mask. I felt like Frankenstein—part kid, part machine. But even on**

oxygen, I could tell I wasn't getting any better. Everything inside me seemed to be breaking down. AIDS was wearing down my liver, my spleen, my kidneys. And fast too.

—Ryan White: My Own Story

When he died, *People* called Ryan "perhaps the best-known of this country's 76,000-plus AIDS fatalities."

Ryan White never surrendered—not to AIDS, not to despair, not to the fearful public passions that his illness once aroused.

—People

I think little Ryan White probably did more to change the face of this illness and to move people than anyone.

—Larry Kramer

Former President Reagan eulogized Ryan in a piece published in *The Washington Post* shortly after Ryan died.

Ryan would probably be embarrassed by all the fuss we are making over him. He did not want to be anyone special. He just wanted to go to school, play with his friends and grow up like every other kid in the neighborhood. But it was not to be.

For reasons which we may never fully understand, Ryan's life was set on a course that no one could predict and which we could do so precious little to affect. How Nancy and I wish there had been a magic wand we could have waved to make it all go away. Ryan White touched our lives in a special way. His ready smile, his youthful innocence, his simple desire to just live his life tugged at our hearts in a way we will always remember. How we wanted to hug him and make him better...

Sadly, Ryan's is not the only life to have been cut short by AIDS. In a most poignant way, he told us of a health crisis in our country that has claimed too many victims. There have been too many funerals like his. There are too many patches in the quilt.

Reagan's hypocrisy did not go unnoticed. In a response to his words, a gay man named David Robinson wrote to *The Washington Post*. As someone who continued to see friends and lovers sicken and die, he was, like many gay men, infuriated by Reagan's words.

> He may not have had a wand, but he had the next best thing: the presidency of the United States during the first eight years of the AIDS epidemic. Reagan could have improved the survival chances of Ryan White and other people with AIDS by speaking out often and forcefully on AIDS. Instead it took him seven years to make a speech about AIDS. In that time, 50,000 Americans contracted the disease, and 30,000 died of it. He could have pushed Congress to spend enough money to fight the disease. Instead, he initially requested no money and then requested insultingly insufficient amounts. Each year Congress had to appropriate more than his administration asked for.
> 
> Reagan could have spoken out about the slow and tangled processes of the FDA and NIH in researching and developing treatments for AIDS. He could have pressed for a clear, explicit, culturally sensitive education campaign to stop the spread of AIDS.
> 
> He could have done many things to alter the course of the AIDS epidemic and save lives, but he chose to do "precious little." That he had the nerve to eulogize Ryan White without first having taken responsibility, and asked forgiveness, for his eight years of inaction is an insult to those who have died of AIDS, including Ryan White.

Others grappled with putting Ryan White's death within the larger context of the tens of thousands of other people who had died of AIDS.

> No other person, living or dead, has so galvanized the spirit of the nation in common battle against this 20th-Century plague. Perhaps, in

the number of his battles, the only loss recorded by young "David" was against the "Goliath" of prejudice and ignorance.

The child is gone, but in the history of our memories is an elder statesman, eloquent beyond poetry and prose in the way he conducted his life.

—Alan Daniels, *Los Angeles Times*

I believe the biggest fear we all live with is to die forgotten. In the gay community we will never forget, never. And while the world mourns the Ryan Whites (and I am part of that world), a thousand others will die never knowing what complete acceptance really means, and I am part of that.

—Daniel Warner, *Los Angeles Times*

How dare you, Joe Public, cry for only Ryan White! He was safe to mourn! Mourn for those dying daily, their deaths hastened by cancelled insurance, exorbitant, unreachable black-market drug prices and a federal policy that ignored the existence of AIDS because it was considered a "homosexual" disease.

—Frances J. Mac Guire, *Los Angeles Times*

Ryan's mission was for us to fight the disease instead of fighting the gays, the drug users and the so-called innocent victims. Everyone is an innocent victim of this disease. We need to find a cure.

—Jeanne White, a year after her son Ryan's death

Four months after Ryan's death, on August 18, 1990, President George H. W. Bush signed the Ryan White Comprehensive AIDS Resources Emergency Act (Ryan White CARE Act) into law. This legislation provided more than $2 billion to help states and communities create and maintain coordinated and comprehensive systems for the care of people with AIDS, particularly poor people. It has since been renewed four times and remains the most important federal source of funding in the fight against AIDS in America, although recently its existence has been threatened by conservative legislators and the drastic cuts ordered by the Trump administration in 2025.

The story of Ryan White is a story of both empathy and the limits of empathy. Ryan himself was unwaveringly empathetic, often connecting his plight to those who weren't like him. But there is something disturbing and cautionary about the fact that it took a straight white teenage boy to die for a number of Americans to start paying attention to the crisis in our midst. There is certainly power in identifying with victims because they are like us, and in being galvanized because of the connection you feel. But if we end up only caring about the people who share our identity, where does that leave us? Ryan White was an incredibly effective symbol who played a role in getting activists some of the attention and funding they needed. But what does it mean that he was the one who could make people care? How much sooner might a treatment have been found if more people had cared in the same way about non-straight, non-white people battling HIV/AIDS?

## Complications

It wasn't AIDS that would kill you. Not by itself. When it went untreated—because the diagnosis happened before the arrival of effective medication or because you didn't know you had HIV or, later, because you couldn't afford or get hold of consistent treatment—HIV opened the door for infections and illnesses that would try to kill you. Your body would become more and more vulnerable to an unpredictable array of symptoms, complications, and opportunistic infections. It wasn't enough to take your freedom and your health. No, AIDS could also take your breathing, your sight, your mind.

When you are diagnosed with AIDS, with a CD4 (or T-cell) count of lower than 200, it means your HIV is at the point where your immune system has stopped protecting you from simple infections. And back when there was no treatment, HIV almost always turned into AIDS, which almost inevitably led to death. As explained earlier, AIDS isn't one single illness: It's an immune disorder that reduces the body's ability to withstand infection. When people talk about someone dying of "AIDS complications" or "complications due to AIDS," it's because AIDS doesn't fire the gun but lets the assassins in the door.

Plagues within a plague—if this sounds like something biblical, that's how it works. Your defenses are down, and your ability to navigate previously normal situations without encountering the risk of illness is drastically reduced. The "complications" below are meant to show some of what suffering from AIDS was like before treatment was found—and what it can still look like now if you are unable to access regular care. In many places around the world, and in some populations within the United States, these illnesses are still leading causes of death for people living with AIDS today. You have to imagine these illnesses as relentless waves of attack: As one is beaten back, another can charge in. The body fights with everything it has . . . but for many, that isn't enough.

Here are some of the things people with AIDS can be up against:

## HIV-related fever

Most people have no idea they've become HIV+ unless they're regularly getting tested for HIV. You can be HIV+ for years without realizing it, even as your body gradually develops the signs and symptoms of AIDS. The lack of initial symptoms is why getting tested for HIV is so important, especially if you're sexually active.

Sometimes people get a bad fever a month after they contract HIV. It's not the end of the world; you might disregard this fever as just another head cold. But it's one of the earliest tangible signs of living with HIV. The lymph nodes in your throat swell up as the body responds to the arrival of HIV in your system. Sometimes the fever passes and health resumes. Other times the fever returns and other things start going wrong.

## Cancer

People with AIDS are much more likely to get cancer. The cancer that is most associated with AIDS is **Kaposi's sarcoma (KS)**, a rare type that had primarily been seen in elderly men prior to the epidemic. Kaposi's sarcoma became synonymous with AIDS partly because of its unambiguous visual markings. People with Kaposi's sarcoma often get lesions—purple, brown, red, or pink marks that blotch across the body as the cancer progresses.

Kaposi's sarcoma forms in the lining of blood vessels and lymph vessels. It manifests first as lesions on the face, arms, and legs. Often for people with HIV, these lesions were the first telltale sign. Their presence made HIV's presence no longer undeniable. You can chalk a fever up to a cold, tiredness to not getting enough sleep. But lesions on your skin can rarely be explained away. You've probably been on this journey for a while, and now your body is making you aware of it in no uncertain terms.

And it isn't just a telltale sign for you or your doctors. If you have a lesion on a part of your body that you can't easily cover with clothing, it's like you're broadcasting to the world that you have AIDS. Best-case scenario, the mark will be a signal for compassion. But more often than not, it is a cause for hostility and/or fear. Our culture likes illness to be discreet, hidden away. People affected by KS are forced to wear their sickness openly—the lesions on the face unmistakable to many by the late 1980s, when newspapers printed images of people living with AIDS whose bodies bore the marks of KS. People would recoil, Jesus's lesson with the lepers all but forgotten.

As with any cancer, the thing you have to fear the most with KS is that it will spread. Bad enough to have KS lesions on the surface or spreading to your mouth or genitals. But it becomes even worse if it goes into your digestive tract or your lungs. At a certain point, the only way to fight it is radiation or chemotherapy—even though you know radiation will make you weaker, more vulnerable to other infections. But what choice do you have?

Sometimes you can make the lesions go away with the radiation or chemotherapy. Sometimes they return. Or there might be a new complication that arises in a deadly form.

> I think one of the difficult things about AIDS is the look of the disease, which frightens and scares most people. You know the lesions and the gaunt look and the pneumonia complications. I think people do have an inner life. When people become so sick, they go look at themselves in the mirror in the bathroom and they have a lot less esteem simply because of the way they look, but their inner life is still them and that's their core. I think people have to make a real effort to get beyond the look of AIDS and to think about the value of people inside.
> 
> —Robin Tichane, AIDS activist and art conservator

\* \* \*

**Cervical cancer** is another form of cancer associated with AIDS. People living with untreated HIV are six times more likely to develop cervical cancer than their HIV– counterparts. Cervical cancer is caused by human papillomavirus, or HPV: the most common STI (sexually transmitted infection), with more than 150 different strains. A body uncompromised by HIV can fend off the infection itself, but with untreated HIV, the body is more vulnerable and the infection can turn into anal and cervical cancers.

You can live with cervical cancer for a long time without realizing you have it. Until the fatigue starts, your appetite stops, and you lose weight without explanation. Sex becomes painful. Your insides hurt. You bleed much more than usual from your vagina without any regular explanation. Because cervical cancer almost always affects women, the connection between AIDS and cervical cancer was slow to be established. The first definitions of AIDS were focused upon the male body.

With **lymphoma**, the AIDS-aided cancer attacks the lymphatic system—ironically, the system that provides white blood cells to fight infection and disease. It might start in one area of the lymph nodes—like your neck, above your collarbone, under your arms, in your abdomen, or in your groin. But from there, it can spread throughout your body—because the lymphatic system exists throughout your body. Imagine a house's sprinkler system being used to burn it down—that's what lymphoma does. The cancer can infiltrate your blood, your brain, your spinal cord, your bone marrow. It can make you want to scratch your skin off . . . and also make you so fatigued that you feel barely able to exist. It can take away your appetite, your vision, your ability to speak.

### Night sweats

You cannot control your body. At night, it reacts like you are out in the sun. Your sweat drenches whatever you wear. It drenches the sheets. You are damp, uncomfortable. *You've wet the bed.* That shame. That discomfort. Night after night after night. You cannot keep the tide within you. You ebb as the sweat rises.

# The Man with Night Sweats
## by Thom Gunn

I wake up cold, I who
Prospered through dreams of heat
Wake to their residue,
Sweat, and a clinging sheet.

My flesh was its own shield:
Where it was gashed, it healed.

I grew as I explored
The body I could trust
Even while I adored
The risk that made robust,

A world of wonders in
Each challenge to the skin.

I cannot but be sorry
The given shield was cracked,
My mind reduced to hurry,
My flesh reduced and wrecked.

I have to change the bed,
But catch myself instead

Stopped upright where I am
Hugging my body to me
As if to shield it from
The pains that will go through me,

As if hands were enough
To hold an avalanche off.

### Thrush

A fungus accumulates on the lining of your mouth. *Candida albicans*—worst drag name ever. She's always there in your mouth, under control, but when you're immunocompromised, she runs all over the place, leaving behind a mess that no mouthwash will clear. You get lesions on your tongue and inside your cheeks. Then they spread to the roof of your mouth. Your gums. Your tonsils. *A cottage-cheese-like consistency.* Scrape it out, it just grows back. Every time you swallow—there's your disease. Every time you taste, if you can taste at all—there's your disease. And that's if you're lucky. If you're unlucky, *Candida albicans* spreads. She will make her way down into your esophagus, so every time you swallow, you will feel like something is stuck in your throat. And she might go even farther, to your genitals, refusing to be ignored.

### Wasting syndrome

Fever. Diarrhea. Weakness. For days. Then weeks. Then more than a month. You lose weight. Far too much weight. Both fat and muscle. AIDS-related wasting syndrome is identified when someone living with AIDS has lost more than 10 percent of their body weight because of the advancement of their condition.

You watch your body diminish; it can't sustain itself. And once the weight is lost, in the days before effective treatment, it likely won't return. The people around you see you shrink. So much effort to walk. Now to stand. To sit up. People who were once two hundred pounds now weigh in at ninety, eighty. *Skeletal:* a word that appears in so many accounts of those who died because of AIDS. *She was just bones. He was so gaunt, sunken. I couldn't believe this was his body, and I could tell . . . neither could he.*

### Pneumonia or *Pneumocystis carinii* pneumonia (PCP)

A bacterial or fungal infection in your lungs. When it takes hold, it's harder to breathe. Your chest tightens. You lose weight. You cough. Your lungs swell, fill with liquid, and it's like drowning on dry land. Pneumonia affects people with weakened immune systems: A nasty cold can turn, suddenly, into something much deadlier.

### Tuberculosis (TB)

People with untreated HIV are twenty to thirty times more likely to develop TB than people without HIV. TB is caused by a bacterium that, given the chance, will infect your lungs. Symptoms include coughing (sometimes with blood, sometimes accompanied by chest pain), fever, weight loss, night sweats. Again, in America this has largely been eradicated by rigorous treatment, but it remains a serious problem elsewhere in the world, where treatments are not as available or affordable.

### Cytomegalovirus (CMV) retinitis

Cytomegalovirus is a common virus—by the age of forty, over half of all Americans have it in their bodies. And usually our bodies keep it in check. But this is not the case in people with AIDS, where CMV often manifests itself in the eyes in the form of CMV retinitis. This is one reason so many people dying because of AIDS lost their sight before they lost their lives.

It might start with blind spots, floating specks of absolute darkness crawling across your vision. Or maybe it starts with a blurring, as if a layer of steam is rising into your eyes and you cannot wipe it away. Then, as the retinitis progresses, the darkness and the blur take over. Imagine that terror. To be struck by a deadly disease, and then to slowly lose the ability to see everyone and everything around you. To lose the ability to navigate the world on your own. To lie in a hospital bed without being able to see where you are or who is with you. To try to live through the dying of that light without feeling doomed.

### Cryptococcal meningitis

Here, a fungal infection attacks tissues covering the brain and spinal cord. It is not your breathing that falters but your mind. With the fever comes confusion. With the nausea comes a profound disorientation, sometimes to the point of hallucination. Possible complications include brain damage, hearing or vision loss, seizures, or death. You feel like you are losing your mind, and that is exactly what is happening.

### Toxoplasmosis

Imagine being a cat owner and finding out that your cat could be carrying toxins that might kill you. Many people with AIDS discovered early on the dangers of keeping their feline companions; often, the cats needed to be sent to new homes, even if the loss devastated the person left behind. The reason? *Toxoplasma gondii,* a parasite spread primarily by cats. Living with advanced HIV meant being vulnerable to what the cats might carry. What might have lain dormant within you for years suddenly becomes active. In the case of people with AIDS, when the CD4 count goes below 100, the parasites are reactivated and cause an infection. In people with AIDS, toxoplasmosis is the leading cause of brain damage. Symptoms that start as headaches, fever, confusion, and bad coordination can escalate to seizures, ocular toxoplasmosis (blurry vision because of severe inflammation of your retina), eye infection that can lead to blindness, and encephalitis, a severe brain infection that can lead to death.

### HIV-related nephropathy (HIVAN)

Disproportionately affecting Black people with AIDS, untreated HIV invades the kidney cells and leads to kidney failure. When your kidneys fail, your body can no longer filter waste products from the blood. Your blood becomes toxic.

### HIV-associated neurocognitive disorder (HAND)

Difficulties with attention, concentration, and memory. Loss of motivation. Irritability. Depression. Slowed movements. And, in more extreme cases, dementia. HAND is a cruel acronym, because in this case, all it does is take and take. People who die with untreated AIDS were, and are, often lost to their loved ones before their actual deaths. Friends could only watch as they were erased from memory, as the people who suffered retreated into an unreachable place. *Can you still hear me? See me? Know who I am?* At a certain point, the questions went unanswered by words and could only be answered by faith. And often there was a strange solace: If they were so far gone that they didn't know what was happening, or who they were, maybe—just maybe—they didn't know that death had come.

## The valley of death
### by Ron Schreiber

John didn't die. he hasn't
died yet. but he's only

rarely coherent, we're
thankful for a smile, a

shard of conversation.
when he screams "no no noo

no no" "go home," we are
glad that he has his voice

back & says actual words
rather than moans. when

he claws at his chest, we
say, "he's trying to use

his hands." today he
may be better, longer

moments of attempted speech.
today he may not

be better. we don't know:
day to day, hour to hour,

it will be short or longer.
his brain will work

or it won't.

## Macular degeneration

Macular degeneration is damage to your vision. Your eyesight becomes impaired; you might be legally blind. Macular degeneration is a common hazard for people in their old age. Having untreated AIDS meant that people were much more likely to experience macular degeneration decades and decades before it was expected.

## Mental health issues

If you're living with HIV or AIDS, you're more likely to suffer from depression and anxiety. This was true in the 1980s, and it's still true today. You might be undetectable and in your prime, but the feeling of being HIV+ can still be a lot for someone to deal with, especially if they're newly diagnosed. It can also exacerbate mental health challenges that were already present. Getting out of bed in the morning might suddenly feel more difficult. Positive status, like any physical health challenge, can affect self-esteem. It may also contribute to panic attacks, insomnia, intrusive thoughts, and suicidal feelings. These issues might lead you down a difficult path into other ones: drug abuse, alcohol abuse, disordered eating. If you don't have the right support system, it can be hard to look after yourself, even though being diagnosed with HIV is a fantastic reason to make your well-being your number one priority. Mental illness isn't linked to the spread of HIV in your body; it's a consequence of living with a stigmatized condition in a world that scapegoats HIV+ people and doesn't want to talk about illness openly.

All living beings are going to experience illness and death. It's part of what it means to be alive. As humans, we tend to spend our lives avoiding this fact. For people with untreated HIV and an AIDS diagnosis, it gets harder and harder to look away as the likelihood of illness increases. The astonishing thing, in the face of all of this, is the desire to live. To know all the ways you could die, and to go on.

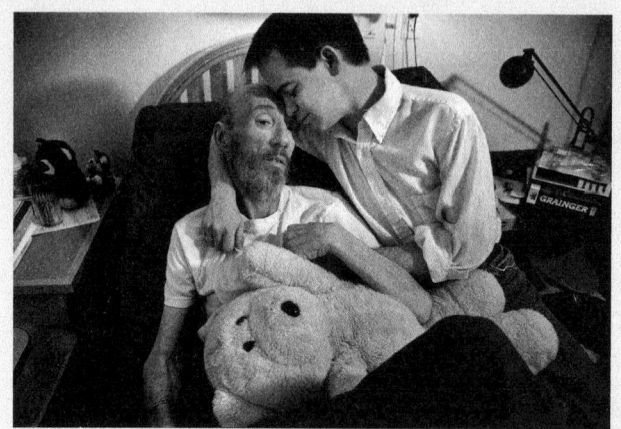
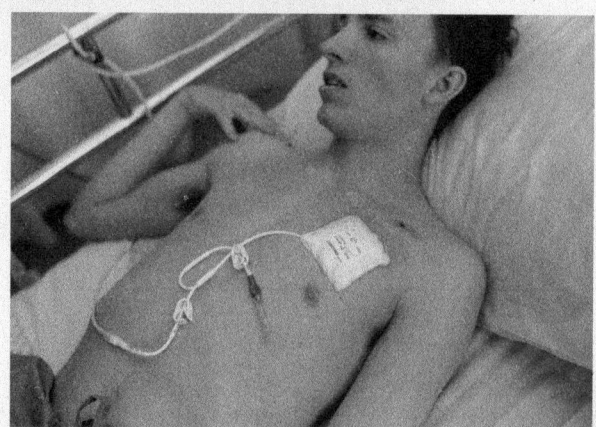
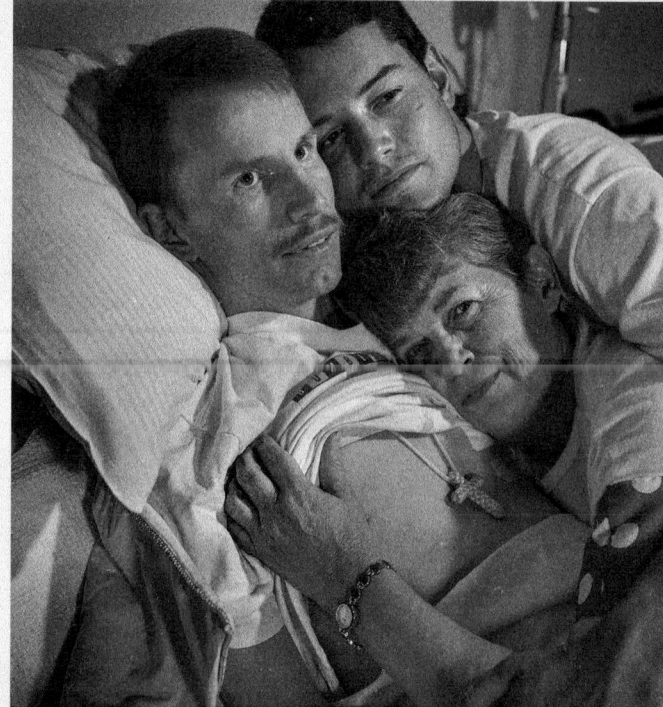

**SOURCE MATERIAL**

# Health Care

## by M.L.

*This piece appeared in* Still Here, *a collection of writing from participants in the Therapeutic Writing Group at New York's Mount Sinai Hospital's Clinic for HIV-Related Concerns. Many of the writings we can find by people with HIV/AIDS come from such writing groups, set up by support organizations, LGBTQ+ centers, and hospitals to help people articulate, document, and process what was happening to them.*

Thank you, so much, dear Hospital. Thanks for your care and attention to my buddy, Shaun.

Thanks for your food delivery staff who would not deliver the meals to his bedside, but left them cooling on trays which they left on the floor outside his door.

Thanks for your cleaning staff who also wouldn't dare to enter his room, but stood outside his door toying with their mops, cleaning only the floor within their arms reach.

Thanks for the endless rounds of students constantly examining him, prodding him and talking about him as if he was already a corpse.

Thanks for the night orderly, the one who looked like a hermaphrodite with one chromosome missing. "A regular greengrocers we have here," he used to quip. "Fruits on this side; vegetables on that side!"

Thanks for the way that you managed Shaun's pain. Thanks for not giving him enough morphine so that he wouldn't become "addicted" during the three weeks prior to his death.

Thanks for the chemotherapy, which he had specifically declined.

He really appreciated waking up that night to find the nurse slipping it into his IV line, telling him it was nothing.

Thanks for treating him like a lab experiment and for not treating him like the loving, caring human being that he really was.

Thank you for not truthfully answering his questions. Thank you for treating him like a child, whose questions were to receive only condescending answers.

Thanks for your lack of civility towards his family and extended family.

Thanks for the lengths of time that you took to answer his buzzer.

Thanks for letting him know that most of his requests for assistance were so tiresome.

Thank you for the heat, which was turned up so high and you could not, would not (?) lower it. Thanks for the incubation of airborne viruses and bacteria.

Thank you for all of this, dear hospital. Your very thoughtful actions drove him from your hellhole into the arms of his loved ones, who gladly nursed him at home through those final days.

Thank you, from the bottom of my heart, for giving me this opportunity.

**SOURCE MATERIAL**

# June 25

## by Essex Hemphill

*So much of what we know about the Black experience of HIV/ AIDS in the 1980s and 1990s is due to the writing, anthologizing, and activism of Essex Hemphill, whose work appears more than once in these pages. His poems were featured in the groundbreaking documentaries* Tongues Untied *and* Looking for Langston, *and his collection* Ceremonies: Prose and Poetry *is a landmark in queer literature. This excerpt comes from the anthology* Life Sentences.

Yesterday, my new doctor, based in short-skirted, fashionable Los Angeles, on trendy, palm-tree-lined Wilshire Boulevard, informed me that I now possess only twenty-three T cells. Needless to say, my face cracked, but I'm a show boy, I learned long ago how to keep things together even under the most strained and pressing of circumstances. I haven't always known how to use this facility, but of late it comes in handy, although I think it costs something internally to hold oneself in check in the face of provocation and overwhelming emotions.

By the end of my visit, I was armed with prescriptions for six different medications, which the pharmacist assured me will not interact violently. Quite frankly, I don't know whether I should calculate my remaining T cells into nanoseconds and minutes, days and weeks, or hours and years.

Some of the T cells I am without are not here through my own fault. I didn't lose all of them foolishly, and I didn't lose all of them erotically. Some of the missing T cells were lost to racism, a well-known transmittable disease. Some were lost to poverty because there was no money to do something about the plumbing before the pipes burst and the room flooded. Homophobia killed quite a few, but so did my rage and my pointed furies, so did the wars at home and the wars within, so did the drugs I took to remain calm, cool, collected.

There are T cells lying dead by the roadside, slain by the guise of friendship, the pettiness and jealousy of minds and talent in the process of wasting to nothingness due to envy, gazing into other yards instead of looking closely at and tending to their own. There are T cells sacrificed between the love and anger my mother and I hold for one another, T cells that have simply exploded due to the decibel of our screeching.

There are countless wasted T cells between my father and me, the result of painful, subterranean silences that I cannot resolve with only twenty-three T cells, nor should I really be expected to, nor should I try, since it was his violence I witnessed and remain scarred from. I am forced to remember him in certain ways, to always see him punching and pushing, slapping and yelling, not because I want to, I just haven't learned how to make so many scars into things of beauty, and I don't know if I ever will.

Actually, there are T cells scattered all about me, at doorways where I was denied entrance because I was a faggot or a nigga or too poor or too black. There are T cells spilling out of my ashtrays from the cigarettes I have anxiously smoked. There are T cells all over the floors of several bathhouses, coast to coast, and halfway around the world, and in numerous parks, and in countless bars, and in places I am forgetting to make room for other memories. My T cells are strewn about like the leaves of a mighty tree, like the fallen hair of an old man, like the stars of a collapsing universe.

That is who I am now, one of *them*, one of *them*. A single strand, a curling leaf, a burning star foretelling grief. I say this only to dispel such gloom. I say this loud to kill death's bloom.

## TESTIMONY

# Robert Levithan

*My uncle's near-death bout with AIDS-related pneumonia in May 1994 was an event he often went back to in his writing. As an AIDS counselor, he was also acutely aware of the physical toll that AIDS took—as well as the resilience of survivors to go beyond this toll.*

## (2000)

The face so caved and drawn . . .

*Will that be me someday? Will that day be soon?* I no longer live in that reality. I no longer wonder daily, hourly how long until I'm the skeletal man swimming in last year's clothes, gamely trying to stand erect in line at the pharmacy.

I don't see these men on the street. I don't see one in the mirror. On the rare occasions when I still find myself visiting someone on an AIDS ward, I do see them in beds—and it's like being pushed into a time warp back ten years, almost twenty, to late nights and terrifying visitations from demented—really demented, as in dementia—friends on their way to save the world or explain my shortcomings or both.

Then I remember it's 2000. I have 658 T-cells not 20 as in 1995.

The faces I see caved and drawn now are due to lipodystrophy, a medication side effect which is almost understood now. These are the ragged masked faces of survival, not death. I noticed myself drawn to one such face just today at the gym, finding the look of that experience attractive—a sign, I hope, that I welcome the ravages, however slight, of my struggles. I now salute my brothers' and sisters' caved or sunken cheeks, battle scars won whether from endurance or luck but rendered beautiful to my expert eye.

Life takes its toll, but it also restores the light in my eyes and my faith, my faith in whatever will happen.

## (1995)

The first time I saw "OI" written in a magazine or newsletter, I couldn't understand what an "oi" (as in "oi vey") would be doing there. Even though I was at least ten years into the AIDS experience, both in community and in my own HIV-positive body, I found myself once more out of the loop. I didn't really *want* to read about OI's—opportunistic infections. They were my greatest fear—they were the Nazis, the McCarthyites, and my worst boyfriends all rolled into one. Most closely, they resembled that recurring childhood nightmare where I fell down the stairs, tumbling out of control, to awaken just before I was to hit the bottom. I would find myself sitting up in bed, gasping for breath, sweat popping from every pore—not sure at first whether the bed or the dream was real.

Last May, when I lay in a hospital bed, gasping and sweaty, I knew what was real. And like almost every feared change or passage in my life, it was not quite or even nearly as bad as I had feared. I found myself in that place of dealing, coping. IVs, pills, and liquids were my job. The simple acts of survival sustained me along with tenderness and care. Oi vey, OI—the time had come: like a bar mitzvah, a divorce, a diagnosis. Pick up the phone, reassemble according to the blueprint or my instinct; open eyes and breathe. Not so very complicated, actually.

## (1997)

I think I may have met a saint at St. Vincent's Hospital in May of 1994. I was having quite a time—hooked up to IVs and watching my new state of enforced quietude with both horror and wonder.

Into my room each day came Carmen, a stout cartoon figure of a Northern New Mexico Hispanic Grandmother. I don't remember her hair—I do remember that she carried the love of the Sangre de Cursos. She was always moving, slowly, pushing a chair, bringing some kind of order to the little room with the too-big bed and too many hard surfaces. It would be morning, not a time for visitors with bouquets of flowers and muffins and tea. It could have been in Spanish or in English— I only know that I thrilled at the sound of her outside my extra large door. In came bright eager eyes and a blanket of peace rested on my pneumonia-filled lungs. Carmen cleaned rooms. She's the Mother Teresa of cleaning women. We spoke about her life—mostly *she* talked, happy to tell me what she was doing as she cleaned. She has been encouraged to become a practical nurse and finally years ago she went to school and moved up the class ladder. Before long she asked for her old job back. Carmen was absolutely solidly sure that she was meant to mop the floors of men and women who couldn't do it themselves.

As I lay there, fully present in my laboring body, I could also feel my safety in the Divine—Miss God had sent me Carmen.

## (2012)

Back in 1994, after two weeks in bed with serious AIDS-related pneumonia, I had not "lost my looks," but I had lost my body. The flesh hung on my thighs. My body had less muscle tone than my energetic 84-year-old father's. I was tired after walking across my small walled garden in Santa Fe.

I decided to see what I could do about it. I remember doing three push-ups one day, twelve leg lifts the next day, and building incrementally until about a year later I was at the gym when a man approached me and said, "You look like you are in good shape and might be able to give me help with this machine." Only then did I realize that I had fully brought back my body.

Although most of the cases of AIDS involved adults, there were babies, kids, and teenagers who were affected. According to the CDC, between 1981 and 2001, there were 9,074 cases in children under the age of thirteen—with 5,257 of them dying. Many of these children were born HIV+ because their HIV+ mothers passed them the virus while they were pregnant. Others were hemophiliacs who had received tainted blood transfusions. For teenagers, there were these causes, but also sexual transmission, either through consensual encounters or sexual violence.

What follow are the stories of three people who had to face off against HIV and AIDS at a young age, told in their own words.

*Doctors told me I would die within two years, which would have meant sixteen....*

# Luna Luis Ortiz

*Luna Luis Ortiz began his journey in HIV awareness as a spokesperson for youth living with HIV at the Hetrick-Martin Institute in 1988. An acclaimed photographer and performer, he has also been part of New York City's house and ballroom community since the 1980s.*

I contracted HIV at the age of fourteen after I had my first sexual experience. It was 1986. Doctors told me I would die within two years, which would have meant sixteen.

I was born in New York City.

In the 1970s, New York was a terrible place. It seemed like every other building on our block was on fire because the landlords were collecting their insurance money and driving away the people who'd lived there for years. So my parents packed up our bags and we moved to Lancaster, Pennsylvania. Lancaster was the opposite of New York City. Everything was green, the sky was blue, the schools were better. I had fields and meadows to run through.

Looking back, it's ironic: I recall my parents not wanting me to go swimming in the public pool in Lancaster, because AIDS was in the news at the time. They were afraid I might "catch AIDS" from the water.

In 1984, we moved back to New York City. The stigma around HIV/AIDS was severe. Whenever I saw anything about AIDS on television, it was always a white person. The media just didn't prioritize people of color with HIV. As a young Latine kid, I never thought HIV would be part of my life.

We lived in Harlem. My mom would tell me to walk the dog over on St. Nicholas Park. I can still hear her voice: "Luna, go walk the dog! He's going to pee all over the place!"

One day, I met a man walking his dog as I was walking mine. I figured he was about thirty years old. We'd bump into each other often, and it became a friendship of sorts. You know how neighbors are. We'd say hi to each other, we'd chat. He used to call me Louie, and I guess it flattered me that he remembered me.

One day in late July, I bumped into him again, but this time, he didn't have his dog with him. We walked together. We ended up in this little, secluded area. There were bushes all around us. I remember my dog running around. The man started touching my knee, and then he was telling me how cute I was. And then it went to a place where I wasn't even sure what we were doing.

That's how it happened.

I was sore when I got home. And scared. I remember being in the bathroom. I remember my mom knocking on the door:

"Everything okay in there?"

I called back, "Yes, Mom!"

But the water in the toilet was red with blood.

By early August, I just felt wrong. My mother is a very "hurry up and get dressed" type of person. She looked at me and said, "Get dressed, you have the flu, we need to take you to see the doctor!"

At first, the doctors thought I had mono—they called it "the kissing disease." But over the summer, my sickness wouldn't go away. My mom and I kept going back and forth to the pediatric unit to work out what was wrong with me.

"Oh, you're still not feeling better. . . ."

"Oh, now you have this symptom. . . ."

"Oh, your glands are swollen!"

"Let's go back to the hospital."

The first week, I had the night sweats. The second week, swollen glands. By the third week, I still couldn't stop sweating and feeling sick all the time.

Not once did I say, "I had sex with someone at the park," because there would be so much shame in that admission. No one suggested I might have HIV. That wasn't mentioned at all.

Finally, they kept me in hospital overnight. They put me in this private room. I'd see the nurse coming, but she'd stop in the antechamber to put on gloves and a mask. I'd lost a lot of weight. I was a skinny kid, but I got so much thinner. I remember being in the hospital room looking at myself in the mirror and just starting to cry. I really thought I was going to die.

They did four spinal taps to check for different diseases. Each time, I had to curl up into the fetal position for them to inject me with a needle. After the last one, the doctor said to me, "Are you homosexual, heterosexual, or bisexual?"

I didn't know what those words meant. I knew "gay" and "straight," and I knew what a "faggot" was, but not these medical-sounding words.

She said, "Do you like boys?"

I didn't answer. I just couldn't.

That's when she went to my mother and told her that we needed to do an HIV test. I guess the doctor had somehow been able to see I'd been penetrated when she gave me the injection.

That was in September. Tests weren't quick back then. In November, they rang. My mom said to me, "Get dressed. They don't want to tell us the results over the phone. We're going to the hospital."

There, they told me, "You have HIV."

Even after the doctor explained it, I still didn't understand what AIDS meant, or what HIV was. Back then, in 1986, HIV tests were new. Everything was so disconnected. No one had any understanding of how to deal with a kid who had something which nobody understood. There were no post-diagnosis support services for me. And of course, in 1986, there was no effective medication.

They told me I was probably going to die by the time I was sixteen years old. We went straight home. Nobody talked about HIV to me. Everything I learned, I had to learn by experience on my own.

Hearing that you're going to die by the time you're sixteen changes you forever. It never leaves you. But it gave me a hunger to live. Between the ages of fourteen and sixteen, I lived a whole lifetime. I needed to be able to say I'd had a fulfilling life, because I was certain I was going to die.

I stopped going to class. My mom thought I was leaving for school each morning, but I'd head into the city and go to museums. If I was going to die, I wanted to see things I'd never seen before. I needed to absorb all the art I could. I'd head downtown and walk around Central Park, loving the sound of the city and the feeling of nature. I'd check out the Old Masters at the Met, or go to the public library—this beautiful old building in Harlem—and read books. I was desperate to access everything that life had to offer me.

It was through my trips to the library that I met Wade and his friend James. And Wade is the one who introduced me to the rest of my life.

It happened like this:

I'd just learned who Marlene Dietrich was. I'd read about her in a book about Marilyn Monroe. I said to myself, *I need to read more about Marlene Dietrich!* I went to the library and saw two other gay kids sitting at a table. It's hard to explain how I knew they were gay—sometimes, we can just identify each other. They were looking at me, and it made me nervous—I hadn't interacted with any gay people yet! I was just by myself all the time back then, figuring out what to do with the rest of my life—a life that I wasn't sure I was going to have.

One of them—Wade—was like, "Hey, come here."

That's how we got talking. Before long, we were speaking about music. He liked Diana Ross, but I was a die-hard Madonna fan.

He was like, "Diana Ross is better!"

I was like, "No way, Madonna is! Diana Ross is so *old*! It's all about the new girls!"

We laughed. That's how we became friends.

Wade took me down to the West Village. He told me about this youth center for other queer kids, which is now known as the Hetrick-Martin Institute. He said, "Miss Luna, you're going to love it there, because there are other people like us."

It was Thanksgiving in 1988. They were doing a dinner for the youth, and you could bring a friend with you, so I was Wade's friend.

I'll always remember that visit. We went up the stairs, took a left, then a right. I walked into the room and was met by this sea of young queer kids, mostly Black and Brown, some white faces too. Everyone was a teenager: you had to be under twenty-one years old. Everyone already knew each other, so I was the new kid, and it felt like everybody was staring at me.

I saw some kids voguing in the corner, and I said to Wade, "What are they doing?"

He was like, "That's called voguing. The sisters vogue. It's amazing."

I said, "But what is it?"

He said, "It's a dance, duh! You know, like that attitude in *Vogue* magazine."

When I remember that day, I think about Dorothy when she arrives in Oz.

You're Judy Garland, stuck in Kansas in black and white, and then you get carried away to Oz, you open the door, and everything is suddenly in full color.

It was instant. I was intrigued by everything. I was absorbing everything. The little rock-and-roll kids in one corner. The voguing kids in another. The punk kids with mohawks. Everybody was just different. Everybody seemed creative and free. Everything that you see and read about what New York City was like in the 1980s—that's what greeted me in that room.

I learned how to get there myself, so I started going to Hetrick-Martin every day. You got connected to a counselor, so I met mine, this young

Latino gay man named Manuel. He was so flamboyant. I loved the way he moved. He was so confident in himself, and that was powerful to me.

I told him I had HIV, and he was like, "Wait, you don't have a doctor?"

He was shocked. I told him that when I'd left the hospital, nobody had contacted us or told me I needed to be receiving care. He connected me to the adolescent clinic in the Bronx, which was designed for young people living with HIV/AIDS. Becoming connected to my community was how I came to be connected to my own health.

Hetrick-Martin was right across the street from the Christopher Street pier. Back then, the piers belonged to the queer community. It was the place to be. Going to the pier was better than going to a club! It was all cement—there was no grass at all, just rocks. The piers were all rotting. We had to be careful, because you could fall into the water if you weren't. The Christopher Street pier was a home for young LGBTQ+ people, specifically Black and Latine folks. If you were popular on the Christopher Street pier, that meant you were popular across New York City. It was our safe haven—and where we came together.

All the homeless kids were there. Back then, there was a *lot* of homeless queer kids. I was still connected to my biological family, but many of us weren't. Sometimes I'd stay out all night just because I wanted to support a friend who didn't have anywhere to go.

All the kids at the Hetrick-Martin were broken into different houses—like cliques. The house system was like having a chosen family of other queer people, and you'd all look out for each other. I joined my first house on the fifth of December, 1988. The house which had been nicest to me when I started coming to the Hetrick-Martin was the House of Pendavis, so that's the one I joined. They introduced me to the voguing scene and ballroom. My house taught me the concept of community, how we support each other, the need for houses and the history of ballroom. Ballroom is a queer subculture of Black and Latine folks rooted in the drag scene in New York. At the balls, different houses compete against one another, walking in categories like "face" (for beauty) or voguing. Suddenly, I was part of something which was bigger than me—and which celebrated me exactly as I was.

Wade's friend James was my first kiss. He was a year or two older than me. We never had sex. I was too scared to have sex, because I was HIV+ and I didn't understand that the risk was different depending on what you did or if you used condoms. It was years before I had sex.

But I figured maybe kissing was okay. James was so sweet about it. The kiss happened in front of his building on 148th Street. He just wanted a peck. He was like, "Give me a kiss!" I was afraid because we were outside, and anyone could have seen us. I gave him a kiss. The second kiss, that was when the tongue slipped in—we were inside the hallway of his building. We didn't really have a crush on each other. It was more like: *You're like me, and I'm like you, let's do this and see what happens.*

You have to remember this all happened before we had any real openly queer heroes. It was just us. There was no other world.

My dad had given me a camera when I turned 13. Initially, I wasn't interested in it, but once I contracted HIV, I started to take photographs. The camera became my voice. Photography became my way to document everything that I was learning.

Taking pictures was about my survival. I used to watch the news and read about AIDS in the papers, but whenever people spoke about AIDS, it was always somebody who was ill. Someone who looked ill. Someone with KS lesions on their body. Every image I ever saw in a magazine to do with AIDS, it was always a sick person, and almost always a white person.

I'd look in the mirror and think: *I'm this beautiful young Brown kid. Let me document this.*

I wanted my family to have nice pictures to remember me by when I died.

\* \* \*

My little sister was my best friend. She was everything to me. Once I'd contracted HIV, our mom would separate us. I dealt with a lot of stigma in the home, even though my parents definitely loved me. I had my own plate and fork. My stuff was always kept separate from everyone else's. And I'm sure my mom was bleaching the toilet bowl with Clorox every time I used it.

My sister was my first ally. She was the first person who I was openly myself around, because I could be a girl when we played together; I could do things I wasn't supposed to do. I think my sister knew I was different from the moment I gave makeovers to all her Barbies, giving them highlights with magic markers and drawing on liquid eyeliner. We'd play this game called Soap Operas in my room. I'd be a Madonna-like character named Cynthia. I'd be a famous singer, and my sister was my best friend, and my mother was Marlene Dietrich. After I contracted HIV, my mom didn't want us to play together anymore because she was scared I'd infect my sister. But we would still play Soap Operas in secret.

My brother was a different story. He was three years older than me. I always felt uncomfortable because he was styling himself as the urban boy, the hip-hop boy. He hung out with the fellas, they listened to LL Cool J, they had boom boxes. We were never that close, because I was just different. I couldn't be one of the boys like he could.

My brother didn't even know I was HIV+ until 1994, which is ridiculous. By that point, I was already in the community. I was doing big things. I was on television. I was already on MTV. I was the "face of AIDS" at that time for Black and Brown young queer people. My brother had no idea.

We were in his car together. I just said it: "There's something I want to tell you: I've been living with HIV since 1986."

He was shocked. His demeanor shifted. He had a young son at that point, and he got nervous about me playing with him.

I'm a good cover-up person. I saw that my brother didn't know how to say what he was worried about: He was scared his baby son would scratch me and somehow get infected. Inside, I was hurt when he said that. But I covered it up and said I understood.

Back in the summer I got infected, I'd take myself over to Riverside Park and sit on the rocks by the water. I was so sick, and the heat of the sun felt so good on my skin. That's where I bumped into him one last time: the man who'd infected me. I told him I hadn't been feeling good, but I never spoke to him again. One time, I saw him at the park with another man. Back then, I thought he was my friend, so I didn't understand why he didn't acknowledge me as they walked by.

Fast forward to 1992. Six years into living with HIV at this point. I'm twenty years old. I used to go the LGBT Center all the time because they stocked this helpful magazine called *The Body Positive*: a pamphlet with all the information you needed to know about HIV/AIDS.

I was picking up the magazine in the little room next to the Keith Haring bathroom. That's when I saw him. I knew he looked familiar but it took me a moment. *The guy from that day in the park. The man he was with.*

I was like, *Wait, that can't be him, he looks so different, only six years later.* But at that time, a lot of us looked frail, because a lot of us were dying. He looked like he was in his final days.

I spoke to him: "You don't know me, but by any chance, do you know anyone named Lee?"

He was like, "Lee! I haven't heard that name in years!"

Everything just started to come up for me then. I knew he was talking about the same man who'd infected me. I asked what happened to Lee. He told me Lee had died, and that he'd known he had HIV when he raped me. I told him I was heartbroken, because of what had happened, because I'd dreamed about confronting him.

And now that wasn't an option.

That's when the panic attacks started. From '92 through '95, I went through some severe anxiety. I lived a lifetime between '86 and '95. I saw everything, and everybody was dying, and I was learning new things about myself, and it was constantly overwhelming.

I think the panic attacks were because the trauma of what had happened to me was finally coming out. I'd been groomed and raped by this man, and it had changed my life irrevocably.

In my childhood, there was nothing in my life which was LGBTQ+. We didn't have talk shows talking about it, and I sure didn't know anything about Harvey Milk or James Baldwin or anything. Everything I was learning, I had to learn alone. He could have become my mentor. He clearly knew I was this new gay kid who had no understanding about life and sexuality and everything that comes with the package of being young and gay. He could have helped me. But instead of being kind, he took my naivety as an opportunity to take advantage of me.

I wonder how different things could have been if the man in the park had been someone different, someone who said, "Let me teach this kid, let me take him under my wing, show him the ropes, keep him safe." Because back then, I had no idea. I just knew that I was different.

The beautiful thing about being LGBTQ+ is that we create our own families to nurture and look out for each other, and I had a really good chosen family when I was coming up. I found my mentors in ballroom. Avis Pendavis was my mother, and Hector Xtravaganza was my father. Hector was the epitome of what it is to be a wonderful gay man in New York City. He was famous for dressing celebrities. The pair of them taught me so much. *This is gay life, this is what you do, this is where you go, this is how you act, this is what you need.* They showed me all the things you need to acquire to be responsible, strong, and powerful. *This is how you become a good person in society to move our community forwards in life.*

Today, I have my own chosen family. And I work at Gay Men's Health Crisis with young people who've recently been diagnosed with HIV. It can be hard not to cry when I hear them speak about their fears. I'll look away because I don't want them to see that my eyes are a little watery.

It's strange: They're dealing with the same things I was dealing with in the 1980s even though nowadays there's treatment and so much more support. They have way more than I did when I was a newly diagnosed teenager! But somehow, it remains similar—especially on an emotional level.

There were maybe twenty or thirty of us at the adolescent HIV/AIDS clinic up in the Bronx. We were all young, and almost all of us were Black or Brown. There was one boy named Calvin who I'll always remember. Calvin was so excited to start taking AZT when it became available. But he got sick. And then he died.

Seeing what happened to Calvin made me afraid to take HIV medication. All the medications had weird names. AZT. D4T. I used to call them the Star Wars Girls, because their names sounded like R2-D2 and C-3PO. Nowadays, doctors are all about measuring your viral load, but back then, that wasn't even a thought. They cared about T-cells. They'd check our T-cells all the time, and yeah, mine kept getting lower, and lower, and lower, and lower.

After Calvin's death, I put off taking medication for as long as possible. I was lucky: I didn't get seriously sick until twelve years into living with HIV. It was 1998. The good drugs were available by then—protease inhibitors—and people were talking about them all the time like they were stopping AIDS. But I was like, "I'm just going to wait and see what the side effects of these new drugs are. I'm still doing good."

But I only had 23 T-cells. A normal amount is between 500 and 1,500! My doctors said to me, "Luna, if you don't start medications now, you are going to get sick and die."

So that's how I finally started treatment.

I remember taking Sustiva and it gave me the craziest dreams. But as a photographer and an artist, I liked that side effect. Life has a way of talking to you, and that's what dreams are.

I can't say I'm a fan of taking medication every day, but it's prolonged my life, for sure. Without medication, I probably would've been dead by

2000 or 2001. The drugs worked really fast. But because I waited so long, even to this day, my T-cells don't go beyond 400. They stay in the 300s.

Every once in a while, I have a moment when out of nowhere I just start crying. I think about everything I had to experience, and everything just hits me. I grew up in a world of just death, nearly everybody I know died, every acquaintance, every person that was a hero to me, every ballroom personality that I'd cheer and scream for.

I've been quoted in the ballroom community as saying we don't grieve enough. We go to a ball, somebody's died, and there'll be a moment of silence for that person. But then it's like, "Okay! Moving on! The next category is . . ." Can we give ourselves a moment to just really feel our feelings together? Can we recognize that the person we've lost was a brother, a sister, a father, a mother? So many of the people who died were the bridges and protectors of our community. It makes me worry about what's going to happen when my time comes. Am I going to be reduced to a Facebook post and forgotten about? Like: *"Rest in peace, Luna*—anyway, let's move on, let's go to the next ball, let's go to the next dance club."

The past is as important as the future. Everybody died. But some of us lived. I have to find the right balance. Half of me is always looking back and feeling sad, but half of me is like, *I'm moving forwards! The future's right there, I can feel it, and I'm going to be 103 years old when I die!*

When I was a kid, I wanted to be an architect. That never happened. My life got turned around and sent elsewhere. It would have been nice to not have grown up living with HIV. But I like who I became because of HIV. It gave me art. I didn't have a voice, and I had to find a voice once I had HIV because I had no other choice. I found my community. It gave me an understanding of the importance of support and guidance. It helped me see myself as a humble servant in life. It's our job to guide the next generation, to make sure they understand what they're capable of achieving.

Maybe I did end up an architect after all.

\* \* \*

Life is a gift.

    I am a face of AIDS.

    I am a voice of AIDS.

    I grew up with AIDS.

    I'm an artist because of AIDS.

    I mean, it's just been my life. My life is AIDS, and it's hard. I can't talk about ballroom and not talk about AIDS, because it was one of the hardest-hit communities, and AIDS is still an issue in that community—period. So it's hard *not* to talk about HIV and AIDS. If you want to talk about voguing, you have to talk about AIDS. Sometimes I get tired of talking about it. Sometimes I feel like I'm always repeating the same story. I wish I could change it.

    But I can't, because it wouldn't be real.

# Derinthia Williams

*Derinthia Williams is one of the "dandelions"—the over 10,000 people in America who were born with HIV. This means she's lived with HIV her whole life . . . and she now helps others navigate this experience.*

I belong to a forgotten-about community of survivors: the children who were born with HIV in the 1990s. Y'all forgot about us. It can be hard for people to understand how we survive, how we thrive. It's not like we asked to be strong. We just have to do it. That's been my story.

From five to eight years old, I had a feeding tube. I knew something was wrong. I was always taking medicine and I wasn't allowed to go to certain places. I knew I was sick, but nobody told me what type of sick I was. They kept it on the hush-hush, like: *Don't talk about this. Don't talk about that.*

I was born in 1991. My mother died when I was four years old. My family told me she'd died from AIDS, but nobody ever explained to me what "AIDS" was, so I didn't know what the hell it meant! There was just so much stigma around AIDS at that time.

I was sheltered from a lot, but not from everything. My grandmother was my sole provider, and she kept me in the house most of the time when I was young. But I saw a lot of drug dealing going on, a lot of womanizing going on. It was my uncles and cousins. My grandmother couldn't prevent it. So I grew up knowing stuff that I shouldn't have known about as a child. I shouldn't have known about drugs. I shouldn't have known about guns. But I did.

When my grandmother left, it had a tremendous effect on me. I had to grow up just that much faster.

Then I'm fifteen years old and I'm in sex ed at school. The teacher's talking to us about HIV and AIDS. I can still see myself in that classroom putting two and two together. Like, "Oh shit, this is what's been going on with my body. Nobody's ever been brave enough to tell me about it. And this is why nobody wanted to talk about it—because it was HIV, and there was no cure." I felt like I'd been handed a death sentence.

Damn. Even the doctors had been hiding it from me. I guess my guardians had told them, "Don't tell her that she has HIV. We don't want problems at school, we don't want people knowing she has HIV."

But then people at school found out anyway.

I was living with another relative by then. I'd been a quiet kid. I didn't rebel. But after everyone found out about me being HIV-positive, my friends acted like they didn't want to know me anymore.

I told my relative I didn't want to go to school anymore. She got mad. She yelled at me, "You're going to drop out. You're going to be a high school dropout just like everybody else." Then she swung at me. She beat me.

A few days later, I did my normal chores like usual. I cleaned her house, I cooked for her kids. Then I packed a bag of clothes and a pair of shoes. I left her home that day and I never went back.

I went to Atlanta. I was free from my abusive relative, but on my own I fell into new kinds of trouble. I got into gangs. I got into selling drugs. I got into things which I knew I had no business doing. I didn't want to go back to the clinic to see the doctor because that meant remembering I had HIV. But if I was on the streets and doing what I wanted, I didn't have to think about it.

It's like: *I don't think about the medication. I don't think about nothing. I don't think about it because if I do, I have to recognize that I have something that nobody else has*—or so it felt. So I ran the streets. I was hardheaded. I was a bad kid, but that was just all the hurt in me. I was only fifteen years old.

The truth was, I felt alone in the world. Everybody I ran with, none of them were HIV-positive. I couldn't talk about it. I kept it secret. People don't understand how it feels to get up every day and have to pop these damn near fifty pills. Okay, not fifty pills. That's me being dramatic. But back then, I took ten pills in the morning, ten pills at night. I was taking so many pills that I stopped caring. And no one around me understood what that felt like.

Once I was on the streets, nobody chastised me about getting my medication. There was nobody to make sure I was taking it. I was in and out of health care while I was on the streets, but I stopped taking my meds. The doctors told me I was going to die if I didn't take them, but I just figured, "Whatever, who cares, I don't want to be here anyway."

I was scared. That's what was really going on. I didn't care about myself enough to take my meds, but I was still scared when I thought about dying. I was scared I was never going to be a mother. I was scared that I was never going to live to see certain ages, especially with the doctor telling me my whole life I wasn't going to live to see 5, then 8, then 10, then 16. "You're not going to see 18. You're not going to see 21. You're not going to see 25."

I got a boyfriend. He told me he was HIV-positive too, even though he wasn't, and we stopped using condoms. I was so mad when I found out he'd been lying about being positive. You don't play with people like that. Disclosing my status can be hard, but you have to give people a choice either way. Not long after, I found out I was pregnant. When I got eight months into the pregnancy, I started to get sick. It felt like I was fighting for my life. I had a terrible migraine. I couldn't eat. I couldn't bear the light. I went to the hospital and found out I had meningitis. The meningitis caused me to have a stroke. I was kept in the hospital for three weeks. I almost died. My body completely shut down on me: the stroke paralyzed me on the right side.

They ran some tests. My T-cell count was two because I hadn't been taking my meds. It was 2007. I was sixteen and pregnant. And I had AIDS.

Something changed in me at the hospital. I started knowing who God was. *Either I get up out of here and go live or I lay down and die.* I chose to get up and live. I started taking my meds, and not long after, my status became undetectable. I started healing emotionally, which was just as important as healing physically. I had my baby. A baby boy. Once I had him, I had something to live for.

Even so, it was hard to stay healthy. It took a long time to work out how to take care of myself and treat my body with the respect it deserves. I was still a teenager, after all. I still didn't want people to know about my status. I'd stop taking my meds, then start again. I'd try to rationalize it: "When I get sick, I'll take them again." All that starting and stopping caused my body to develop resistance to some of the medications. I nearly lost my life trying to be like everyone else. I didn't know that I could be whatever I wanted and still take medication. I had no one in my life to show me that it was possible.

It was only in 2019 that I got my status properly under control. I was in my late twenties by then. I said to myself: "Yo, Derinthia, smell the freaking coffee, you've got to take care of yourself for real this time."

I do HIV/AIDS advocacy work. I can't be sitting up here telling other HIV-positive people to make sure they're undetectable when my own ass ain't undetectable. I've been undetectable for six years now. And my T-cell count is through the roof these days! Higher than it's ever been. It feels good as hell knowing that. With a high T-cell count and an undetectable viral load, I don't get sick as much. These days, it's one pill a day, not twenty. I'm just glad science has woken up and given us one damn pill versus all those damn pills.

Having HIV can still feel like a heavy-ass weight on my soul. But *living* is the priority for me now. Not just surviving. My life might have gone differently if my family told me about HIV from the start, if I hadn't had to work it all out on my own. But my family didn't have the education they needed to educate me. So I was left with secrecy, silence, and shame.

It's been a long road. Today, I'm chill. I'm a mother. I'm a business owner. I'm heading back to school. I feel good. I'm drop-dead gorgeous. For sure, life gave me lemons, but I made myself some lemonade. I'm thirty-three this year and I don't plan on going nowhere. For a long time, I didn't want to be involved with HIV/AIDS. I tried to push HIV away. I was raised not to talk about it, but I can help others by speaking out. Voiceless people still have voices. They just don't know how to use them, because nobody ever showed them.

I work with positive women who are pregnant. Most people don't realize that for positive folks, HIV is not our biggest problem. It's people stigmatizing us. It's not knowing our worth. It's staying connected to good health care. We got housing problems. We got financial problems. We got parenting problems. HIV isn't the brunt of my problems. I'm not defined by HIV.

I don't live with HIV; HIV lives with *me*.

I didn't meet anyone else who was openly HIV-positive until I was twenty-seven years old. My friend Antoinette was the first person I met that was born positive. When it came to my HIV status, I'd felt so alone in the world up to that point.

I was at Antoinette's house one day, and she was like, "Listen to this poem by Mary Bowman." She put on a video of Mary reading a poem called "Dandelion" about her experience growing up with HIV.

I listened.

And I was like, "Yo, that's it. That's exactly it."

We started talking about how there wasn't a space for people who were born with HIV. Antoinette and I started an organization to connect other people like us. We named it Dandelions, after Mary's poem. There are so many more dandelions out there dealing with the kind of stuff I went through. Dandelions are little weeds at first, but they push up through the cracks in the sidewalk. I want everyone who was born with HIV to know there are spaces in this world for them. There's a lot of us out here. There are more than 10,000 Americans who were born with HIV.

Antoinette and I are trying to find every last one of them. So they'll know they got a space. So they'll know that other people are here who can really understand.

## Kalee Garland

*Kalee Garland has been called a "stigma warrior" by Poz magazine for her tireless work speaking out as a woman who was born with HIV. She uses her Instagram account @aidsbaby86 to share her story and raise HIV awareness.*

When I was seven, my mom took me to my favorite deli. There was an old nickel jukebox in the corner, and whenever we went, my mom would give me a quarter to pick some songs. I was drinking my chocolate ice cream soda, eating my potato knish, when my mom said to me, "Kalee, you and I have got a bug. It's a bug called HIV."

And then she started to cry.

I thought about Magic Johnson. I was too young to know much about HIV or AIDS, but I'd seen him talk about how he was HIV-positive. It was an infomercial on TV. It ended with him turning to the camera and saying, "HIV—it can happen to you."

*It's happened to me.* Mom was still crying. But then the song I'd requested—"Stand by Me"—came on the jukebox, the music filling the diner like a message from an angel.

It was 1993. AIDS was still new to the world. And here I was, a young kid from San Diego, recently diagnosed with HIV, along for the ride.

I had a lot of bruises when I was a kid, but I just assumed it was because I was such a tomboy. Anything my older brothers did, I wanted to do too. I thought the bruises on my arms made me look pretty badass, but my second-grade teacher ended up calling Child Protective Services. She thought I was getting beaten at home.

When Child Protective Services concluded that nobody was abusing me, I was referred to the doctor for a physical. They thought I had leukemia. I had to go into the hospital to have bone marrow taken out of my back for testing, but the results didn't yield anything. It took them a while, but eventually they worked out I had immune thrombocytopenic purpura. ITP is a disease that elderly people get. When you have ITP, you don't have enough platelets in your blood, because your white blood cells attack them. And when you don't have enough platelets, you bruise and bleed really easily.

You can imagine the doctors' conversation. "Wait a minute, how come this kid has ITP when she's not eighty-five years old? Shit, she needs an HIV test."

My test came back positive. And so did my mom's. That's when she took me to City Deli and told me we were both HIV-positive. That's when my life changed.

Through the Elizabeth Glaser Pediatric AIDS Foundation, my mom managed to get me a place on a drug trial at the National Institutes of Health in Washington, DC. It was a big deal. Elizabeth Glaser was a woman who contracted HIV after receiving a blood transfusion when she was giving birth to her daughter in 1981. Her daughter, Ariel, contracted HIV too. Ariel died from AIDS complications when she was seven years old—the same age I was when I joined the trial. The Glaser Foundation was set up to improve research on children and AIDS. Over the years, the work of the Glaser Foundation has helped reduce new HIV infections in children in the United States by more than 95 percent and more than half globally.

The doctors told me I only had seven T-cells. They put me on medication immediately. I hated it, because it made me feel sick all the time. I remember puking in airplane bags every time we flew over from San Diego to DC.

At the NIH, there were constant tests and examinations. Each morning, the doctors would tell me what was going to happen that day. "You're going to do a CT scan. You're going to have cognitive tests. And then you'll go to the eye doctor and have your eyes dilated and inspected." Every single part of my body was examined and touched. The doctors wanted to see how my body was affected by AIDS and the effect of all the experimental medication on my body. Because I was one of the first test subjects they had.

I was always in a hospital bed. Or on an examination table. Or in an MRI machine. The CT machine was the worst because it sounded like a jackhammer and you had to be inside it for an hour every time. It was all exhausting, but I liked the doctors. I was curious about everything that was happening. I liked learning about my body. The doctors were humble enough to say if they didn't know if something was going to work or what would happen. It was hard to hear that the medications were going to make me better, especially because they made me feel so sick. It was so confusing to be a kid with AIDS because I'd be feeling perfectly fine before I took my meds but then the meds always made me feel horrible. One time while we were in DC, my mom and I went to the National Mall to see the AIDS quilt when it was laid out for everyone to see. It filled the whole lawn. My mom was overwhelmed. She kept crying. It was definitely a sad occasion. But I felt comfort when I looked at all the panels too. I saw so much love in them. *These are memorials for people who went away way too soon. But people loved these people. And that love goes on.*

*Hey,* I thought, *I'm not gone yet. I'm right here.* Suddenly, it felt like all these people who had died of AIDS were angels at my side. They had my back.

There was always a layover on the flight from San Diego to DC. I used to love looking through the glossy magazines at the newsstand at the airport. I'd get the *National Geographic* and flip through the pages until I found an image of somewhere beautiful. Later, inside the CT machine, I'd tune out the noise by picturing things. I'd say to myself, *Time to think about the Great Blue Hole in Belize.* I'd envision the deep blue water ... the green reef that runs in a circle around it. ... *I am no longer being prodded and poked like a guinea pig. I'm not a science experiment. I'm somewhere else. Somewhere beautiful.*

Breathing. Relaxing. Meditation. These skills didn't just help me survive the hospital. They helped me deal with my regular life back in San Diego, at school where no one knew I was positive. From kindergarten through eighth grade, I hated school. Like, I just couldn't get away from those people. If I felt unhappy, I could go somewhere else in my mind. I could become a space cadet. I had some friends, but the friendships felt one-sided and false. At school, no one knew I was HIV-positive, and that made it feel like they didn't really know me at all.

At the Institutes, all the children would stay with their families at the Children's Inn across the street. There were lots of other families taking part from all across the world. There was a playroom full of toys, and going to the playroom was always the silver lining at the end of a long day of getting poked and prodded. All the kids' parents would gather in the living room. They'd speak about their communities, where they came from. Parents never realize how much children hear. It was by listening to their conversations that I learned just how HIV could be seen as a bad thing. *Don't tell anyone you're positive because something bad will happen to you, people will hate you.* . . .

I'd hear stories from the other kids too. Some of them had been shunned by their communities for being HIV-positive. Being HIV-positive wasn't any different from the fact I had blond hair. It upset me to learn about the intolerance these kids had to deal with back at home. I hated that I was powerless to stop it.

When I was twelve, the doctors at the NIH started me on the protease inhibitor trial. I had to take twelve pills, three times a day. The first time I took them, they dissolved in my mouth, and it made me gag. The trial was tough. They were giving all the kids the same dosage of medication as they were giving to fully grown men. There was a little girl on the same treatment regimen as me, and one day, I saw her walk into a wall because the pills were making her go blind. I was so scared of going blind.

I started hiding my medication after that. I might have been a guinea pig for the Institute, but I still had authority over my body. When they found out, nobody pinned me down to the hospital bed to squirt medication directly down my throat. Instead, I got kicked off the trial and sent back to California.

I went to live with my dad after that. I was often sick, but life went on. By the time I was at high school, it was second nature not telling anyone about my HIV. The other kids at school were going on dates, but my romantic life was totally nonexistent. I was worried. *How do I go beyond kissing? How do I tell someone? How will they react if they found out about my status?* It was so heavy carrying my HIV around like a secret, but I thought it would feel even worse to put that secret on someone else. I was scared that if I did tell someone, it would become the hottest gossip ever. So I stayed in the closet. I didn't say a word.

Throughout my teens, I got infusions of white blood cells to restore strength to my body, but my T-cells were staying low. Between the ages of sixteen and eighteen, I was hospitalized with meningitis four different times. The final time, I only had one T-cell, and the meningitis was in my brain. At the hospital, the nurses had to shave my hair off to put a shunt in my brain to drain the fluid. I had a shaved head and I weighed 88 pounds. People would stop and stare at me when I walked down the street. I remember wishing I had a mirror to hold up so they could see their own faces staring back at them. If they had a loved one going through what I was going through, they wouldn't want them treated the way I was treated. All I was doing was trying to live my life and stay as healthy as I could.

Turning eighteen was the light at the end of the tunnel. I wasn't a child anymore. After the meningitis, it took two years to get back to a weight where I could get my period. When I was well enough, I started college. One day in health class, the professor spoke about sexual health, and everyone started discussing what they knew about HIV. So I raised my hand and said to the class, "I'm Kalee and I have AIDS." It was a spontaneous decision: I couldn't silence myself anymore. It felt good to no longer keep HIV separate from my "regular" life. I made friends who were cool with me being positive. Anyone who wasn't cool with it, I just didn't see them. I didn't put myself around them. That's exactly the way I wanted it.

My health continued to improve. The medication got easier. Eventually, I became undetectable.

HIV is just part of who I am. HIV lives in my body. I can't change that. I just want to be a good host. I feel empowered now that I'm older. It's like I'm living for my younger self.

HIV is an acronym and the H stands for *human*.

# TIMELINE

## 1983-1986

### January 1983

Sometimes a giant leap in scientific knowledge can happen because of the smallest of snips.

On January 3, 1983, a French doctor, Willy Rozenbaum, cuts a small sample from the lymph node of one of his patients and sends it to Dr. Luc Montagnier, the director of the Viral Oncology Unit at the Pasteur Institute in France. Like so many others at the time, Rozenbaum's patient is suffering from a disease that has yet to be definitively named, caused by a source that is yet to be found. Montagnier's team, experts on retroviruses, gets to work—and in four short months reveals to the world that they have isolated a retrovirus that has never been seen before. They call it LAV (for lymphadenopathy-associated virus). They say further study is needed, but this is the breakthrough that the medical detectives need in order to solve the mystery of the disease.

### March 1983

"If this article doesn't scare the shit out of you we're in real trouble."

So begins Larry Kramer's front-page essay in the *New York Native*, a gay community newspaper. It is a landmark alarm call, meant to cut through any denial community members may have about the illness that is striking them.

He ends with a list of twenty dead men he knows, and a warning:

"If we don't act immediately, then we face our approaching doom."

## April 1983

One of the legends in AIDS research is Dr. Mathilde Krim, a research scientist who dedicated herself to the fight against AIDS. On April 27, she joins forces with Dr. Joseph Sonnabend, Dr. David Baltimore, AIDS activist Michael Callen, and philanthropist Mary Lasker to create the AIDS Medical Foundation (later the American Foundation for AIDS Research, or amfAR), which will provide money for AIDS research that is largely being ignored by governmental funding. Krim puts up $100,000 of her own money to start the organization and soon becomes one of its best-known representatives. At the start, because of the stigma of AIDS, the organization cannot have any signage for its office, but over time it becomes a fundraising powerhouse, especially after Krim joins forces with famous actress Elizabeth Taylor, who becomes one of the most vocal advocates for AIDS research at the height of the epidemic.

## May 1983

On May 2, 1983, 10,000 people in San Francisco and 5,000 people in New York march in the first public demonstration by people with AIDS.

"It wasn't clear how society was going to respond," organizer Hank Wilson later tells *SFGate*. "We also didn't know how our own community was going to respond in terms of rallying to the support of people who were sick."

But people *do* show up, creating an annual tradition that many cities will emulate. In San Francisco, marchers carry candles down Market Street, from the Castro to the Civic Center, a symbolic journey from a gay homeland to a governmental hub.

"It was incredibly quiet," Wilson recalls. "We knew people were dying, and we wanted to do something very serious that would touch people emotionally."

## August 1983

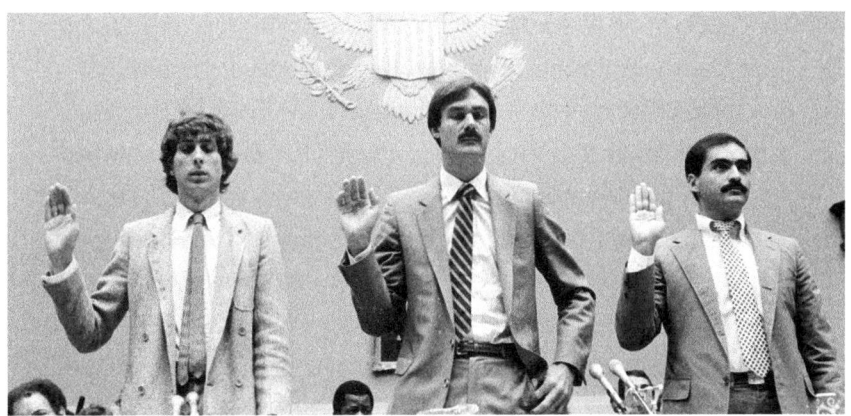

Left to right: Michael Callen, Roger Lyon, and Anthony Ferrara testify at congressional hearings on the federal response to AIDS, August 1, 1983.

On August 1 and 2, the US House of Representatives Subcommittee on Government Operations invites Michael Callen, Roger Lyon, and Anthony Ferrara to testify about their experiences living with AIDS.

Callen tells the members of Congress:

> The effect of being told that I was immune deficient was devastating. I called my parents and said "I am going to die." I was not hospitalized until the summer of 1982, when I was diagnosed with cryptosporidiosis, which is one of the qualifying opportunistic infections according to the CDC definition of this syndrome.
>
> I was hospitalized for over a week with what is known as the wasting syndrome. It was the lowest point of my life. I was convinced from everything I read and heard that I was going to die. But I recovered from that specific infection, and I was rehospitalized in the fall of 1982. They suspected pneumocystis pneumonia. I had a bronchoscopy performed and other tests. It turned out to be bronchitis. But my story really illustrates one of the consistent stories for people who have this syndrome. So little is known.

When my doctor indicated to me in December of 1981 that I was immune deficient I said, "What does that mean?" And he said, "We don't know." So now a lot of people who are being told they are immune deficient are simply waiting, waiting for the next infection.

Now, I have come to believe that I am going to beat this disease. I no longer think that I am going to die. But it is very difficult when you pick up newspapers or turn on the television and you hear that no one has fully recovered from this syndrome, and that 80 percent of those diagnosed with the syndrome are dead after 2 years.

So I guess that is my story—waiting around for infections, checking myself every morning for Kaposi's sarcoma lesions and waiting for information about this disease to be forthcoming.

Ferrara testifies:

I do my best to do as much as I can to dispel misconceptions about the disease. People don't have to be afraid to be in the same room with us, people don't have to be afraid to swim in the same swimming pool. I believe that gay organizations across the country should be given more information concerning guidelines that can be disseminated to the gay community in terms of—in terms of ways that gay men can protect themselves from the disease, rather than causing the paranoia and hysteria that the information that has been disseminated so far caused.

And Lyon makes a plea:

I came here today with the hope that this subcommittee would be able to do everything possible to halt the spread of this disease. AIDS has been called the number one health priority of the Nation. It certainly is my No. 1 priority.

I came here today with the hope that this administration would do everything possible, make every resource available—there is no reason this disease cannot be conquered. We do not need infighting, this is not a political issue. This is a health issue. This is not a gay issue. This is a human issue. And I do not intend to be defeated by it. I came here today in the hope that my epitaph would not read that I died of red tape.

Lyon dies a year later, at the age of thirty-six.

## September 1983

On September 28, the DC Coalition of Black Gays and the Whitman-Walker Clinic hold what the *Washington Blade* calls "a first-of-its-kind AIDS forum for black and Third World Gays" at a nightclub where the Black queer community often gathers. Forty people attend and discuss everything from medical issues to religious and moral issues pertaining to the illness.

The *Blade* reports, "As one person pointed out, most slides used in presentations on the symptoms of Kaposi's sarcoma . . . depict the lesions characteristic of that disease on a white person's skin, and I wondered what the lesions would look like on dark skin." Another speaker, Wes Clark, an aide to Senator Edward Kennedy, observes that "the media does not portray [people with AIDS] as non-white," even though at this point 40 percent of people with AIDS are Black.

## September 1983

When Dr. Joseph Sonnabend opens a clinic in Greenwich Village in New York to treat people with HIV/AIDS, he faces eviction from his office building, with other occupants saying such a clinic will create an unsafe environment and lower their property values.

Rather than move, Sonnabend fights back. With the help of Lambda Legal, a law organization specializing in LGBTQ+ issues, and the New York attorney general's office, *People v. West 12 Tenants Corp.* becomes the nation's first HIV-discrimination lawsuit.

A New York court issues a preliminary injunction in 1983 that bars the eviction. The neighbors on the co-op board appeal but eventually settle. The clinic stays put, and stays open for many years, helping thousands of people with HIV.

## May 1984

On May 4, 1984, Dr. Robert Gallo of the National Cancer Institute, a part of the National Institutes of Health, announces in the journal *Science* that he and his team have definitively identified the retrovirus that causes AIDS. Initially the virus is named HTLV-III, because Gallo believes it is related to other leukemia viruses his lab was studying. Later the name will change to HIV.

Gallo receives a patent for this work in 1985, and the identification of the virus is integral to creating the first antibody tests to discover its presence within patients. (The tests are antibody tests because doctors can identify only the proteins bodies manufacture to try to combat the virus, not the virus itself.) The twist in the tale arrives when it is discovered that what Gallo identified as HTLV-III is the same retrovirus Dr. Luc Montagnier at the Pasteur Institute identified as LAV. And later it is revealed that Gallo's team used a sample from Montagnier's study (either accidentally or deliberately) in their own work. President Ronald Reagan of the United States and President François Mitterrand of France have to negotiate a settlement by which half the proceeds of these discoveries will go to each country.

Whatever its provenance, the world now knows the retrovirus causing AIDS. The next task is to discover how to stop it.

## September 1984

Among the creators of the performing arts, playwrights are the first to deeply engage in writing about AIDS and bringing stories about AIDS to the public. This is not particularly surprising, considering the great overlap between the queer community and the theater community, which will both be devastated by the epidemic. But it also speaks to the cowardice of the movie and television industry, where the sharing of such stories continues to be rare (with some notable exceptions).

The first play in the United States to openly address AIDS is *The AIDS Show*, which premieres on September 6 at the Theatre Rhinoceros in San Francisco. The play is based on the experiences of its cast—to them, "AIDS" represents *Artists Involved with Death and Survival*.

More plays follow. On April 22, 1985, Larry Kramer's autobiographical play *The Normal Heart* premieres off-Broadway, showing the bumpy, messy origin story of AIDS activism. Two weeks later, William Hoffman's *As Is* becomes the first play about AIDS on Broadway, deeply affecting audiences who watch a gay couple navigate the rough waters after one of them becomes sick. These works will be the foundation of a large theatrical body of work about AIDS, including Cheryl West's *Before It Hits Home* (1991), Tony Kushner's *Angels in America* (1991 and 1992), Paul Rudnick's *Jeffrey* (1992), Paula Vogel's *The Baltimore Waltz* (1992), and Jonathan Larson's *Rent* (1993).

## September 1984

*Money for AIDS, not for war.*

This is the demand at the heart of the first recorded act of civil disobedience to confront AIDS, vocalized by the Enola Gay "Faggot Affinity Group," an offshoot of a larger protest outside the Lawrence Livermore National Laboratory, a center for the research and development of nuclear weapons located in Livermore, California.

As the antinuclear protestors rally at Livermore Lab's gates, the Enola Gay members—roughly ten in number—stand in two rows and empty vials of blood onto the road that leads to the facility. As they do, they chant:

> *blood is holy*
> *blood is sacred*
> *workers that come this way*
> *will cross the blood of gay men every day*

Then the men prick their fingers and rub them against dollar bills, some bearing the Enola Gay slogan "Gomorrah for tomorrah."

Decades later, Enola Gay member Jack Davis will tell *48 Hills*, "This was really a statement. . . . Gay blood was considered dangerous. And here we were, pouring it out on the road. But it wasn't meant to be a threat. That never even crossed our minds. It was more about saying, 'We are here.'"

## October 1984

On October 10, 1984, Dr. Mervyn Silverman, the public health director for the city of San Francisco, announces that fourteen of the city's gay bathhouses will be closed in the name of public safety—the climax of an intense debate where public safety has been weighed against individual freedom.

San Francisco's bathhouses had long been a social and sexual sanctuary for the gay community, private establishments where desires could be explored and camaraderie could flourish. When AIDS hit, it posed a profound dilemma. On the one hand, officials and some members of the gay community argued that since HIV was transmitted sexually, one way to stop it would be to make it harder to have unprotected sex. On the other hand, many gay people and civil libertarians pointed out, it was wrong to patrol a person's consensual sexual behavior, and there was a serious double standard at play—while the disease could be transmitted just as easily by straight sexual contact, only gay establishments were being targeted.

Controversially, when the city ordinance banning certain sexual activities in bathhouses passed in April 1984, Mayor Dianne Feinstein announced that police officers would be sent into the bathhouses to patrol the sexual practices. For a community that had long been forced into the shadows and shamed, this felt like a sinister step backward, with spies invading what had once been a safe and open space.

Activists argue against the ruling, saying that bathhouses also act as community centers, and that the right thing to do isn't to send in spies or close spaces but to use those spaces to distribute condoms and information about preventing the spread of HIV.

Decades later, activist Harry Breaux compares the closing of the baths to what it would be like to queer people if the internet were shut off today: "Our lines of communication in the war on AIDS were severed here in this city. The solutions were in our faces and Dr. Silverman knew it (information, condoms, sanity), but Mayor Dianne Feinstein exercised her power from the basis of her fear, interests and prejudice."

There are no easy answers here, and the actions will continue to be debated. It was not until January 2021 that the restrictions were formally rescinded.

## March 1985

The first HIV test is approved on March 2, 1985—and the first "patient" to receive it is America's blood supply. Up to this point, there has been no way to screen blood for the presence of HIV, because no one has known what to look for. But once the teams from the Pasteur Institute and the National Institutes of Health identified it, an ELISA (enzyme-linked immunosorbent assay) test could be created, and HIV+ blood could be identified and removed from the blood supply. When the FDA (Food and Drug Administration) approves the first commercial HIV ELISA test, it's been four years since the start of the crisis. The test is designed to screen blood for the national blood supply. The number of people who've contracted HIV because of transfusions is at the time comparatively low—*Time* magazine reports that, as of April 1985, only 142 of the roughly 10,000 Americans with AIDS contracted HIV through a blood transfusion. The fact that the first HIV test was invented to ensure the safety of the blood supply feels like proof that the establishment is more interested in protecting its own interests than helping the most at-risk people, those already sick and dying. But it also shows a growing awareness among government officials and scientists that HIV/AIDS isn't going to quietly disappear.

Blood donation centers and other custodians of the blood supply act quickly. The test begins to be implemented in April, and even though it is imperfect and oversensitive at first, it errs on the side of false positives, not false negatives—so even though uncontaminated blood is thrown out, contaminated blood does not go unnoticed. On the first of August, a little over three months after testing began, it is announced that the nation's supply of blood for transfusions is HIV-free.

This is understandably a triumph for hemophiliacs and others who rely on blood transfusions to stay healthy. But it is too late for the thousands of people (including Ryan White) who have already received blood transfusions prior to August 1985, and who will soon find out they have AIDS because of infected blood.

The existence of a test is viewed as a mixed blessing for high-risk populations, especially once the problem of false positives is corrected. On the one hand, confirming the presence of HIV takes away some of the mystery of why people are sick. On the other hand, there still isn't an effective treatment, and there are significant concerns for the civil liberties of people who test positive. Within six months of the first ELISA testing, Colorado becomes the first state to require that its health department be given the name, age, sex, and address of anyone who tests positive. While the state vows to keep the information confidential, organizations like the American Civil Liberties Union (ACLU) warn that this could easily be the first step that leads to people who test positive being forcibly quarantined or in other ways stigmatized and segregated.

The existence of the test raises one of the most fundamental questions people who suspect they might be HIV+ will face: Is it better to know, even if there's no treatment to be had? Or is it better not to know, and to keep your status out of other people's hands?

## June 1985

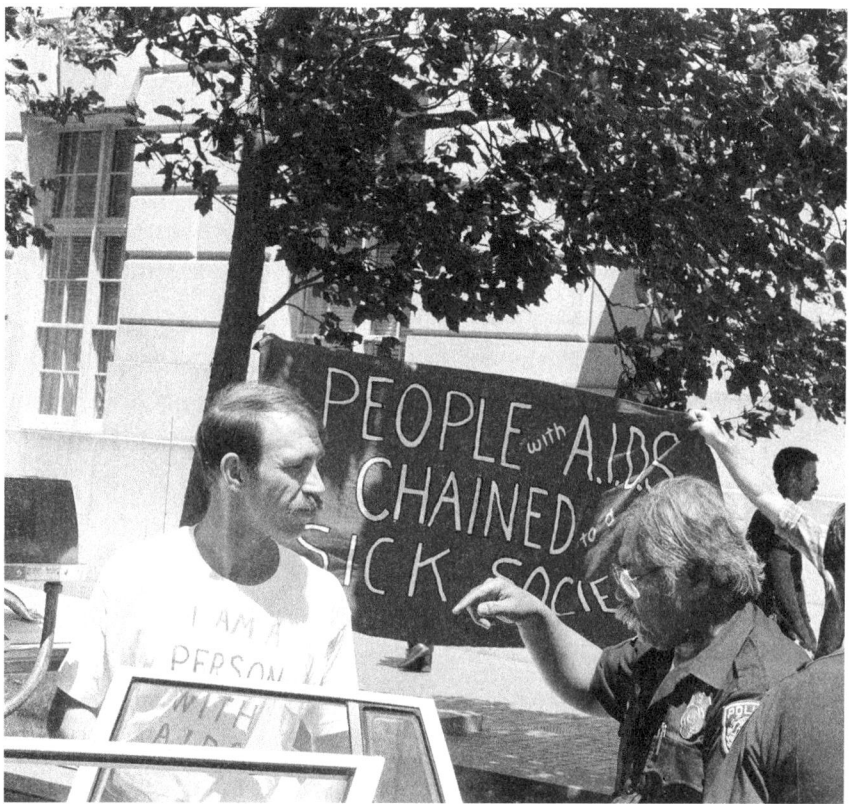

Wearing a T-shirt that proclaims *I am a person with AIDS* and holding a sign that reads *PEOPLE with AIDS CHAINED to a SICK SOCIETY*, activist John Lorenzini chains himself to the door of the San Francisco office of the US Department of Health and Human Services, demanding funding and attention from the government for the fight against AIDS. He is the first HIV+ person to make such a protest. As officials, officers, reporters, and bystanders look on, he demands that the head of the office come down and talk to him—which he does, allowing Lorenzini to make his case. Then federal officers cut through the heavy chain that links the activist to the doors. He's arrested . . . but then promptly released, because the police have no protocol to deal with a person with AIDS in jail.

This act of civil disobedience will be echoed in the later work of ACT UP and other activists. The district attorney refuses to press charges against Lorenzini, and he continues to be a voice in the AIDS community until his death in 1990.

## November 1985

On November 11, 1985, 34 million viewers sit down to watch *An Early Frost* on NBC. It is the first major movie, on TV or in theaters, about AIDS. In many cases, it is the first time American viewers let a fully drawn story of AIDS into their homes.

The movie is about Michael, a Chicago lawyer (played by Aidan Quinn) who leaves his lover and heads home to his family to tell them he is gay and that he has AIDS. While his mother and grandmother are supportive (after the shock wears off), his pregnant sister is worried she may "catch AIDS" from being around him, and his father says he doesn't recognize his son anymore. But over time, the family comes together—when Michael nearly takes his own life, his father intervenes. And the film clarifies for its viewers how AIDS can and can't be transmitted. In the end, Michael returns to his lover and to his life in Chicago, vowing to fight on. It is about as promising an ending as an AIDS narrative could have in 1985. (Although, it must be noted, another person with AIDS dies in the course of the movie, to show viewers the full impact of the disease.)

Getting the movie to the small screen has not been easy. The script went through thirteen rewrites, and the network was clear that Michael and his lover could say affectionate words to each other . . . but could not come into any physical contact. ("We wanted neither to romanticize the homosexual relationship nor hit it with a sledgehammer," network executive Steve White tells *People*.)

Beyond the ratings, the movie is a critical success, receiving a record fourteen Emmy nominations. But the reaction isn't all positive: NBC estimates that it loses over $600,000 from advertisers pulling out . . . and then another $1 million when the movie is re-aired in 1986.

To the creators of the movie, the advertisers are beside the point.

Says Ron Cowan, one of the gay cowriters of the movie, "We want viewers to say, 'That could be my brother, my friend, my son.'"

Later, his cowriter and partner, Daniel Lipman, will talk about a letter he and Cowan received from a young man with AIDS telling them about how his father, who had rejected him, came to his hospital room and watched *An Early Frost* with him. "By the end of the film, the father was laying in bed with his son with his arms around him."

It has this effect on some of the 34 million viewers . . . but there won't be another film centering on a gay person with AIDS that garners the same amount of attention until *Philadelphia,* starring Tom Hanks, comes out in 1993. There won't be a comparable movie about women's experiences of AIDS until *Something to Live For: The Alison Gertz Story* airs on ABC in 1992, a dramatization of the life of Ali Gertz, who contracted HIV as a teenager.

## November 1985

On November 15, 1985, the Reverend Steve Pieters prepares to tell his story to 20 million people. A pastor of a largely LGBTQ+ congregation, he has been sick since 1982, and even though his prognosis is bleak, his doctor has told him, "If there is one in a million survivors, why not believe you're that one in a million?"

Although Pieters is not in the same studio as his host, his interview will run live. He has insisted on it, out of fear that his words will be edited down or not shown at all.

The fact that Pieters is on a talk show is not unusual. But the particular talk show he's on *is* unusual. Pieters is about to become the first person with HIV/AIDS to ever speak on a Christian televangelist's show about their experience.

The host of *Tammy's House Party* is Tammy Faye Bakker, the wife of superstar televangelist Jim Bakker. And for five minutes, she makes the radical gesture of showing Pieters nothing but kindness and compassion. From the very start, she says Pieters "generously allowed us to talk to him today."

When Pieters talks about how accepting his parents have been of his identity, Bakker broadens it to say, "Thank God for a mom and dad who will stand with a young person. They're still your boy, they're still your girl, no matter what happens in their life, and I think it's so important that we as mom and dads love through anything, and that's the way with Jesus, you know. Jesus loves us through anything."

And Pieters, in front of 20 million Christian viewers, gets to say, "Jesus loves me just the way I am, I really believe. Jesus loves the way I love."

Toward the end of the interview, Bakker tearfully looks into the camera and addresses her viewers. "How sad that we as Christians—who are to be the salt of the earth, we who are supposed to be able to love everyone—are afraid so badly of an AIDS patient that we will not go up and put our arm around them and tell them that we care."

Later on, Pieters would recount how people would "come up to me through the years and say that my interview with Tammy Faye helped them come out or even saved them from suicide, by helping them realize they could be gay and Christian, or that God was not punishing them with AIDS for being gay."

## December 1985

In 1985, the Reverend Carl Bean and other members of his Unity Fellowship of Christ Church found the Minority AIDS Project in Los Angeles, the US's first community-based HIV/AIDS organization established and managed by people of color.

Bean's path to activism is lit at least in part by the light of a disco ball. A young gospel singer who knew from an early age that he was gay, Bean was approached by the legendary record label Motown in 1977 to record a cover of Valentino's "I Was Born This Way." Unintimidated to be out and proud while singing the song's lyrics ("I'm happy, I'm carefree, and I'm gay; I was born this way"), Bean saw the single hit the dance charts. Three decades later, it would inspire Lady Gaga's use of the phrase in her own gay anthem, "Born This Way."

Having always felt a calling to the ministry, Bean left Motown and was ordained, particularly with the hope of bringing Black gay people and others who'd been marginalized by Christianity to a place where they felt they belonged. In 1985, he founded the Unity Fellowship of Christ Church in Los Angeles, and by year's end, the Minority AIDS Project had begun, since Bean and other church members saw the pressing need to care for their impacted brethren... and also to spread the word in a community that still didn't understand how hard HIV/AIDS would hit them.

As Bean said to the *Los Angeles Times* in 1989, "AIDS took the cloak off for the world that homosexuality exists, especially for minorities. People who wanted to think there was no such thing as a gay Black man or a gay Latino had a rude awakening."

## March 1986

On March 18, 1986, *The New York Times* publishes an op-ed piece by renowned conservative thinker William F. Buckley Jr. that says, among other things, that women intending to marry men with AIDS should be sterilized. Then, in what becomes one of the most famous images of conservative disregard for people with AIDS, Buckley writes, "Everyone detected with AIDS should be tattooed in the upper forearm, to protect common-needle users, and on the buttocks, to prevent the victimization of other homosexuals."

With these comments, which clearly hark back to both the Nazi practice of tattooing concentration camp victims and the larger history of eugenics, Buckley joins the ranks of conservative commentators making homophobic, bigoted comments against a group of people fighting illness. Others would ultimately include Reagan communications director and future presidential candidate Pat Buchanan ("With 80,000 dead of AIDS, our promiscuous homosexuals appear literally hell-bent on Satanism and suicide"); televangelist Jerry Falwell ("AIDS is not just God's punishment for homosexuals, it is God's punishment for the society that tolerates homosexuals"); televangelist and future presidential candidate Pat Robertson ("I think people in the gay community, they want to get people. They'll have a ring, and you shake hands, and the ring has a little thing where you cut your finger.... Really, it is that kind of vicious stuff, which would be the equivalent of murder"); and

Senator Jesse Helms ("I call a spade a spade, a perverted human being, a perverted human being").

These comments are not made on social media; there is no social media at the time. Instead, Buchanan and Falwell, like Buckley, publish these thoughts in major newspapers. Robertson discusses his ludicrous gay ring conspiracy theory on his television show, *The 700 Club*. And Helms makes his comments while addressing the US Senate in 1987, introducing an amendment that prohibits the use of any federal money to "encourage, condone or promote" homosexual sex. (The amendment is approved.)

Over time, Buckley, Helms, and Robertson will try to distance themselves from their comments to some degree. But none of these men will be able to erase these words from their obituaries. Fittingly, their hateful words will work like a tattoo on all their legacies.

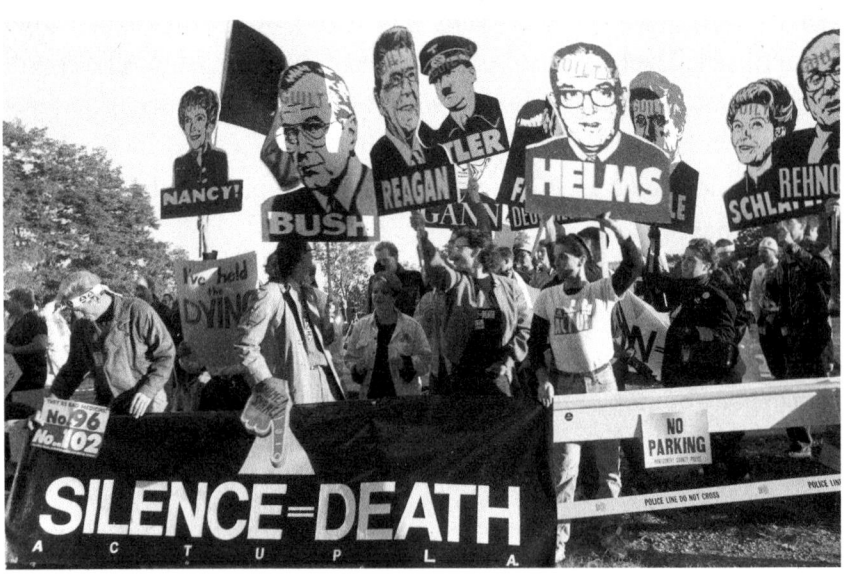

### October 1986

By October, the Centers for Disease Control reports that Black and Latine people are increasingly bearing the brunt of AIDS as the numbers grow. Of the people with AIDS who have been counted in national reporting,

25 percent are Black (even though only 12 percent of the general population in 1986 is Black) and 14 percent are Latine (even though only 6 percent of the general population is Latine). Among women, the statistics are much higher: 51 percent of all females with AIDS are Black and 21 percent Latine. When it comes to children with AIDS, 58 percent are Black and 22 percent are Latine, which means that the incidences of AIDS in Black and Latine children are 15.1 and 9.1 times, respectively, greater than the incidence for white children. When it comes to transmission from mother to child, 90 percent of cases are in Black or Latine families.

At its 1986 conference, the American Public Health Association holds a plenary session on AIDS. The plenary—a meeting of lots of delegates from all across the conference—doesn't feature a single speaker of color, despite clear evidence that AIDS is increasingly affecting Black and Latine people. Craig Harris is in attendance at the plenary. He's a gay Black man who's living with AIDS, a writer and activist who's appeared as a commentator on Black TV shows to discuss the rising threat of AIDS in the Black community. Before anyone in the audience can realize what's happening, Harris rushes the stage. He declares, "I will be heard!" as he takes the microphone from the San Francisco health commissioner. After his protest at the absence of people of color from the American Public Health Association plenary on AIDS, Harris cofounds the National Minority AIDS Council, which rallies for greater awareness about the impact of AIDS on communities of color across the country.

## October 1986

Dr. C. Everett Koop, the US surgeon general under President Ronald Reagan, is nobody's idea of a liberal radical. But he ends up being the loudest voice in Reagan's administration in the fight against AIDS—simply by telling the truth and sticking to it.

When Koop was nominated to be surgeon general in 1981, he was a polarizing choice. An evangelical Christian with an outspoken stance against abortion, the pediatric surgeon had never worked in the field of public health. Democratic members of Congress blocked his nomination for months, calling him "Dr. Kook" and fearing that his fervent religious beliefs—including the belief that homosexuality was wrong—would impede his medical judgments. *The Boston Globe* warned that Koop was a "dogmatic Christian fundamentalist with the kind of tunnel vision that limits bureaucrats of any ideological stripe."

But that, it turns out, is not how Koop approaches his job. In forty years as a surgeon, he has seen only two cases of Kaposi's sarcoma . . . so when, shortly after his confirmation, he is told of twenty-six cases that have emerged in San Francisco, he understands this is a problem with potentially epidemic implications. As the number of cases increases, he realizes "if there ever were a disease made for a surgeon general it was AIDS." Republicans who once cheered his appointment are critical as he starts to talk about proper AIDS prevention (as well as the dangers of smoking, angering the powerful tobacco lobbyists). For years, the Reagan administration keeps him out of conversations about AIDS policy, even though he is supposed to be "America's top doctor." He is deliberately kept off Reagan's executive task force on AIDS until 1985, and even after that, he is told not to rock the boat. Koop realizes the best way to get his message out is to issue a report. He chooses to write it himself, drafting it in his basement with only a few members of his staff after speaking to a wide range of experts. After seventeen drafts, he unveils it on October 22, 1986.

*Surgeon General's Report on Acquired Immune Deficiency Syndrome* tells the truth (as best as it was known in 1986). It talks frankly about how HIV is transmitted (anal and vaginal sex, drug injection) and how it *isn't* transmitted (kissing, touching, using the same utensils). While it states that the best method of staying safe is abstinence from sexual activity, it also advocates for condom use among sexually active couples and suggests that sex education should begin as early as third grade.

People who are deeply involved in the fight against AIDS hail Koop's report, which he supports with numerous appearances, looking very authoritative in a military-like uniform and a Lincoln beard.

As Jeffrey Levi of the National Gay and Lesbian Task Force later tells *The Atlantic*, "It's hard to understand how desperate those of us who were affected by the epidemic were for the validation by a mainstream public health official.... We were totally unprepared for the nature of the conversation because it was so positive and so forthcoming."

Koop writes in the report's foreword: "At the beginning of the AIDS epidemic many Americans had little sympathy for people with AIDS. The feeling was that somehow people from certain groups 'deserved' their illness. Let us put those feelings behind us. We are fighting a disease, not people.... The country must face this epidemic as a unified society. We must prevent the spread of AIDS while at the same time preserving our humanity and intimacy."

Predictably, conservatives freak out, condemning Koop and the report (even burning him in effigy during some protests). Famous conservative Phyllis Schlafly denounces the AIDS report for looking "like it was edited by the Gay Task Force" and promoting "safe sodomy" to children. Koop's response? "I'm not surgeon general to make Phyllis Schlafly happy. I'm surgeon general to save lives." As he tells the *New York Times* reporter Maureen Dowd, some critics "seem more concerned with homosexual genocide, and with things like William Buckley's suggestion that AIDS victims be tattooed, than with the human tragedy.... I don't like to see people excoriated in the midst of illness because there's some other part of their life style that people don't like."

Around 20 million copies of the surgeon general's report are distributed—not by the Reagan administration, but by members of Congress, public health organizations, and parent-teacher organizations. Koop is still frustrated by the Reagan administration's messaging. Its "America Responds to AIDS" campaign focuses only on abstinence and stays entirely away from the question of safer sex. So when Congress asks the surgeon general to go directly to the people, he accepts the assignment. In May 1988, a pamphlet titled *Understanding AIDS* is sent to 107 million American households, the largest public health mailing in history up to that time. Printing it requires the use of 20,900 miles of paper.

On the front page of *Understanding AIDS,* Koop writes: "Some of the issues involved in this brochure may not be things you are used to discussing openly. I can easily understand that. But now you must discuss them. We all must know about AIDS." In clear, nonjudgmental terms, the facts are given to the American public, with sentences like: "The AIDS virus can be spread by sexual intercourse whether you are male or female, heterosexual, bisexual, or homosexual. This happens because a person infected with the AIDS virus may have the virus in semen or vaginal fluids. The virus can enter the body through the vagina, penis, rectum or mouth. Anal intercourse, with or without a condom, is risky. The rectum is easily injured during anal intercourse."

Equally important are statements like this, which aren't sexually explicit at all but speak to Koop's underlying vision: "Who you are has nothing to do with whether you are in danger of being infected with the AIDS virus. What matters is what you do."

According to follow-up surveys, over 80 percent of the people sent the brochure read it. It is the largest single act of AIDS education in the disease's history. Even though it is condemned by those who want to keep AIDS education quiet, it conveys what it wants to convey to a lot of people in the comfort of their own homes, where they can draw their own conclusions.

Koop never sees his work in fighting AIDS as being in any way oppositional to his beliefs. He later writes in his memoir that his position on AIDS was "dictated by scientific integrity and Christian compassion." In a different essay, he will say, "My whole career has been dedicated to prolonging lives, especially the lives of people who were weak and powerless, the disenfranchised who needed an advocate."

Or as a former colleague tells *The Washington Post* upon Koop's passing in 2013 at the age of ninety-six: "He was a born-again Christian and conservative Republican who said to me . . . 'I have my own biases, but we don't base public health policy on our biases; we base it on science. We don't play politics with people's lives.'"

Perhaps the most famous phrase to come out of AIDS activism is SILENCE=DEATH, created in 1987 by the six-person collective of Avram Finkelstein, Jorge Socarras, Chris Lione, Charles Kreloff, Oliver Johnston, and Brian Howard. Its stark equation resonated: When lives are on the line, indifference and inaction can be just as deadly as hate and fear.

It was not enough for those directly affected to be the only ones to speak. It took a wide range of people—many but not all of them queer—to speak truth to power, and to put their bodies on the line when power wouldn't listen. Tactics could differ. Some approaches were more polite than others. Some activists wanted to work within the system, and others wanted to overthrow it. It was far from a unified front . . . but the one thing that every activist could agree upon was that silence wasn't an option.

*You don't know how we're living,
you don't care that we're dying. . . .*

# Young People Schoolin' Other Young People: Zines, Raps, Comics, and Beyond

Early on, young people weren't thought of as at risk of HIV unless they had acquired it through blood transfusions or through natal transmission. By the late 1980s, scientists realized that people who developed AIDS in their mid-twenties may have contracted HIV during their teenage years, whether through sex or drug use.

This new information meant that many teenagers were living with HIV without realizing it until years later, when they finally began to show signs of AIDS. Under the radar, HIV was spreading among young people, both straight and queer, who weren't being tested or informed about this risk.

Many trailblazing young people cared deeply about the AIDS crisis and rose up to help make friends and peers aware of it. Sure, there were safe-sex ads on TV and, in places where it was allowed, safe-sex education in schools. But with zines, raps, and comics, teens weren't just the target audience—they were also often the creators.

The AIDS and Adolescents Network of New York campaigned for the lives of young people affected by HIV/AIDS. This flyer advertises a protest against Resolution 33, a policy to teach abstinence-first sex education in New York City schools in 1993. The AIDS and Adolescents Network argued that abstinence-based policies were unrealistic and caused more harm than good in preventing the spread of HIV/AIDS among New York youth.

## Youth Activist Zines

The Youth Education Life Line—or YELL for short—was an organization of young people speaking to other young people about HIV/AIDS. YELL (shout it) began as the youth wing of ACT UP New York. Like ACT UP, YELL met at the place now known as the Lesbian, Gay, Bisexual & Transgender Community Center on West Thirteenth Street in Manhattan. Members of YELL went to protests and took part in civil disobedience to raise awareness of the injustice of HIV/AIDS. The group produced several zines throughout the early 1990s, explaining their activism and providing templates for young readers to undertake their own. YELL zines were full of information about safer sex and drug use, and unlike most examples of AIDS awareness materials, they were written by young people, *for* young people. YELL's mission was to fight against the political powers that controlled research and pharmaceuticals; they insisted that, as young people, they deserved access to free condoms and needle exchanges. Unlike most examples of youth-focused HIV/AIDS awareness in this time, the *YELL* zine was loudly and happily political in its flavor, directly naming the inequality and injustice that shaped the official response to HIV/AIDS.

Zine culture is about a DIY approach. Unlike big magazines, zines are designed and self-published by a handful of people, working for free, doing it for fun and because they care about what they have to say. Zines are put together by the people who design them, often in their bedrooms or at the local library, then photocopied, self-published, and self-distributed. In the 1990s, it was typical for zines to be cut-and-pasted together by the creators rather than designed on a computer. Photocopied and stapled into a booklet, a zine isn't focused on making money; it's about a punk ethos and an authentic voice. Zines were an important platform for people to talk about HIV/AIDS without having to conform to the opinions and needs of big organizations and corporations. The pages of *YELL* are filled with a combination of typeset and handwritten columns and features answering questions about civil disobedience or risk-reduction behaviors, as well as testimonies from young people about their experiences.

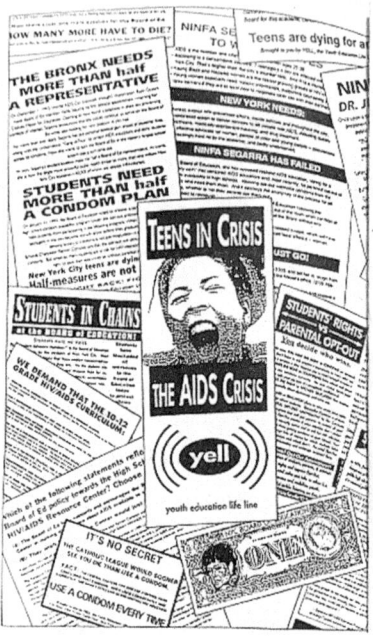

## Who is yell?

Youth Education Life Line is the committee of ACT UP that focuses on teen issues in the AIDS crisis.

We are a body of diverse, articulate, in-your-face activists fighting for students' rights to comprehensive AIDS education, free condoms, dental dams, and clean needles in the New York City schools.

Our members represent a cross-section of the multicultural society we live in today: women, men, queers, straights, young and old, HIV+, HIV-, ethnic and other minorities. We do not discriminate.

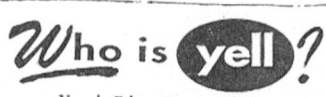

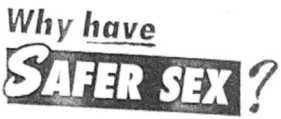

The HIV virus can *only* be transmitted by exchange of infected blood, semen, vaginal fluids and breast milk. So protect yourself with latex every time.

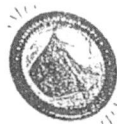

USE LATEX CONDOMS — natural skin condoms don't protect you
USE LATEX OR REGULAR SARAN WRAP FOR DAMS
USE WATER-BASED LUBE WITH NONOXYNOL 9 — baby oil or vaseline on a condom makes it break

| NO RISK | |
|---|---|
| • Kissing - Hugging | • Cruising |
| • Talking Dirty | • Visual Turn-Ons |
| • Masturbating | • Abstinence |

| LOW RISK |
|---|
| • Vaginal or anal sex with a latex condom and a water-based lube with Nonoxynol 9 |
| • Sex toys - with a condom if you share them |
| • Oral sex with a latex barrier |

| HIGH RISK |
|---|
| • Any vaginal or anal sex without a condom |
| • Oral sex without a latex barrier |
| • Sharing unclean needles or works |

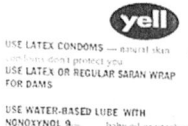

### we demand: — the youth education life line

• comprehensive, non-judgmental AIDS education for students at all grade levels in all schools.

• free access to condoms and dental dams for all students, with or without parental consent, in both junior and senior high schools.

• needle exchange and drug treatment on demand for teenage injection drug users (IDU's).

• mandatory sensitivity training for all faculty and school staff to help meet the needs of youth who are HIV-positive or at risk for HIV infection.

• an elected student representative on the NYC Board of Education with voting rights to advocate for AIDS education.

• responsible AIDS awareness reporting by all teen-oriented media (e.g. magazines, radio, TV) to provide safer sex and safer drug use information.

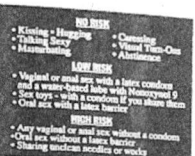

Don't forget:
• Always use a condom when you fuck, give or get a blow job, or use a dildo, vibrator and other sex toys.
• If you can't find condoms in your school, call the High School HIV Resource Center at (718) 935-3900.
• Never let anyone pressure you into doing something you don't want to do. It's your body, your choice.

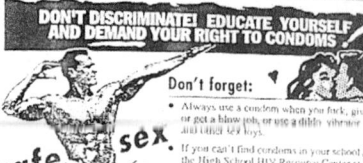

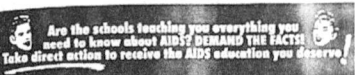

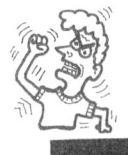
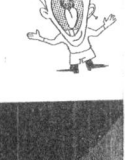
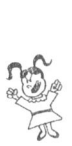
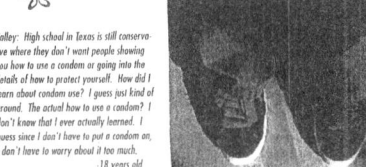
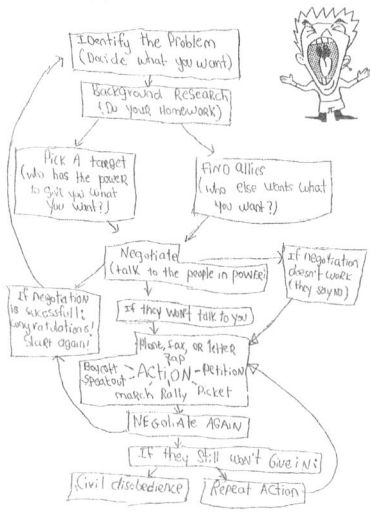

YELL was far from the only zine made in response to HIV/AIDS in this period. Zines of this kind were often darkly humorous, with biting names like *Diseased Pariah News* and *Infected Faggot Perspectives.* If these titles seem distressing or shocking, it's because they were meant to provoke a reaction. They were a rebuttal to a mass media that tended to either ignore or stigmatize the trials of people living with HIV/AIDS. For many people associated with AIDS, morbid humor became something life-affirming in the face of a society that didn't seem to care if you lived or died.

If silence equaled death, then it was important to make young people understand that they weren't alone in their fears and anxieties about HIV/AIDS. The aim of the game was for young people to help other young people talk about their concerns, while empowering them to understand the simple actions they could take to protect themselves from HIV. These lessons remain important today, even though HIV is now easily treatable.

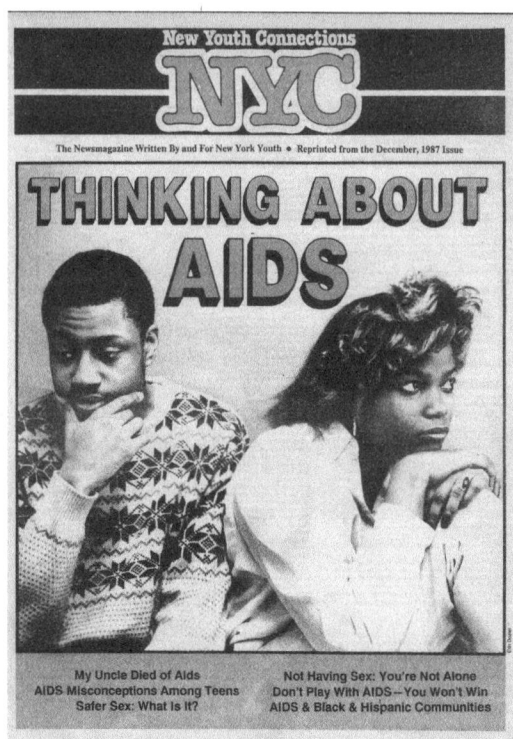

*New Youth Connections* was a monthly newspaper in New York City in the 1980s and 1990s targeted at and written by young people. The December 1987 edition was dedicated entirely to HIV/AIDS. The editorial for this issue complained about the lack of HIV/AIDS education in New York schools, suggesting that "waiting until high school to teach the facts about sex and AIDS is like teaching a nine-year-old to walk."

"Everybody is scared of this disease. It kills!" says Jasmine. "Nobody really wants to get AIDS. Now you are finding out that there are condoms that are not safe. I'm scared and I'm not doing anything."
—*New Youth Connections*, December 1987

So, in 1996, the youth of New York City are delivering this message: "You don't know how we're **LIVING**, YOU DON'T CARE that we're **dying**. SO, YOU'LL NEVER EXPECT IT WHEN WE KICK YOUR *&!%#@* IDEAS **out**!"

## Teen Raps and Music

In 1995, the rapper Eazy-E died from AIDS complications. Eazy-E was born in the mid-1960s in Compton, a suburb of Los Angeles. In the 1950s, Compton was a middle-class Black neighborhood, but by the

# Young People Schoolin' Other Young People

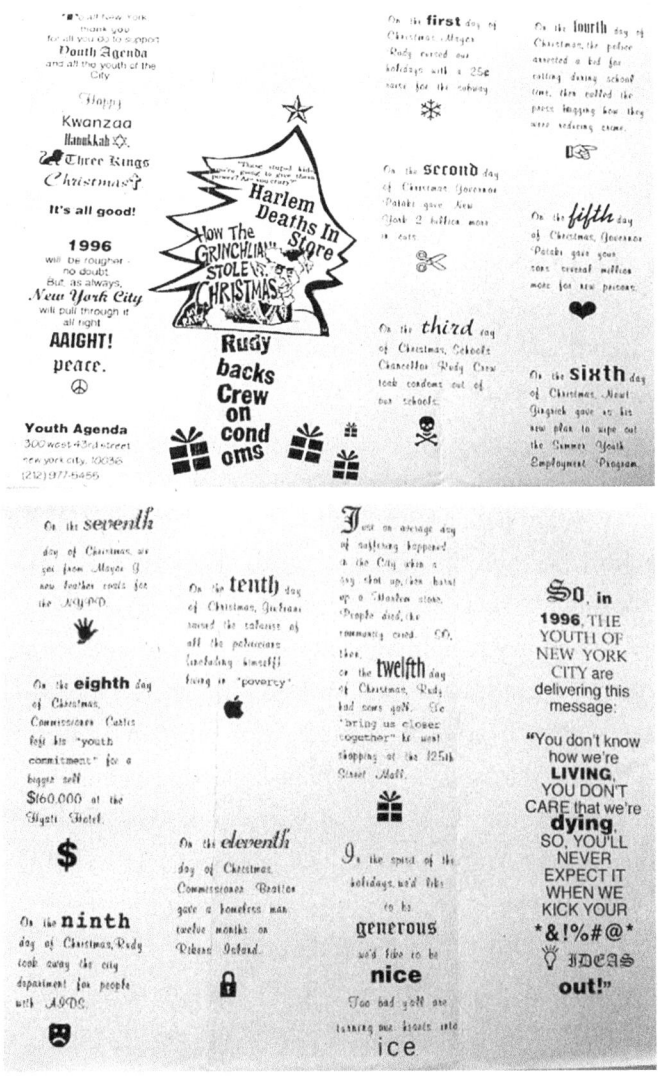

This pamphlet was created by the organization Youth Agenda. It riffs on "The Twelve Days of Christmas" to draw attention to inequalities in New York City, including those regarding HIV/AIDS.

time Eazy-E came of age, it was associated with drugs, deprivation, gang violence, and a high crime rate—one of the "most dangerous cities in America." In his youth, Eazy-E dealt drugs to survive before becoming famous as a member of N.W.A, a notorious rap group with links to gang warfare in Compton. By the early 1990s, Eazy-E was no longer in a gang; he was famous as a musical entrepreneur in the hip-hop scene.

In 1994, Eazy-E was hospitalized and diagnosed with AIDS. He made amends with Ice Cube, another rapper and his longtime rival, and composed a public statement announcing his diagnosis to his fans. His wife, Tomica Woods, stood in front of a crowd of journalists in tears as his friend Ron Sweeney read out his statement:

> I'm not religious, but wrong or right, that's me. I'm not saying this because I'm looking for a soft cushion wherever I'm heading. I just feel I've got thousands and thousands of young fans that have to learn about what's real when it comes to AIDS.

Eazy-E died a month after his diagnosis. His death drew attention to the risk of HIV among young Black men. Youth organizations had already been working hard to reach this population. Young people wrote "teen raps" to be performed in schools to address the presence of HIV/AIDS and the things that young people needed to do to protect themselves, particularly those in big cities. The hip-hop girl group Salt-N-Pepa even included a reading from a play about AIDS on their album *Very Necessary*, which was released in 1993. The following year, the group released a remixed version of their 1991 song "Let's Talk About Sex" called "Let's Talk About AIDS" to raise awareness of HIV/AIDS among their young fans. In the intro, Salt talks about how the group has been fighting AIDS for a long time, saying that the best cure is "not to get it and not to spread it." She then introduces a group of young people from Boston who are involved in AIDS education, calling them "young people schoolin' other young people." This is followed by a dialogue in which a young woman expresses shock and fear after finding out she's HIV+ and may have AIDS. Her boyfriend speaks, but when she tells him about her diagnosis, he rejects her. The aim was to make it clear that HIV/AIDS was an issue for teenage girls to take seriously—particularly urban youth of color associated with Salt-N-Pepa's radio-friendly hip-hop style.

* * *

The raps created by young people to spread awareness about HIV/AIDS might not have had the same polish as Salt-N-Pepa's, but they're a great example of teens with conviction trying to talk to their peers and wake them up to the reality of AIDS.

---

**TEEN RAP #2**

YOU GOT PEOPLE WALKIN 'ROUND
WORRIED AND AFRAID
WITH CRAZY IDEAS
ABOUT THE WAY YOU GET AIDS

WELL YOU SURE CAN'T GET IT
FROM THE FOOD YOU EAT,
FROM THE AIR, FROM MOSQUITOS
OR A TOILET SEAT

BUT WHEN PEOPLE ARE SCARED
THEY CAN BE QUITE CRUEL
AND HERE'S ONE THING
I HOPE YOU LEARN IN SCHOOL

THAT PEOPLE WITH AIDS
ARE PEOPLE TOO
THEY NEED LOVE AND CARE
LIKE ME AND YOU

BUT IF YOU USE DIRTY NEEDLES
OR YOU'RE HAVING SEX
WHEN IT COMES TO AIDS
YOU KNOW, YOU COULD BE NEXT

SO TAKE CARE, BE CAREFUL
YOU BETTER WATCH OUT
THINK ABOUT WHAT YOU'RE DOIN'
WHEN THE LIGHTS GO OUT

AND IF YOU DON'T HAVE A CONDOM
WHEN IT'S TIME TO PLAY
YOU'D BE A WHOLE LOT SMARTER
JUST TO -- WALK AWAY,
WALK AWAY, WALK AWAY

THIS IS DJ SMALL. FOR MORE
INFORMATION ABOUT CONDOMS
AND SAFE SEX, CALL THE SAN
FRANCISCO AIDS FOUNDATION AT
863-AIDS

---

This teen rap was part of an HIV/AIDS awareness project led by the San Francisco AIDS Foundation in 1989. The project was put together by a combination of HIV/AIDS workers, educators, and teenagers.

## Comics

Many of the comics produced about HIV/AIDS were targeted at American teenagers from the late 1980s onward—a time in the crisis when people were more and more aware of the long incubation period of HIV, which meant that teenagers could contract HIV without even realizing it. But comics had played a role in AIDS awareness from the first years of the crisis. Howard Cruse was a pioneering figure in the gay comic scene. Born in Alabama and the son of a preacher, Cruse founded Gay Comix in 1980. The company published a variety of comics that explored LGBTQ+ themes and issues. By 1983, Cruse was working with

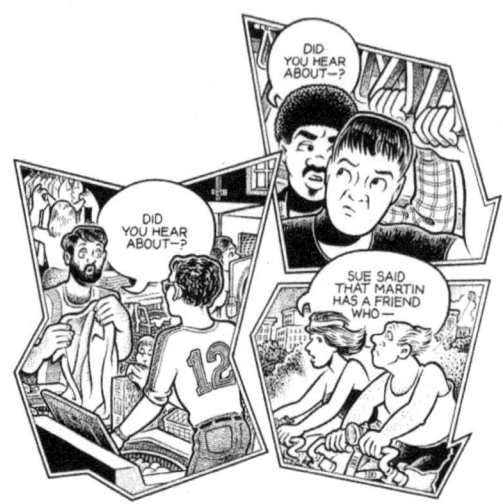

A detail from one of the first comic strips about HIV/AIDS: *Safe Sex* by Howard Cruse. The comic strip was circulated in 1983 and provides one of the first examples of "safe-sex" discourse.

the Committee on Safer Sex, a branch of Gay Men's Health Crisis that promoted knowledge and behavior to reduce the risk of HIV/AIDS. Cruse's *Safe Sex* is an early example of the use of comics as an accessible platform to not only provide information about HIV/AIDS but explore the effect the unfolding crisis was having on affected communities—before many others cared.

Youth-made zines like *YELL* often included comics—comic strips were a familiar format to communicate basic knowledge about HIV/AIDS. They could make it simple to understand. *YELL* even made a comic book to address the issue of HIV/AIDS in young people who were growing up in foster care, *The Foster Kid's Guide to HIV Testing*. By the early 1990s, a number of young people in the foster care system were the surviving children of HIV+ parents who had died from AIDS-related causes. There was a lot of pressure on these young people to know their own HIV status. Today, that might seem logical—if you're living with HIV, you need to know about it so you can start treatment. But what if there was no treatment? What if being known to be HIV+ could put you in harm's way? Too often, the state undermined the rights of these young people to consent to being tested and sharing the results with medical professionals. Often, the state reserved the right to control information about a positive test, which meant that caregivers and caseworkers could be made aware of the test results without the permission of the person in question. The state could demand that teenagers in the foster care system submit to taking a test simply because they were gay or because they were presumed to be sexually active.

*The Foster Kid's Guide to HIV Testing* explained these issues. It encouraged some of the most vulnerable young people in society to understand their rights and how to navigate a cruel system. Testing for HIV is important, but everyone deserves to be empowered in this process—not dehumanized.

Zines and comics are still powerful art forms, but nowadays, they're as likely to circulate through viral images on social media as in print form.

Social media is a powerful space for young people to help other young people understand the ongoing reality of HIV/AIDS today. Raised in Missouri and a student at San Diego State University, Zach Willmore was only nineteen years old when he was diagnosed with HIV in early 2023. Willmore became popular on TikTok after he began to post about his diagnosis and treatment through a number of lighthearted and informative posts.

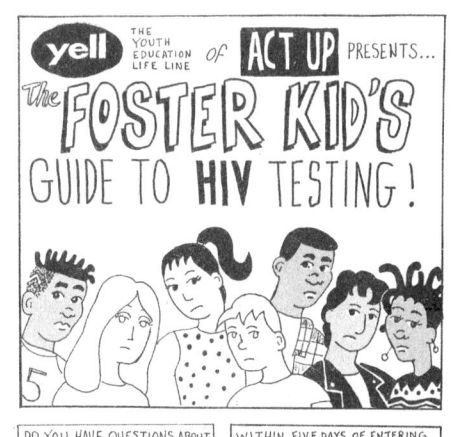

*The Foster Kid's Guide to HIV Testing* was made by YELL in the 1990s.

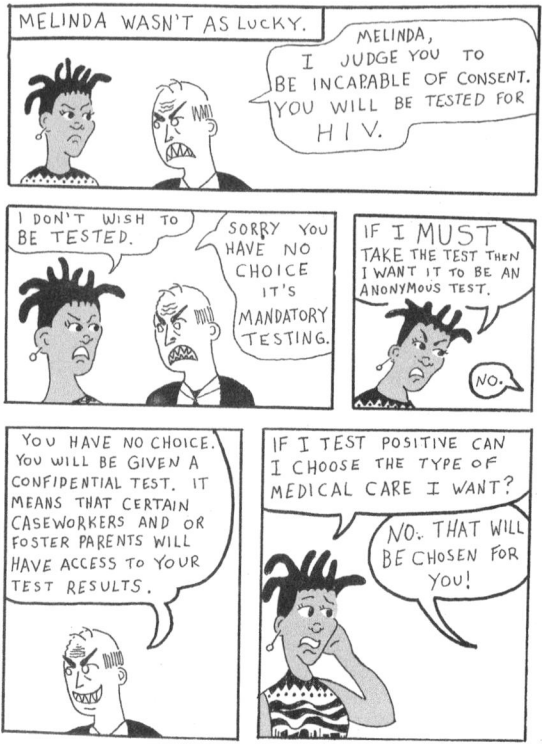

*The Foster Kid's Guide to HIV Testing* is a record of an important issue that is easily forgotten today. Many young people were in foster care because their parents had died from AIDS-related causes.

"It's Friday, February 17. I'm nineteen years old. And yesterday I found out that I got diagnosed with HIV," Willmore said as he put on makeup in the inaugural post of his TikTok video "diary."

After his diagnosis, Willmore was able to start treatment quickly, and so his HIV status became undetectable and untransmittable. Willmore's diary-style use of TikTok amassed nearly 2 million followers. He received a homophobic backlash in the comments section for his supposedly irreverent attitude about what had happened to him—but having a sense of humor has always been an essential survival strategy for people at the front line of the HIV/AIDS epidemic. Maybe these trolls just didn't like the fact that Willmore felt comfortable being queer, camp, and happy in his body. Some people want HIV+ people to hide away in shame about their condition, but Willmore's TikTok became a platform for sharing the ups and downs of his journey, making HIV visible and relevant for his generation.

> **People are scared of the unknown. Information is power, so I really wanted to help people understand.**
> —Zach Willmore to NBC News

With a topic as scary and isolating as HIV/AIDS, humor is powerful. Honesty is radical. The controversies around Willmore's posts are a reminder that silence will only create more silence and lead to new cases of HIV. The opposite of silence is connection. And young people deserve the opportunity to connect with other young people about the issues they are going to be confronted by in their lives.

## *How to Have Sex in an Epidemic* and the Denver Principles

In the early 1980s, Richard Berkowitz is a young hustler with a specialty in S&M. He is no stranger to (easily treatable) sexually transmitted infections, which have been increasingly part of the price of being sexually active in the gay scene in New York since the late 1970s. Then AIDS comes along. In 1982, he learns he's living with AIDS. His doctor, Joseph Sonnabend, introduces him to another patient, Michael Callen, a singer-songwriter, and the pair begin discussions about how they can help people learn about AIDS and how to reduce risk. Berkowitz and Callen don't trust the medical establishment to help the gay community, because the American Psychiatric Association classified being gay as a disorder until the mid-1970s.

In May 1983, Berkowitz and Callen self-publish a pamphlet for the gay community called *How to Have Sex in an Epidemic*, drawing on Sonnabend's medical expertise. They're sure that the most realistic way to help gay men navigate the new risk of AIDS is to acknowledge that there's nothing inherently wrong with gay sexuality. They want to help their community find ways of living and loving that can survive the crisis, that will limit risk, and that don't depend upon approval from the establishment. They write:

> Sex doesn't make you sick—diseases do. Gay sex doesn't make you sick—gay men who are sick do. Once you understand how diseases are transmitted, you can begin to explore medically safe sex.
>
> Our challenge is to figure out how we can have gay, life-affirming sex, satisfy our emotional needs, and stay alive!

Berkowitz and Callen want people to understand that different sexual acts carry different levels of risk when it comes to sexually transmitted infections (including HIV, although they aren't aware of how HIV works when they write the pamphlet). They recommend that gay men use condoms if they have anal and/or oral sex. Before AIDS, condoms were associated with protecting people from getting pregnant, rather than protecting gay men from infections. If your sex life doesn't involve anything that can create a baby, why bother with condoms? AIDS is changing that, and Berkowitz and Callen want to make that change seem sexy rather than bad.

The pamphlet becomes a pioneering example of how to be sex positive while staying safety conscious. The pamphlet will go on to be regarded as key to how we understand safer-sex education. Berkowitz and Callen aren't right about everything: They didn't set much store by rumors that AIDS was caused by a specific virus, instead suggesting that promiscuity itself was overloading the immune system. Once HIV was identified in mid-1983 by scientists in France, this theory was disproven. But much of the advice in the pamphlet remains sound. If you want to help people protect themselves, you need to make safer sex seem *sexy*, not like a punishment.

> Not all gay men are well-educated and well-off; not all gay men can afford the benefits of proper health care. What we as a community must do is to make available vital information about how diseases are transmitted so that each of us can make <u>informed</u> decisions about our lives.
> What's over isn't sex—just sex without responsibility.

In June 1983, Callen and Berkowitz travel to the fifth annual National Lesbian and Gay Health Conference, which is being held in Denver, Colorado. At the conference, they take part in a panel led by Bobbi Campbell, one of the best-known early AIDS activists. The panelists agree to establish a political network of people with AIDS—and also agree that this is how they want to be known: not as *AIDS victims* or *AIDS patients*, but as *people with AIDS*.

At the end of the conference, Callen, Campbell, and Berkowitz come onto the main stage with eight other gay men who are all also living with AIDS. They unfurl a banner that reads *FIGHTING FOR OUR LIVES*.

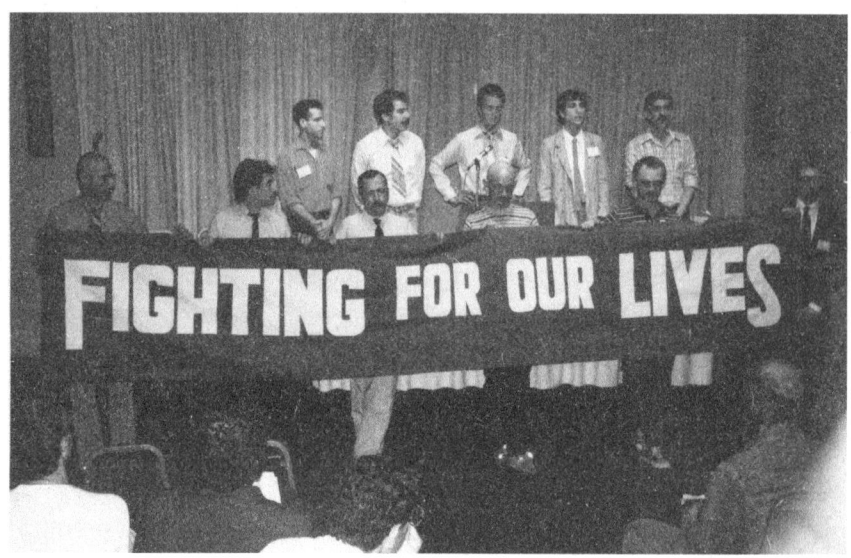

As the crowd in the room takes in these four words, the men begin to speak. They take turns reading a statement that was quickly drafted.

It begins:

> We condemn attempts to label us as "victims," a term which implies defeat, and we are only occasionally "patients," a term which implies passivity, helplessness, and dependence upon the care of others. We are "People With AIDS."

As the room watches, they read a manifesto that becomes known as "The Denver Principles"—a declaration of the rights of people with AIDS. These principles will become the foundation of the AIDS activist movement.

Inspired by the women's rights and gay rights movements of the

1970s, the Denver Principles represent a powerful and provocative voice of defiance in a world that remains happy not to think about AIDS. That day in Denver, eleven activists make an unapologetic demand that Americans recognize that people with AIDS have an inalienable human right to live without discrimination, prejudice, and scapegoating. The Denver Principles change the language we use to talk about AIDS—not just with the term "People With AIDS" but also by calling for people with AIDS to be central in national conversations about AIDS policy and care, to be taken seriously as leaders in the response to AIDS. And they demand recognition that HIV+ people have a right to empowering, fulfilling, and responsible sexual and emotional lives; to receive care without prejudice; to have privacy; to be able to consent to any future treatment program with knowledge, power, and free choice.

The final principle voiced on the stage that day in Denver in 1983 is the right of people with AIDS "to die—and to LIVE—in dignity." Some of these activists will die within weeks of their action at the conference. Within two years, the majority will be dead.

Callen dies from AIDS complications in Los Angeles in 1993. Today, Berkowitz is the sole surviving member of the eleven men behind the Denver Principles. Their work in the early years of AIDS was not only pioneering but life-changing—their guidance for gay men's sexual health set a precedent for how to convey sexual and reproductive health advice, and their role in the Denver Principles made a huge impact in giving people with AIDS the dignity they demanded.

# How to ACT UP When SILENCE=DEATH

The Lesbian, Gay, Bisexual & Transgender Community Center in Manhattan is a sprawling building on a tree-lined street in the West Village. The building was built before the Civil War and lived several lives as a grammar school and a culinary school before it became "The Center" in 1983. Today, young queer people still flock there. You can see them outside, smoking cigarettes, or in the foyer, using the space as a safe location to charge their phones and use the Wi-Fi. Now as then, the Center is a beacon for LGBTQ+ people in the city, and in the late 1980s, it became an essential meeting ground to discuss what could be done about AIDS. The Center was around the corner from St. Vincent's Hospital, which housed the city's first AIDS ward, accommodating many of the thousands of AIDS cases erupting across the population.

One day, Keith Cylar went to the Center. He worked downtown as a therapist and social worker. He was distressed: He was seeing the impact of AIDS on Black gay men firsthand—AIDS was affecting his clients, and it was affecting his inner circle. One year previously, his lover had died, and not long after, Cylar found out he was living with HIV. The Center was a great place to get information about HIV/AIDS. Cylar was looking through a display of flyers and posters when he noticed one about ACT UP. It said ACT UP was a new group focused on using nonviolent forms of direct action to make more people care about finding a solution to the AIDS crisis.

ACT UP: AIDS Coalition to Unleash Power.

There were men hanging out nearby, all dressed in leather jackets. Cylar liked their style; they looked intriguing. He was so curious about the leaflets and these leather-jacketed men that he followed them into one of the Center's meeting rooms and found himself at his first ACT UP meeting:

> It was the black leather jackets that pulled me into the room. . . . I became part of a community and I watched my community disintegrate. . . . I wanted to keep people from dying. I needed to fight against this thing that was killing us and killing me.

ACT UP was birthed out of the fires of fear and fury among LGBTQ+ people in New York as AIDS decimated the city's gay population in the mid-1980s. Between 1987 and the early 1990s, ACT UP grew into a powerhouse of AIDS activism. ACT UP members were responsible for passionate and provocative actions to draw attention to big issues: free access to contraception in schools to reduce new HIV diagnoses among teenagers; getting potential treatments out of the testing stage and into people's bodies; enabling HIV+ people to be eligible for health insurance; redefining AIDS to better include women's symptoms. ACT UP members ran needle exchanges with injection-drug users to help this population reduce the risk of either contracting or passing on HIV by providing them with clean needles—an action seen as illegal and immoral at the time, leading to the arrest of ACT UP activists who took part in this radical, urgent action. Cylar, for example, went on with fellow activists Charles King, Eric Sawyer, and Virginia Shubert to found Housing Works, a New York City–based nonprofit that sees homelessness, AIDS, and drug addiction as connected issues that need nonjudgmental compassion.

ACT UP began spontaneously. It was March 10, 1987, at the Center. That evening, an angry bespectacled man stood before a crowd in one of the Center's meeting rooms and expounded his rage. Larry Kramer was a writer and activist—he'd been a notorious figure in the gay community in New York for a decade, perceived by many as slut-shaming gay men for their voluminous sexual activity in the 1970s. As mentioned earlier, he was one of the first gay journalists to ring alarm bells about the rise in AIDS cases in the early 1980s.

He wasn't supposed to speak that day. The meeting was part of a regular speaker series, and the author Nora Ephron had to reschedule at short notice, so Kramer stepped in.

At that point, the city had seen more than 30,000 AIDS diagnoses. Too much of the city government's response was rooted in the idea that AIDS was a niche concern—something that might still just blow over if you looked the other way.

Kramer knew it wouldn't blow over.

"We have not yet even begun to live through the true horror," he began. "As it has been explained to me, the people who have become ill so far got ill early; the average incubation period is now thought to be five and one-half years, and the real tidal wave is yet to come: people who got infected starting in 1981. You had sex in 1981. I did, too. And after. Last week, I had seven friends who were diagnosed. In one week. That's the most in the shortest period that's happened to me."

Avram Finkelstein was in the audience at the Center that evening. Like most early members of ACT UP, Finkelstein was a white gay New Yorker whose whole understanding of the world was changed irrevocably by the impact of AIDS on his community. For many gay men after Stonewall, AIDS was their first life-or-death political awakening. Finkelstein and his gay male friends had been meeting once a week to discuss how to deal with AIDS, how to make people care, and how to cope with the loss of so many friends and lovers. Finkelstein's boyfriend died from AIDS-related causes in the very first years of the crisis, even before the word "AIDS" had been decided upon. It was a harrowing experience—a time when total panic among health care professionals was the order of the day:

> They wouldn't bring him food in the room. They left it in the hallway. They wouldn't even pick up his trays when we put them back

in the hallway. It was masks. It was gloves. There was blood underneath his bed from a previous patient. They didn't clean it. We brought in cleaning supplies and cleaned the room. He was terrified, and it was terrible.

Finkelstein and his friends were part of the New York art scene. Most of them grew up in left-wing Jewish households—families that had immigrated to America to escape antisemitic persecution in Europe. In 1986, Finkelstein and his friends started creating political posters to draw attention to AIDS in public. Their goal was to find an image that would immediately grab people's attention. The men settled upon the pink triangle: the image employed by the Nazis during the Holocaust to brand LGBTQ+ people. Finkelstein and his friends flipped the pink triangle upside down and captioned it with two words and a symbol to drive their message home: SILENCE=DEATH.

Finkelstein suggested to his friends that they go hear Kramer speak rather than holding their regular private meeting in someone's apartment. He'd become intrigued by Kramer's perspective on AIDS after reading his writing in the *New York Native*.

Kramer told everyone in the audience from the right-hand aisle to the left wall to stand up. As two-thirds of the crowd stood in the low-ceilinged room, Kramer gestured to them and said, "At the rate we are going, you could be dead in less than five years. Two-thirds of this room could be dead in less than five years. Please sit down."

His point was brutal: AIDS was decimating the LGBTQ+ community in New York, and nowhere near enough noise was being made.

Kramer was a divisive figure with a famously dogged temper. That day at the Center, he articulated a shared feeling of outrage and fear. Like an overflowing drain, the emotion in the room gathered into something powerful. That collective anger became a fuel that drove the creation of a new political group—an organization that *fought back* rather than begging for crumbs from those in power.

As one of the founders of Gay Men's Health Crisis, Kramer understood that community-led responses were important. Groups like Gay Men's Health Crisis could be bureaucratic and slow-moving. The atmosphere in the room that evening was rooted in the sense that something had been missing for queer New Yorkers who were angry about AIDS. That missing something was now present, rippling through the room and galvanizing the audience to sit up.

Something louder.

Something bigger.

Something that would bite back.

Kramer asked the crowd:

*Do we want to start a new organization devoted solely to political action?* The answer came back loudly: YES.

Two days later, about three hundred people gathered again at the Center and discussed what this new organization might look like. Their goal was to act quickly: to take control as best they could of an unbearable situation.

Sometimes, things fall apart. Other times, they fall together. The initial shape and objectives of ACT UP were clarified rapidly over the course of a few short meetings. The name ACT UP was thrown out by somebody in the crowd and won support. Unlike some of the other AIDS groups at the time, ACT UP was not interested in pleading for greater accommodations for people affected by AIDS. It was about challenging the powers that be directly and unapologetically.

Not asking nicely for change, not waiting around as people got sick and died, but getting out onto the streets and demanding it.

Soon after this first meeting, ACT UP's first action took place. On March 24, 1987, more than two hundred members of ACT UP descended on Wall Street in Lower Manhattan during the morning commute with a number of different demands. ACT UP argued that drug companies were motivated by greed rather than a sincere aim to abate the suffering of people with AIDS as soon as possible. They argued that drug companies and the FDA were moving much too slowly and that new drugs needed to be put into people's bodies as soon as possible—even if they weren't yet approved by the FDA. They argued that it was cruel that drug companies were using placebo trials for new AIDS drugs: double-blind studies that meant only 50 percent of a sample group would receive the trial medication while the remaining 50 percent would receive no treatment at all. On Wall Street, ACT UP called for AIDS to be treated as a national crisis. That meant ending placebo trials, maximizing the availability of any promising drug, and curbing the price of these drugs to make them as affordable as possible. At this first protest, ACT UP also called for a massive national education campaign to make people understand HIV/AIDS, and for the immediate improvement of legal protections for people with AIDS to end the savage neglect and discrimination they were experiencing.

Wall Street is the center of the country's finances and plays an extraordinary role in the global economy. Causing a nonviolent disruption in this part of the city was a way to demand the attention of the rich and powerful. As police acted in response to this new group of activists and struggled to get a handle on the protest, protestors sat in the street and refused to move. The voices of the activists became united as one, their chants climbing above the noise of the financial district around them:

*Release the drugs! Release the drugs! Release the drugs!*

An effigy of the commissioner of the FDA, Frank Young, was installed in front of Trinity Church—intended as a symbol of neglect and greed. A homemade placard called out the president, reading, *REAGAN GUILTY OF CRIMINAL NEGLECT.*

*We are angry! We want action!*
*We are angry! We want action!*

Activists handed out copies of a recent article by Kramer from *The New York Times* to passersby, along with leaflets that declared: *AIDS*

*IS EVERYBODY'S BUSINESS NOW.* The police attempted to remove protestors from the road to release the flow of traffic. Eventually, seventeen of these activists were arrested for civil disobedience after traffic was stopped in one of the busiest and wealthiest areas of the world for several hours.

*We'll never be silent again!*
*We'll never be silent again!*

They weren't. This first action on Wall Street was a threshold. Once it had been crossed, a new community of activists was created. Lifelong solidarities were formed. The grief and fear of a group of people who had been ignored—a group of people who were dying—was redirected into radical displays of outrage, into a life-or-death demand for things to change.

Said Kramer:

> These are men and women, some barely in their twenties, who have a comfort with their homosexuality that I never had at that age, and a desire to be politically active that, at such a young age, for such large numbers, is actually historically new and important in the ongoing struggle for gay rights.

A few days before the Wall Street action, the FDA announced that a drug called AZT would be made available for people with AIDS.

But the price was set by its manufacturer, Burroughs Wellcome, at up to $12,000 a year for a course of treatment, at a time when the median income in the US was just over $30,000 a year for a household. In 1987, this made AZT the most expensive drug ever sold. Many people with AIDS, especially those who were unemployed because of illness, were making far less. As *The Washington Post* noted, "Even patients whose private insurance pays 80 percent of the costs can pay up to $200 each month out of their own pockets."

AZT was thought to be one of the most promising drugs to stop the progression of AIDS. It's impossible to overstate how meaningful that was. At that time, AZT represented a light at the end of the tunnel—a drug that might stop the relentless pace of death among almost everyone diagnosed with AIDS. People were infuriated that access to this drug was hindered by bureaucracy, which meant lives were being squandered. They argued that access to AZT was being controlled in favor of the profits of pharmaceutical companies, and to the detriment of people living with AIDS.

In December 1987, Burroughs Wellcome reduced the price of AZT by 20 percent. The company had previously justified the high price through their assumption that it would be of value for only a limited proportion of the population. It took almost two years to get Burroughs Wellcome to lower the price once more. On September 14, 1989, ACT UP infiltrated the New York Stock Exchange, with protestors chaining themselves to a balcony. The protest was so disruptive, it caused trading to cease on the floor. No trading meant no money flowing in the global economy. And money talks. A few days later, Burroughs Wellcome agreed to reduce the price of AZT again, by a further 20 percent. The lower price was still far from perfect. Profits were still being made out of the desperation of people with AIDS. But it was more proof for ACT UP that their strategies could work. It showed that the world could be changed by nonviolent civil disobedience, by the adrenaline of people who had nothing to lose but their own lives, with so many members of ACT UP living with AIDS themselves.

AZT wasn't the remedy that everyone wanted it to be—or the remedy the price tag implied it was. In fact, none of the early trial drugs would prove very useful in the fight against AIDS. AZT turned out to be devastatingly toxic, even fatal. But in the mid-1980s, getting access to AZT and other drugs was a symbol of hope. By calling for faster access to new drugs and condemning the extortionate pricing of the only approved one, ACT UP was demanding that pharmaceutical companies act with the urgency that the crisis required.

Treat the crisis as a crisis. Treat people affected by AIDS as the experts they are, rather than as pariahs or hapless victims. *Give us the best chance of staying alive.*

Many of the first members of ACT UP were white gay New Yorkers on the front line of the impact of AIDS on the city's gay community. As ACT UP gained recognition as a political force, its majority-white and majority-gay membership would seem problematic. One of the early Black members, Allan Robinson, remembers his frustration as a Black person in the space:

> I kept my distance. At the first meeting I attended, there were about 500 mostly white men present. An energy in the room made me go back, again and again. There were so few Black and Brown men in the organization that people kept approaching me. . . . I would hear them referring to us as this generic thing, "people of color." I realized that there were people there who didn't even know Black people. I would actually hear other Black and Brown people refer to our people as if they were talking in the third person. Outside all of my criticism, I found an energy in the organization that was frankly exciting. That energy helped me deal with the loss, anger, and the frustration with societal indifference I was encountering.

Robinson noted that the other ACT UP leaders were "always looking to me to be 'the Black man.'"

> I noticed very early on that had it not been for the health crisis, many of the white men I came in contact with would not think twice about returning to their old misogynist ways. As white men, they would not think it was their responsibility in life to change the status quo with regards to racism, sexism, and certain other social concerns in this country. One of the things I picked up, especially among the upper middle class, is that they were goddamned angry. They were

angry because they thought they had everything—trips to Brazil, and Fire Island, hanging in the clubs, boyfriends, drugs, money, and living perhaps on 81st Street and Central Park West. They were angry because they were being treated like everybody else.

Before he died in 1991, Robinson told B. Michael Hunter:

> I was active in ACT UP and concerned about AIDS even though I knew I was HIV-negative, at least that's the way I tested. Then, in the spring, I tested HIV-positive. I didn't exactly handle it the way I thought I would—I was shocked. I went off. I stressed out, and felt empty, lonely, and detached. I was asymptomatic but I still considered suicide—I even wrote out a note. Real drama, real, real drama. I made myself dream a solution. I realized that I had lost touch with who I was. As far as I'm concerned, there would still be life, there would still be consciousness. Also, there are people in my life that really care about me, that I love. I really enjoy living, trees, touching and I love all sorts of physical things. I think I said to someone that I was going to live to spite a couple of people. Life is my birthright, it is the earliest and fondest wish of my parents. I created new dreams and even envisioned myself as some stunning, unfettered, lovely 80-year-old man, with an adobe home in the Southwest surrounded by men in love. As Black men, when we view ourselves holistically, HIV really doesn't mean that much. It means as much as everything else—racism, poverty, inadequate health care, homophobia, etc. I think to heal ourselves of all of this, we must continue to talk to each other.

Robinson remained close to ACT UP despite his reservations because he saw that the adrenaline that powered the group was rare. Things were happening. Robinson became one of many Black and Latine members of ACT UP who helped lead life-changing and life-saving actions. Think of Katrina Haslip, a Black woman who found out she had HIV when she was incarcerated in the mid-1980s. During her time in prison, Haslip worked as a librarian and coordinated a group of prisoners to advocate for better services for prisoners living with AIDS. When Haslip was released, she broke her probation to take part in an ACT UP protest and went on to play a pivotal role in getting the Centers for Disease Control to change the definition of AIDS-defining illnesses to ensure that women's experiences were included.

ACT UP is most associated with its founding and actions in New York City. But the organization quickly spawned subgroups or chapters that addressed the different contexts of AIDS in other parts of the US: Louisiana, Philadelphia, San Francisco. Always intended as a democratic, organic organization shaped by the various diverse goals of its members, ACT UP spread throughout the country and across the world. At its height, there were ACT UP chapters in London, Paris, and Puerto Rico.

But adrenaline only lasts so long. You can't remain at crisis pitch forever. By 1992, the energy of ACT UP had started to deflate. As activists died, the turnover of new members struggled to sustain the momentum of what had been lost. ACT UP's strength had always been the diversity of its members, but infighting became a weakness after the deaths of many of the organization's most well-known and well-respected members.

As activist Emily Nahmanson told the ACT UP Oral History Project:

> Dead. A lot of people were dead. I mean, people were just dying and dying and dying. And, you had people coming in with these second generation of ACT UP tee shirts that were just wrong—that they bought—almost, like they bought it at the mall. There was shit going on here in San Francisco, with ACT UP Golden Gate and ACT UP San Francisco and there was the treatment people and the activist people and there was the inside the system people versus the outside of the system people. And I think that the energy just—people were just exhausted.

The biggest moments in ACT UP's history took place between its founding at the Center in 1987 and the arrival of combination therapy in the mid-1990s. The multiple voices and perspectives that shaped ACT UP were its strength—the organization was never monolithic—but would later contribute to its collapse. The demise of some ACT UP chapters often came down to disagreements about how to move forward after so much loss. By the mid-1990s, the surviving longtime members were just burned out after witnessing so much death.

Life in ACT UP was an endless roller coaster of funerals and protests, highs and lows, energy and exhaustion, direct action and periods of illness.

Love and vigilance. Life and death.

Some ACT UP chapters remain active today. Still largely led by HIV+ people and people with a lived proximity to the crisis, these groups remain focused on the ongoing needs of people affected by HIV/AIDS and the connections between AIDS-related injustice and other forms of inequality and oppression in society. ACT UP New York continues to meet on a weekly basis at the Center on West Thirteenth Street in Manhattan.

The flyer from the first ACT UP demonstration in March 1987 read:

> NO MORE BUSINESS AS USUAL!
> Come to Wall Street in front of Trinity Church
> at 7 AM Tuesday March 24 for a
> MASSIVE AIDS
> DEMONSTRATION
> To demand the following

1. *Immediate release by the Federal Food & Drug Administration of drugs that might help save our lives.*
   These drugs include: Ribavirin (ICN Pharmaceuticals); Ampligen (HMR Research Co.); Glucan (Tulane University School of Medicine); DTC (Merieux); DDC (Hoffman-LaRoche);

*AS 101 (National Patent Development Corp.); MTP-PE (Ciba-Geigy); AL 721 (Praxis Pharmaceuticals).*
2. *Immediate abolishment of cruel double-blind studies wherein some get the new drugs and some don't.*
3. *Immediate release of these drugs to everyone with AIDS or ARC.*
4. *Immediate availability of these drugs at affordable prices. Curb your greed!*
5. *Immediate massive public education to stop the spread of AIDS.*
6. *Immediate policy to prohibit discrimination in AIDS treatment, insurance, employment, housing.*
7. *Immediate establishment of a coordinated, comprehensive, and compassionate national policy on AIDS.*

*President Reagan, nobody is in charge!*

**AIDS IS THE BIGGEST KILLER IN NEW YORK CITY OF YOUNG MEN AND WOMEN.**
**Tell your friends. Spread the word. Come protest together. 7 AM ... March 24 ... You must be on time!**
**AIDS IS EVERYBODY'S BUSINESS NOW.**

*The AIDS Network is an ad hoc and broad-based community of AIDS-related organizations and individuals.*

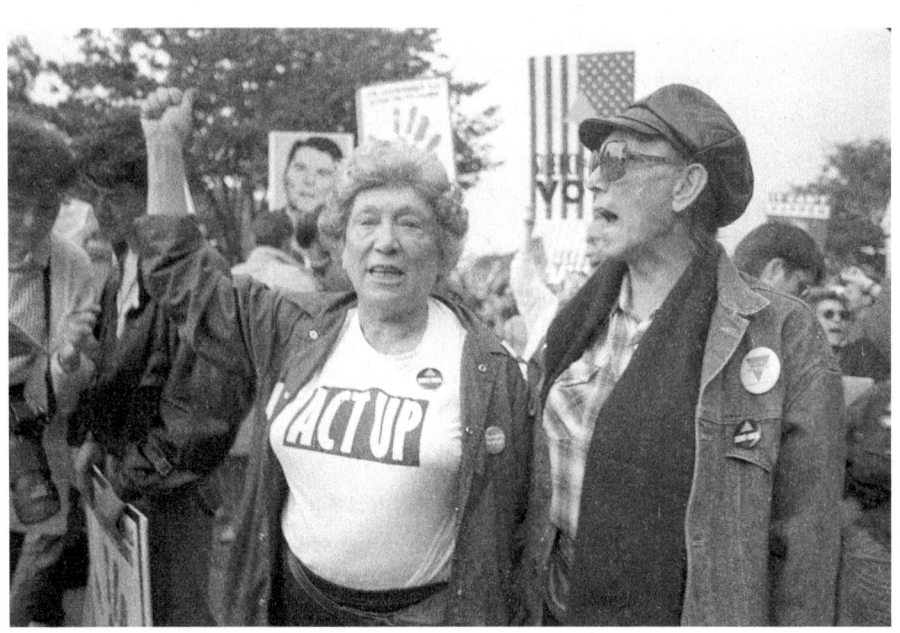

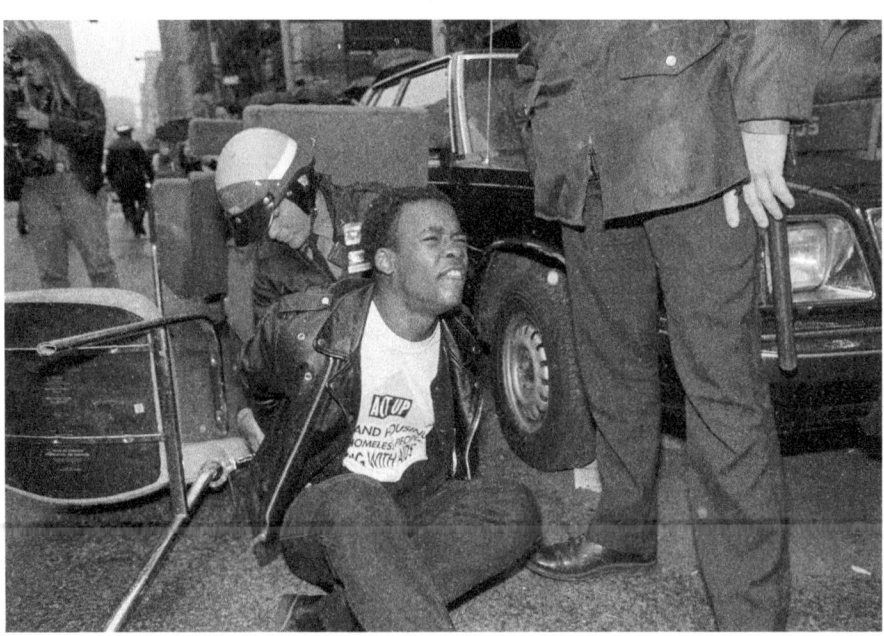

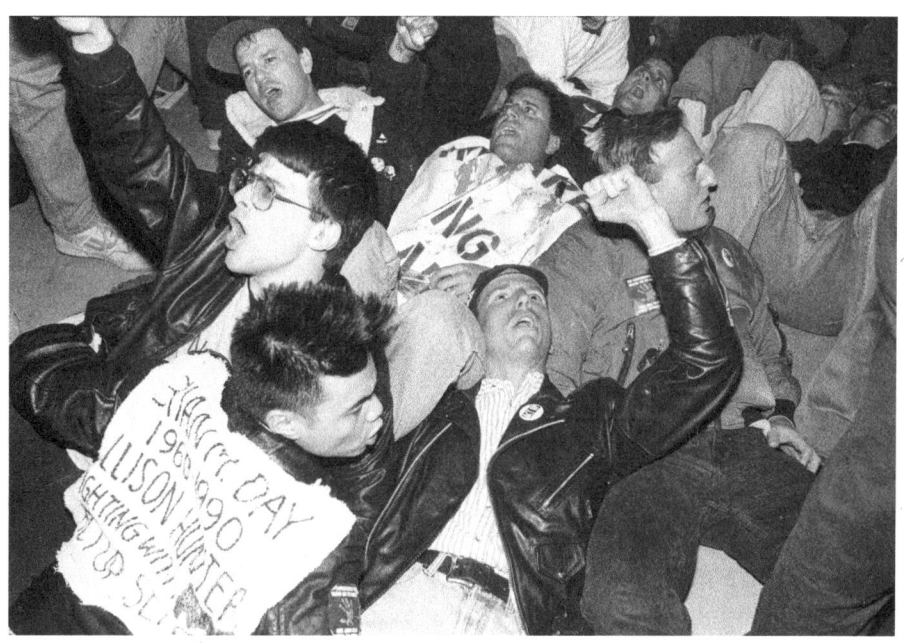

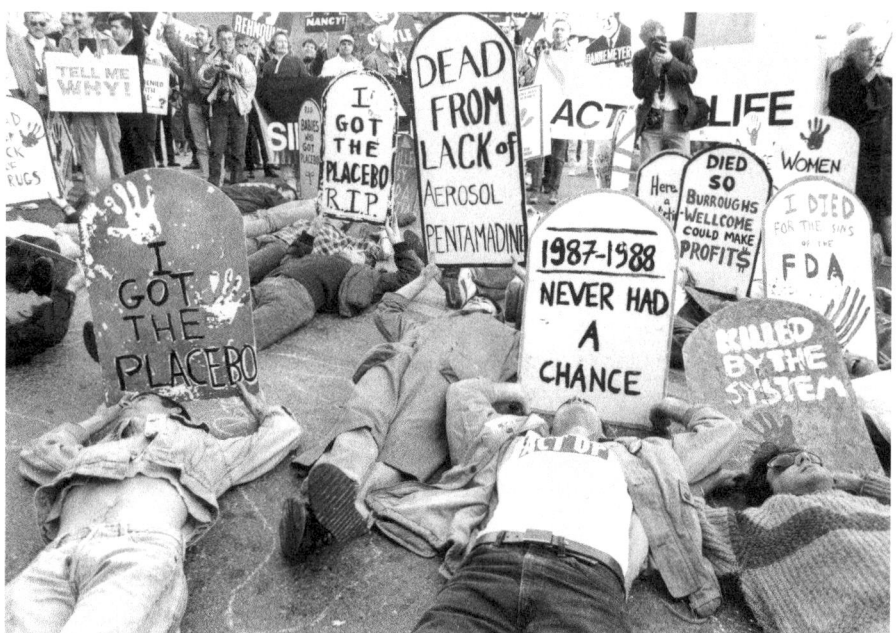

# Peggy Sue

*Some members of ACT UP were still in their teens, skipping out on the more typical touchstones of American teen life to protest. It was a lot to learn at once, to be at the height of living and at the same time be surrounded by dying. Peggy Sue is one such activist, whose own identity was forged in the fire of AIDS protest.*

Peggy Sue was still only a teenager when she went to her first ACT UP meeting in San Francisco in the autumn of 1989. She'd come up from Belmont, a small city twenty miles south of the city, to join her best friend, Jason, who'd moved up to the city after they'd finished high school. For two young queer kids from the suburbs, San Francisco held the promise of belonging.

When Peggy Sue met Jason, she'd never met a gay kid before, not in sleepy Belmont.

Sometimes, you meet someone, and your life changes.

Peggy Sue says:

> I felt like an outsider. The classic tale, right? I was fifteen and he was sixteen. My whole life, I knew I did not belong in this suburban nightmare place. I was severely bullied as a child, so by the time I was a teenager, I was just looking for my people.
>
> I met him through our mutual friend, Tammy, who was very cool. She was the first person I knew who had a car. She knew Jason from somewhere and introduced me to him. We bonded immediately. He was the first beautiful person I liked who liked me back. And that meant a lot to me.

He was shiny and the golden boy. His mother had kicked him out. I did not care why, although it ended up that he'd been caught dealing drugs to local kids. My mom was very permissive, so I was like, "Jason, come move in with us!" So he did. He lived in my house with me and my mom and my sister for a couple of years. Looking back, I gave him roots and he gave me polish and shine.

We had our own language. And it was that deep need I felt to belong, at a time in my life that I reflect upon now as a deep sense of weightlessness, a longing to fit someplace. It was painful to be so solitary and so alone in my white-bread, middle-class upbringing, longing for something I couldn't even name. I knew I didn't belong in the suburbs. I knew one day I would make it to the big city. And here came Jason: the shining blond, my knight in platinum armor.

We did everything together. I represented stability for him. My mom saw him as her son. With the innocence and desperation of two teenagers in the middle of the suburbs, we just clicked.

Twenty miles up the road in San Francisco, there were new cases of AIDS every day, but down in suburban Belmont, it was another world. These worlds collided when Peggy Sue and Jason met Darlene.

When we were sixteen, Jason and I performed in a local production of *The Rocky Horror Show* in Belmont. I played Magenta. Jason played Rocky, of course. And there was this beautiful, legendary trans woman named Darlene, who was performing in a neighboring production in Berkeley. Darlene played the lips that sing "Science Fiction/Double Feature" at the start of the show.

Darlene died in 1987. We all went to the funeral, me and twenty other people from my local band of misfits. Her family had dressed her in her coffin in male clothes and deadnamed her. She'd died from HIV. That was maybe two years before I found my home with the ACT UP movement and my people, two years before I came out as a lesbian. Until that moment, I hadn't really understood the

> stigma. I was in my own privileged little world, but staring at Darlene in the coffin, I really began to understand the ramifications of HIV and transphobia.
>
> Because I did not know that person in that coffin at all. I did not understand the name she'd been given. That was just Darlene to me.
>
> That was my first time as a human being who understood a little bit about the rest of the world as opposed to being a child. It was absolutely shameful to me that these people who purported to be her family did what they did. It was disgusting. We all knew it was disgusting.
>
> That was my first taste of it. Like, *What the fuck is going on here?*

Peggy Sue's political awakening at Darlene's funeral would shape her for years to come. High school ended, and college was the ticket to leaving Belmont behind her. Peggy Sue enrolled at a college in Santa Cruz at the age of seventeen. Before long, she knew she wanted to join Jason in the city. She struggled to adapt to college and didn't like being told what to do. After the Loma Prieta earthquake hit in October 1989, with Santa Cruz at its epicenter, Peggy Sue made her move. She was nineteen years old.

> My parents weren't pleased. By then, they'd already learned not to try and control anything I did, but they still tried to talk me out of it. I was like, "Nice try. I'm done. Bye."
>
> Jason had moved up to the city already and discovered ACT UP. I was like, "I've got to join that motherfucker! College is terrible, I hate it! Let's go!"
>
> So I quit and went to join him.
>
> After that, we were glued at the hip. I rented a room on Henry Street for six months, and eventually moved in with Jason and one of his gazillion boyfriends. We used to play pinball together, go to ACT UP meetings together. We got arrested together at demonstrations. There wasn't one without the other really. One happy image I have of the pair of us is laughing until we almost cried. We were

walking up Castro Street past Eighteenth to Nineteenth and up to Twentieth Street, and I had this stupid little joke book—you know, a booklet with fifteen pages of really stupid jokes. I just remember we were convulsing with laughter reading it out loud together. So dumb.

When I remember Jason, I remember laughter.

ACT UP San Francisco met once a week at the Women's Building on Eighteenth Street. Peggy Sue and Jason became part of the community of regular attendees—activists and organizers from across the city who were desperate to create noise about AIDS.

ACT UP was just the perfect vehicle for me to plug into. It was like this ready-made family. I knew when I first saw them. With my crazy nineteen-year-old brain, I asked no questions about the normality of my life choices at this time. It was just like, "Oh, of course I quit college and moved to the city and joined a bunch of political queers and hold a wheat pasting assembly line in my living room to fight AIDS." (We used wheat paste to stick up flyers raising awareness of AIDS around the city.) That just became a normal day for me.

Today, I have wonderful children in my life. It amazes me how quickly they learn new information and understand what to do. It was like that when I joined ACT UP. There was nothing more natural in the world to me than taking myself and my deeply disaffected feelings of otherness and fury to this wide-open field of brilliant, angry, queer badasses. Everyone at ACT UP was just like, "Oh yeah, come in, come in!"

I didn't question shit because I'd just come out of college; I was still not even really a fully formed adult and now I meet this movement which embraces me wholeheartedly. Nobody ever spoke down to me. It didn't even occur to me until like ten or fifteen years ago that Jason and I were so much younger than everybody else, because we were treated like comrades immediately.

So I went from the learning environment of college to this fully formed unit of people who loved each other and took care of each other and sometimes died together. I got to wear black leather, be a badass, yell at people, go up against the cops, and learn how to be a public speaker and how to write a press release and how to talk on camera and how to try and save people who mattered. ACT UP was where my adulthood really started, this world of death, glamour, gallows humor—and the most ecstatic joy I had ever seen. It was my coming out. It was my introduction to "sticking it to the man." It was rebellion. It was fury. My sexual identity—my orientation—my social stratosphere—my political understanding—all of it emerged at once.

Peggy Sue got an entry-level job at a bank to pay the rent while simultaneously maximizing the time she could spend helping with ACT UP, sticking up posters and taking part in demonstrations to agitate for people affected by AIDS. In whatever free time she had after all that, she'd go drinking and dancing with Jason, sneaking into the bars because they were both still under the legal drinking age.

San Francisco at the time was extremely affordable and the hub of all queer everything, at least in my little baby eyes.

An average week went like this: Wake up on Tuesday, go to my stupid job, answer the stupid phones. Have lunch with my hot girlfriend, who of course dumped me six months into the relationship because I didn't know what the fuck I was doing. Get off work at seven o'clock, go home, grab a piece of pizza, go to a direct action group, an affinity group meeting at my house or at someone else's house, stick up flyers until two in the morning about the next action, go to sleep, do the same thing on Wednesday. On Thursday, right after work, I'd go to the ACT UP meeting at the Women's Building with the other hundred miscreants. Afterwards, we'd go dancing at Chaos, the local ACT UP nightclub round the corner. Wash, rinse, repeat on Friday and Saturday. Then, on Sunday and Monday, I'd catch up on sleep; we'd figure out the next action we were going to do, and I'd Roplex posters every night.

I really believed that this routine was going to be the rest of my life. Because I had nothing to compare it to. Have a shit job, do ACT UP stuff, sometimes have a girlfriend, Roplex assembly-line parties in my house every night. Meetings. That was it. I thought that was going to be my whole life. Because not only were we young, but we didn't know what was going to happen the next day. None of us thought we were going to see thirty, much less get married.

We all thought we were going to die. Some of us did.

Peggy Sue and Jason became ubiquitous as some of the youngest members of ACT UP San Francisco. They were often at the front of the protests, calling out for justice, leading chants, doing whatever it took to get attention to AIDS.

Jason and I were foot soldiers for ACT UP. We were together in practically everything. We were always at the weekly meeting at the Women's Building. Between fifty to a hundred people would gather in a large room. ACT UP was ruled by consensus, which meant it could be difficult to reach any kind of meaningful decision unless everybody agreed. At every meeting, there was always lots of planning, lots of talking, lots of ranting—a lot of disparate opinions and a lot of people wanted their say. They got it. I don't think there were ever any snacks or refreshments at all, even though each meeting would last three or four hours. Sometimes I can't believe I did that every week! But it gave me purpose. I loved being at the meetings with my people. There were no polite edits. If someone had died, we said their names. Nobody held anything back. That's what kept us motivated, kept us going: the truth of it all. The losses continuously informed the fight. And when there were no more losses, there was no more fight.

Peggy Sue was often involved with affinity groups—subcommittees of ACT UP formed to address certain issues or carry out certain actions.

> I have been a fighter for the underdog since I was a small child. Fairness and equity has mattered to me my entire fucking life. And I could not handle the way politics were shaking out. I needed a place to vent my rage. I was well-known for screaming at large political demonstrations because I was loud. Very loud.
>
> Affinity groups were small, self-contained pods of people—maybe six, ten at the most—choosing to create and enact a direct action during a demonstration. A group of us would make a plan prior to a demo: what kind of civil disobedience or lawbreaking we were going to engage in. And then we'd enact our plan. So it was just a small group of people not acting officially in the name of ACT UP, although the media and the police never made that distinction.
>
> Nonviolent protest was central to ACT UP. You'd go limp every time you got arrested. We were inspired by the civil rights movement and the women's movement and the labor movement—all the movements that came before us which engaged in nonviolent civil disobedience. We encountered lots of violence at the hands of the authorities. But we also were not stupid enough to hit a cop—ever. Of course, the police said we did, but I never did. I wanted to sometimes! But I didn't. Because I like my teeth and my face.
>
> Sometimes we got arrested for civil disobedience. We knew this was a risk, so we knew we had to have lawyers. We had a lot of community-based attorneys and community-based AIDS service providers who supported us. A lot of large firms did pro bono work for us. When any of us got convicted and ordered to do community service, the deal would be that the AIDS service organization appreciated what we were doing, so they'd just sign off and say we'd done our five hundred hours.

Peggy Sue's willingness to put herself in dangerous positions, to risk arrest by taking part in direct action, was because being part of ACT UP meant being constantly confronted by the reality of AIDS-related death. Understanding Peggy Sue's experience in ACT UP means reconciling the joy that adrenaline could bring—the excitement of belonging to a community of outsiders who wanted to change the world, the importance of pleasure and happiness—with the trauma of this period.

> The joy and the death, the hurt and the pain are inextricably linked. I can't talk about one without the other because the death informed the joy. The cloud of imminent death never dissipated. Ever. Knowing that people were going to die informed how hard we had to live, how deeply we pursued joy. It was this cloud that almost required me to seek out the highs because we all knew the lows were going to be really fucking low. They're forever linked in my mind.
>
> I was at the deathbed of one ACT UP member. His name was Peter. He got really sick and was in a hospice. Jason and I went to go see him. We'd taken him out to the beach a couple of times to bring him some joy, but then one day, we were in the room with him at the hospice and he was having trouble breathing.
>
> He just died. Stopped breathing. It was real clear to me that his spirit was gone from his body, because that dude lying there wasn't Peter.
>
> He was maybe twenty-eight. Maybe twenty-five.
>
> The worst part is that it wasn't surprising at all. The numbness was almost instantaneous. As soon as I got started in ACT UP, it was like, "Okay, people are definitely going to die." My job was to endure it.
>
> My old-school gay male friends from that time who are still around have story after story after story like Peter. It's not the grief Olympics—nobody wins a medal for having more friends who are dead. I didn't lose any lovers. But eventually I did lose my best friend. And an ex-girlfriend. Because it wasn't just AIDS that killed people living with HIV, it was substance abuse too. HIV drove them to substance abuse, and sometimes that killed them.
>
> It was deeply damaging to everyone I knew, myself included, to

witness the absolute fragility of life alongside the intentional lack of action from the majority of the populace in response to our dying. Like, not only did people I love die, but the general populace seemed kind of glad they were dying.

This pall of death and disease was inescapable, and nobody knew how or why somebody would die or not die. It was like this giant fucking pinwheel of death!

Peggy Sue and Jason got tested for HIV regularly—you could say it was part of their politics as activists to take their status seriously.

In the early 1990s, Jason's test came back positive.

Jason found out he was HIV+ when he was twenty or twenty-one years old. It wasn't a surprise for either of us. After the news, we just kept soldiering on like it just was a blip and we had to keep doing what we needed to do.

It's hard to explain, but his HIV status somehow felt negligible to us, because it seemed like everyone was HIV+ by then. It didn't change how I thought of him. And, of course, Jason had a not particularly unique ability to ignore things he didn't like and didn't want to deal with. I assume he told me because he had to and then he just went on with his life. I think he figured he would get it anyway. And why worry about it? There were a lot of fatalists in our circle. Not seeking death and not celebrating death by any stretch. But also not being surprised by it. HIV was everywhere.

As Peggy Sue saw the effects of HIV and AIDS on her inner circle, her commitment to making noise about AIDS-related injustice only got stronger.

Peggy Sue was one of the "Sansome Seven"—a group of activists who were arrested at an ACT UP action during the Sixth International Conference on AIDS, which took place in San Francisco in June 1990. ACT UP San Francisco organized actions to coincide with the conference—not disrupting the proceedings of the conference itself. Each of these actions focused on a different AIDS-related issue, including calling attention to the invisibility of women in medical approaches to AIDS, which remained framed through male experiences. On June 19, Peggy Sue was gathered with six other activists at the Immigration and Naturalization Service (INS) on Sansome Street for that day's action. Their target: to alert people to the fact that HIV+ foreigners were banned from entering the country.

In 1987, the INS had added HIV to the federal list of "contagious and loathsome diseases"—essentially forbidding HIV+ people to enter the country. This law was deemed immoral by many activists, who argued that the restriction undermined the credibility of the United States as the host of an international AIDS conference. In 1989, an HIV+ man named Hans Paul Verhoef was stopped and detained after the INS found AZT in his luggage. Verhoef had traveled to America to represent the Dutch HIV Foundation at the National AIDS Forum in San Francisco. His detention caused an uproar in the international AIDS community. Activists like Peggy Sue and Jason argued: How can you hold an international conference on AIDS in a country that forbids entry to foreigners living with HIV?

The INS responded to public outcry by providing only a temporary waiver of the ban, solely for the conference.

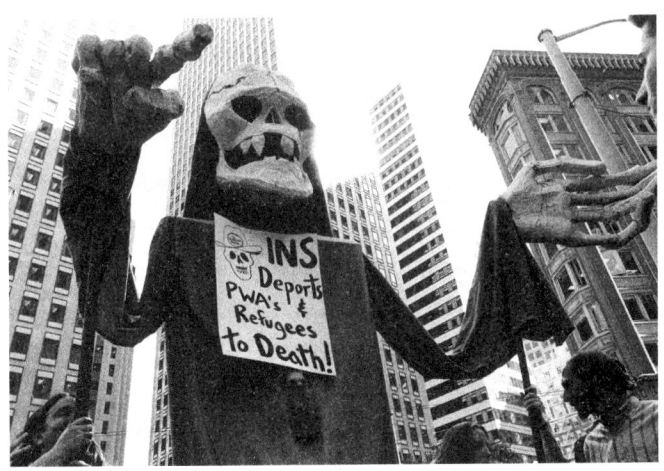

> The ... protest was replete with drums beating a marching cadence and activists from ACT UP chapters all over the country walking behind two huge American flags sewn together, backwards and upside down, with "Smash Nationalism" scrawled across the stripes. A police spokesman called the protest "noisy and raucous."
>
> —*Bay Area Reporter,* June 21, 1990

Peggy Sue remembers:

We had an international stage: thousands of people came to San Francisco. The conference was happening during Pride Week. . . . I don't know who thought that was a good idea but it was extremely convenient.

That week is set in my memory. There were San Francisco police officers directly at the barricade and then federal police who have no accountability process—and much larger clubs, by the way—in front of the building. So there were two sets of police.

The seven of us planned to push past the San Francisco Police Department and get into the building, the Federal Building. We jumped the barricade, but instead of doing anything, the SFPD were basically like, "Go ahead!" Later on, we realized they must have known that the federal police with their giant clubs were waiting.

They grabbed me and knocked the crap out of me.

The seven of us got arrested and charged in federal court. Two of us were convicted of "interfering with the duties of federal offices" and the rest of us were acquitted. A big reason for the acquittal is because it was all on video. That video was played during the trial: the seven of us rushing the police and then I disappear into this giant pile of cops, who were hitting us so hard with their clubs, aggressively raining down blows. I was acquitted because the video proved I didn't really do anything and mostly the cops just beat the shit out of me.

The furor around the Sansome Seven drew greater attention to the punitive treatment of HIV+ travelers. But the ban on HIV+ visitors wasn't formally lifted until 2010, despite attempts to repeal it over many years. Peggy Sue's acquittal in federal court offered her a sense of vindication, galvanizing her to continue to protest for the lives of HIV+ people, refusing to shut up and simmer down like the police department wanted.

> We were like annoying little gnats. We never went away. We were constantly drawing attention to AIDS and, say, the fact that women died five times faster than men because of the fact they didn't let women into clinical trials because we had menstrual cycles.
> We plugged away. Over and over.

As this was going on, Peggy Sue continued to feel empowered to explore her sexuality. Pleasure—friendship, camaraderie, and sexuality—was a powerful antidote to a world filled with the noise of AIDS-related death and injustice.

> I'd slept with boys in high school and I always found it kind of gross. I guess I just didn't understand that there was any other option. When I got to the city in 1989, I dated androgynous or feminine lesbians. But that wasn't right either. I was like, "Well, this is also boring. I guess I'll just never be truly happy."
> But then I went to an ACT UP demonstration in Chicago at the end of 1990—or maybe the beginning of 1991. Me and four out-of-their-minds gay men drove all the way from San Francisco to Chicago. Thirty-two hours nonstop in a van. Why we drove, I don't know. When we got there, it was dawn. The sun was just coming up. I remember seeing it rise above some Chicago fountain. And there she was, silhouetted by the rising sun—this super butch, crew-cut tall-drink-of-water dyke in Doc Martens. I was like. "Oh! Oh!" We went to the protest together.
> At the demonstration, the police chased us. I thought San Francisco police were bad? Holy fucking shit! The police in San Francisco at least knew a little bit about gay people and had established

> procedures to deal with large demonstrations, but the police in Chicago had no organization. They just ran around hitting us! There was no line. There was no riot gear. They were just chasing us.
>
> We hid together in a bathroom in a restaurant and ended up making out. I went home with her for the weekend. And suddenly, I was like, "I'm a dyke, I'm a femme, I love butches!" I realized, *Okay, now I'm really gay, now I understand what I want—perfect.* And my love affair with butch women has never faltered, not once, since that day. All because of a chance meeting in Chicago for no other reason than I was in ACT UP San Francisco and she was in ACT UP Chicago.

The good memories sit alongside the bad. As ACT UP lost momentum in the mid-1990s with the arrival of treatment, many activists and HIV+ people found themselves unmoored. Post-traumatic stress disorder (PTSD) has become a familiar term to describe the problems of people who survive terrible experiences when those experiences are finally over. It's not an exaggeration to say that many of the people on the front line of the worst years of AIDS in America were suffering—are still suffering—from PTSD. People with PTSD are more likely to face difficulties with anxiety and depression as their life enters a new phase after the trauma and they work to live beyond it.

If you've spent your youth on the front line, your friends dying around you as you endure extreme prejudice, what do you do when the war is over?

Here, Peggy Sue's story separated from Jason's.

> Jason had a drug and alcohol problem, as many of us did. Jason had got married to his boyfriend in a friend's backyard. It was beautiful and perfect, but I don't think it lasted that long, because the drugs got in the way. This was the early 1990s: it wasn't an official or legal marriage. But they exchanged rings and everything. In 1996, he'd been sober for a while, thanks to 12-step programs. But then he went off the wagon and broke into his now-ex-husband's house to steal stuff to sell so he could buy more drugs.

Around this time, my ex-girlfriend killed herself. She was HIV+. She died right around the last time I spoke with Jason directly. He was about to go to jail for stealing a bunch of shit—I assume the theft was to support his drug habit. In that final conversation, I knew I couldn't talk to him anymore. I loved him. I will always love him. But at that point, it was no longer safe to do anything but love him from a distance. So I did. At a very long distance. Because addiction robbed him of everything, including his life. And I certainly couldn't save him.

It broke my heart. It still breaks my heart. To not see so many of these people become adults. To not get to watch them grow old is really painful. The waste and the loss. The privilege of watching people age. You take it for granted until an epidemic wipes out a bunch of your friends when they're twenty years old.

In that last conversation I had with him, Jason was high and he was stupid. He lasted eight more years. Maybe ten. It's fuzzy because it's so painful. At the end, he was on the streets, living in filth. He died at his mother's house near Sacramento. His ex-husband cleared out his single room in some dumpy hotel in San Francisco—he'd been back in the city for that whole time and I hadn't known.

It took me a long time to let go of the idea that I should have saved him. HIV killed him—HIV and poor life choices from addiction. I intertwine HIV and addiction as killers because they're reflective of each other. They both killed him.

I dream about him a lot. I owe most of who I am to him, I think.

Because if I hadn't known him, my life would have been a 100% different trajectory, no question. I would have probably been one of those old ladies who came out when she was forty which . . . God help me, no thank you.

Peggy Sue is now far older than she ever thought she'd get to be, back when she was a teenager. She remains in the Bay Area and remains active in many causes, still in touch with many of the other surviving ACT UP members from that time.

Even decades later, her years on the front line reverberate.

> One day it was just over. Cocktails in, boom! People stopped dying and everybody went on with their lives. But collective trauma is collective trauma, right?
>
> We were all collectively traumatized together. Watching people die.
>
> I think it stained my soul somewhere.
>
> It wasn't just the trauma that people were dying. It was the fact that people in the prime of their fucking lives were kicking the bucket for no goddamn reason that anybody could discern. It was constantly devastating.
>
> To watch people over and over get cut down ... *inhumane* doesn't even begin to cover it.

## "Stop the Church"

I'M JESUS CHRIST. I'M PRO-CHOICE. I SUPPORT A WOMAN'S RIGHT TO CHOOSE. AND I AM ABSOLUTELY IN FAVOR OF CONDOM USE. I THINK THAT ALL LESBIAN AND GAY CATHOLIC TEENAGERS SHOULD BE TAUGHT ABOUT HOW TO HAVE MORE AND HEALTHIER SAFE SEX.
—Ray Navarro, dressed as Jesus Christ

The tenth of December 1989. It's Christmas on Fifth Avenue. The windows of department stores are lit up with festive scenes. Christmas carols blast out from Saks Fifth Avenue: invitations to spend money, be happy, max out your credit card on expensive toys and gadgets.

Nearby, people are gathering around St. Patrick's Cathedral for the start of Sunday Mass. A handful of people turns into hundreds of people. Then thousands. It's cold—so cold you can see your breath. The people outside the cathedral are shouting now. Their voices call out against the din of the city, rising above the tinny carols and grinding traffic:

*Teach Safe Sex! "Just say no" is not enough!*
*Act up! Fight back! Fight AIDS!*
*Our bodies! Our Lives! Our right to decide!*
*O'Connor loves gay people . . . if they're dying of AIDS!*

They're protesting about Cardinal John O'Connor's stance on HIV/AIDS and abortion rights. Inside the cathedral, O'Connor continues leading Mass. O'Connor has been the archbishop of New York since 1984—a spiritual leader of the city's Roman Catholic population. In 1987, O'Connor was appointed by President Reagan to join the Presidential

Commission on the HIV Epidemic—and rather than advocate for safer sex and effective treatment for people with AIDS, O'Connor has used his position to argue against the distribution of condoms and has maintained that gay sexual activity is a sin in the eyes of God. The numbers of cases of HIV and AIDS-related deaths have soared in the city throughout the late 1980s, but O'Connor refuses to tell his congregation how to protect themselves because it contradicts the doctrine of the Catholic Church. Protestors argue that his condemnation of condoms is tantamount to complicity in the deaths of people for whom transmission could have been prevented.

O'Connor won't even advocate for condom use between gay men, even though sex between men doesn't have anything to do with the conception of new human beings. Were the cardinal of New York to say he thinks it's okay for gay men to use condoms, it would imply that he thinks it's okay for people to be gay. And right now, in 1989, that's unthinkable.

From his position of power, O'Connor successfully sued the city to exempt the Catholic Church from laws meant to prevent discrimination against lesbian and gay people, and he lobbied hard against other antidiscrimination civil rights laws. He has also banished the gay Catholic group Dignity from holding meetings in the cathedral and been outspoken in his loathing of homosexuality, even while the church has supported the care of people with AIDS in its hospitals.

A poster advertising the protest.

The use of prophylactics is immoral in a pluralistic society or any other society.

—Cardinal O'Connor

Sometimes I believe the greatest damage done to persons with AIDS is done by the dishonesty of those health-care professionals who refuse to confront the moral dimensions of sexual aberrations or drug abuse.

—Cardinal O'Connor

Don't blame the Church if people get a disease because they violate Church teaching.

—Cardinal O'Connor

I'm not going to argue that too many condoms are defective, or improperly used, or induce a false sense of security, so that kids end up with AIDS or a venereal disease or get pregnant. Those arguments are absolutely true, but there's a much more critical argument about pushing condoms on kids: It's wrong! It's corrupting thousands of kids. It's telling them they have no personal moral responsibility for their actions. It's telling them that the only real sinners are those who deny them condoms. It says: "It's not your fault if you get AIDS or give someone else AIDS. It's the fault of those who try to push moral values down your throats—those killers—those Catholic priests and bishops, those Protestants and Jews and Muslims who believe in Divine Law and personal responsibility."

—Cardinal O'Connor

Outside St. Patrick's Cathedral, the protestors chant and shout. The police jostle them, constraining the crowd within the security barriers to avoid disrupting the flow of traffic and Christmas shoppers, and to keep them separate from the worshippers arriving at the cathedral. One protestor, wearing a leather jacket adorned with balloons, twirls and calls themselves a guardian angel of safer sex. Another wears a cardinal hat to mock O'Connor.

One man, Ray Navarro, is dressed up as Jesus Christ, a crown of thorns atop his head. A protestor records him—this pretend Christ, right here on Fifth Avenue—and he declares that God is pro-choice and supports the use of condoms. He says he wants gay and lesbian Catholic teenagers to have access to education about safe sex so that they can have lots of sex. This strange Jesus Christ makes camp jokes about his sex life with the disciples and suggests that he's on his way to Canada after the protest is over to smuggle new AIDS drugs to distribute among those in need. Navarro's performance is deliberately provocative and iconoclastic—a subversive attempt to challenge ideas about what the real Jesus would do if he was around in the 1980s as people living with HIV/AIDS fought for health care, freedom, and measures to prevent the further spread of HIV among American youth.

Later, Navarro removes his costume and speaks directly to the camera about the motivation behind his participation in the protest:

> We're protesting Cardinal O'Connor's refusal to advocate safe sex practices, the use of condoms, the complete ignorance of the Catholic Church with respect to HIV transmission, the issues facing people who are living with AIDS.
>
> ... I'm a residual Catholic, I'm here because I find that the church's intolerance of sexuality throughout the ages has historically placed lesbian and gay people at a complete disadvantage in terms of actually getting our existence affirmed. As a Latino person, I'm here because I think it's really important that ACT UP and WHAM communicate to the Latino population—90 percent of whom happen to be practicing Catholics or semipracticing Catholics. We need to communicate to people that we aren't anti-Catholic, we aren't antireligion. We're against a political bureaucracy which is known as the Catholic Church.

... As an HIV+ person, I could have gotten HIV into my system when I was a teenager. It could have been my first or second sexual experience. And if I had had safe sex taught to me—sure, I knew about contraception but I didn't know about protecting myself against diseases. And if that had been something that was taught to me when I was fifteen, then I might not be in the position I'm in now, which is ... my health could be better!

... Every time that a Catholic priest stands up there and tells people not to use condoms and abstinence is the only solution, not only are they enforcing hypocrisy, but they're encouraging homophobia, and that's why I'm here today.

Navarro is an artist who moved to New York in 1988 from California and joined ACT UP. The protest against O'Connor has been organized by ACT UP and Women's Health Action and Mobilization (WHAM!), a group campaigning against the Catholic Church's stance on pro-choice issues.

Navarro is twenty-five years old when he's dressed as Jesus Christ outside St. Patrick's Cathedral in one of the biggest Christmas shopping areas in the country. Underneath his white robe, he's wearing a thick puffer jacket and heavy-duty gloves to survive the chilly December day. In the following months, Navarro will lose his hearing and vision as an effect of AIDS-related illness. He will die eleven months later, in November 1990, at the age of twenty-six.

Navarro's trajectory isn't unusual for members of ACT UP. People in ACT UP don't have a lot to lose, and in a way, that makes them powerful. Many members of the organization are living with HIV. Many have already lost loved ones to AIDS. And many members of the New York chapter—like Navarro—will not outlive the main life span of the organization, which will only be active from 1987 until the mid-1990s. The presence of death is terrifying, but it is also an incredible motivation to make change happen. Members of ACT UP behave like superheroes— they take drastic, difficult, sometimes ridiculous actions. As ACT UP member Emily Nahmanson put it: "After all, what's the worst that can happen? Well, the worst that can happen is you die. Well, guess what? People were going to die anyway."

Nahmanson was only seventeen years old when she joined ACT UP as an undergraduate student at New York University. She came out as a lesbian shortly after arriving in the city, and she found herself taking part in ACT UP meetings and demonstrations after befriending some members at the NYU Lesbian Rap Group. After the Rap Group met, she would go for beers and popcorn at a nearby college bar, and people would talk politics. "Stop the Church" is Nahmanson's first ACT UP demo. She is part of Operation Ridiculous—a group intended to parody Operation Rescue, an antiabortion group connected to the church.

> We dressed up in clown makeup, specifically to go and get in the face of the Operation Rescue people, who were at the "Stop the Church" demonstration. So, all these crazy antiabortion fanatics. So, we dress up in clown makeup, and we're Operation Ridiculous. This is actually another brilliant, brilliant genius move on our part. So, we're on Fifth Avenue, there's thousands of people there. It's the most fabulous, insane energy to happen, I think, in the AIDS activist movement. We had worked so hard to get there. It was just going off incredibly well. My sister and all her friends came down from Barnard to march in the street with her picket signs. . . . So, we went onto the side street, and we took a cab down the block, and had the cab go through and come down Fifth Avenue. And here we are—five or six people in clown makeup, busting out of a cab. And once they saw us come out of that cab, we were gone. We were gone. We were arrested so fast. And here I am, standing in the back of a paddy wagon with all these people with all this clown makeup on.

Several protestors attempt to burst into the cathedral to disrupt the Mass, but the police prevent them from entering. Earlier on, however, another group of protestors successfully infiltrated the service by pretending to be worshippers.

As O'Connor begins his homily, these protestors come out from the pews and stage a "die-in"—dozens of them dropping to the floor in the cathedral as though they are already dead. Once they hit the ground, they lie silent, refusing to move. Meanwhile, other protestors begin screaming from the pews: "You're murdering us!" and "Stop it! Stop it!"

Die-ins are a frequent tactic of ACT UP, modeled after other civil rights protests. By going limp as though dead, the protestors are able to nonviolently resist arrest while also forcing onlookers to recognize the fact that every day more and more people are dying without sufficient attention or care. At "Stop the Church," the die-in is dedicated to the memory of the 100,000 people who have died by this point. Obituaries often use euphemisms, because there is so much stigma attached to dying because of AIDS, and many of the people dying are already marginalized because of their sexuality, skin color, nationality, and socioeconomic status.

Even as body after body falls to the ground, O'Connor continues. "We must never respond to hatred with hatred," he tells the congregation. He ignores the fallen and ignores the cries of the living . . . a pretty apt symbol of his approach to stopping AIDS.

Michael Petrelis hadn't intended to go to the demonstration that day. By the late 1980s, he'd had plenty of experience of activism. In the late 1970s, he was a teenager living in San Francisco, connected to gay rights activism; he attended the vigil for Harvey Milk when he was assassinated in 1978. By the early 1980s, he was twenty-one and back in New York. He started to see his friends die before the illness was even known as GRID, let alone AIDS. In 1985, Petrelis was diagnosed with Kaposi's sarcoma—a sure sign of HIV infection. He was told to expect to only be alive for six months to a year. By the time Petrelis joins ACT UP at the end of the decade, he is regarded as something of a loose cannon. As he said later in his ACT UP Oral History Project interview, "People felt I was too angry, too over the top and—you know, look, I guess I did set myself up as an isolated character for whatever reason." Because nobody wants Petrelis around to help with their participation at "Stop the

Church," he turns up alone and makes his way into the cathedral. When Cardinal O'Connor ignores the die-in, Petrelis decides to take a different kind of action from the tenth row.

> I started screaming, "Stop killing us." I repeated: "Stop killing us" at the top of my lungs. . . . Because the Catholic Church had a lot of influence over public policy regarding AIDS prevention and . . . was stopping the distribution of condoms.

Just like Navarro, Petrelis grew up in the Catholic Church. All too well, he remembers the intolerance he faced as a gay man in that environment. His memory of mistreatment turns into anger. And that anger finds a focus in the failure of the Catholic Church to help stop the spread of HIV/AIDS among vulnerable young Catholics. As he told the Oral History Project:

> Some people were going into the aisles and sitting down or laying down on the cold tile. And, I remember I wanted to be heard. And I didn't want to do a sit-down action. So, I stood up on the pew where I was, and started screaming.
>
> "O'Connor, you are killing us. You are killing us!" And I couldn't hear myself, because there's this cacophony of competing voices from the parishioners saying the prayer—I don't remember which prayer it was—ACT UP demonstrators trying to read their state—reading their statements, trying to be heard. I do remember hearing noises of the boots of the cops on the tiles, you know? Which I thought was kind of surprising because there was so much of this noise. And, standing up and screaming, "O'Connor, you're killing us! Just stop it, stop it!" And then, an usher for the church came over and asked me to sit down. I said, "No, I'm not going to sit down!" He goes away and then came back and said, "Please sit down." I got down in a little bit. Stood up again, started screaming again. This time, there was a policeman who came over to me and said, "You're

going to have to sit down." I said, okay. Sat down, and got up a minute or so later, doing it again. And I guess it was at that point, I went into this thing of well, it's a Fellini movie. Listen, I'm half Italian, so I felt like this was fine. This was more than fine for all of the surreal aspects of this. And I eventually was pulled down from standing up on the pews screaming, by two cops. They got me into the aisle. They put the handcuffs on me, and they're leading me out, and as they're leading me out, this fellow says, "Well, who are you?" and everything. And I said, "Why do you want to know?" It turned out to be a reporter from the *Times*. And he quotes me the next day and everything.

Tom Keane is another ACT UP member present at the cathedral. He and his friend decide not to attend the service wearing their ACT UP T-shirts. They dress down, pretending to be a pair of Italian tourists. As the die-in happens around them and the screaming starts, the cathedral organist plays music to try to block out the noise of the protestors.

Keeping calm, Keane makes his way to take Communion.

I put my hands out, and suddenly I have the Communion wafer in my hands, and the priest says, "This is the body of Christ," and I say, "Opposing safe-sex education is murder." Then I sort of—I didn't really know what to do, and I think in some sense, some part of me was sort of saying, "Well, fine. You guys think you can tell us that you reject us, that we don't belong, so I'm going to reject you." So I took it and I crushed it and dropped it.

During Communion, the wafer represents the body of Jesus Christ. Worshippers are passed the wafer by a priest, and through this exchange, they believe they are consuming the body of Jesus. It's one of the holiest things you can do as a Catholic. Crushing the wafer is perceived as a sacrilegious act.

A total of 111 protestors are arrested, 43 from inside the cathedral.

Those who have fallen dead to the floor remain dead as they are carried out on stretchers. Congregants are aghast. Outside, more protestors cheer.

The actions of Petrelis and Keane and others were provocative and extreme, and that changed everything. The protest became mired in controversy and turned into a mainstream talking point—how could these crazy protestors have the audacity to be so disrespectful? It might be better to ask why the protestors felt they had so little to lose that this kind of action was their best option. And hey, no one was hurt. No windows were smashed. No one died—except those who were dying because of AIDS.

But of course, this coverage drew more attention to the ACT UP cause than ever. The protest became major news, receiving attention across the country and around the world. But it was less a direct decision and more a consequence of what happens when activists are desperate to be heard, when more "respectful" actions just get ignored, when people have been mistreated by powerful organizations because of who they are.

Neither Keane nor Petrelis was exactly applauded for his bravery afterward. While some in ACT UP saw the protest inside the cathedral as laudable, many others were disgusted by the intrusion into a religious service, especially during Communion. Ann Northrop, an ACT UP member who took part in the protest, recalled, "Many, many gay people and straight people and all sorts of people hated this action and thought it was absolutely horrible. And, within ACT UP, it was a huge debate. There were so many people within ACT UP who never liked that demonstration and thought it was an awful thing to do."

Coverage of the protest wasn't kind—the media basically asked, *Who are these crazy people and why are they being so offensive toward one of the most important religious leaders in the country?* And it wasn't like the protest solved anything overnight. But perhaps public opinion shifted: ACT UP members were invited to speak to news reporters and gained a place at debates on television. If these members were often treated like they were crazy, it still meant that ACT UP was able to put its agenda and concerns on a bigger public stage than it had before.

Three decades later, in 2019, ACT UP member Northrop was interviewed by the website TheBody. She noted that while the action was viewed as a terrible thing at the time, ultimately it was a boon to the activists, putting ACT UP on front pages around the world. She talked to one gay man whose mother, after seeing a report of the action, called him to say, "I used to think that gay men were weak and wimpy, and after this demonstration, what I realized was that gay people are strong and angry." Reflected Northrop, "It showed the world that we were angry and that we wanted them to pay attention."

The thing is, ACT UP never officially planned to enter the cathedral, out of respect for the people who used it to worship. Even so, some members argued that protesting *inside* the cathedral, rather than outside, was a necessary provocation. By causing havoc and outrage—without resorting to violence—ACT UP drew attention to the role of the church in the accelerating number of new HIV cases and AIDS-related deaths. Internal disagreements in ACT UP about the right and wrong tactics of "Stop the Church" are also a clear example of tensions that rippled, not even under the surface of the organization. These tensions were powerful and connected to the organization's success. But they also played a role in ACT UP's starting to unravel in the early 1990s.

Most members of ACT UP were gay men and lesbians. It's easy to forget that so many of these members were Catholic—they'd grown up in Catholic communities and been rejected by their families and churches when they came out as queer. This was particularly true for Latine members, who also represented an urban demographic in the city that was increasingly hard-hit by AIDS across the 1980s. The "Stop the Church" protest is the most notorious and iconic episode in the history of ACT UP. If the protest was meant as a confrontation with the Catholic Church, it's important that this confrontation was initiated by people who *belonged* to that church. People who'd grown up in the

Catholic Church and struggled for acceptance in its spaces—as queer people, as HIV+ people.

Does the fact that the protest against the Catholic Church was initiated and accelerated by Catholic members of ACT UP make it more or less controversial?

> To many parishioners, the recent invasion . . . was an act of desecration. But to Christopher Hennelly, a former seminarian among those arrested, . . . it was a prayer for self-preservation.
>
> "The strongest prayer I've ever made in my life was on the floor of St. Patrick's," he said.
>
> —*The New York Times,* January 3, 1990

# Milo Miller

*Milo Miller is one of the founders of the Queer Zine Archive Project, an amazing online archive of zines made by LGBTQ+ folks. They live in Milwaukee, Wisconsin. As a punk involved in zine culture from the early 1990s to the present day, they remain a passionate advocate for grassroots activism and the power of queer community building today. Here they talk about the roots of their activism and a particular high school challenge they faced.*

When I was seventeen, growing up in Milwaukee, I was passionate about abortion rights activism. I'd keep watch at reproductive health centers to protect visitors from antiabortion protestors. I met a bunch of people who were connected to ACT UP Milwaukee through doing this. It was the early 1990s. I joined ACT UP Milwaukee myself when I was a senior in high school, and it was through ACT UP that I found the power to come out as queer. ACT UP gave me a place to put my energy, and through that energy, I began to live a more authentic life. When you're able to be open with yourself, you can be more open with other people.

I remember the stigma about AIDS firsthand—"You don't want to talk to him, he's got AIDS!" When I was a teenager in the 1990s, our society still seemed to think being gay was a bad thing. I was taught that being gay meant you had AIDS, you were diseased, you were sick. That's how it felt. So if you were gay in high school in the 1990s, you might as well just be in the grave already. It was empowering to join ACT UP because there were no other openly queer young people at my high school. Queer teenagers might as well just not exist. I found other queer folks through ACT UP and gained a community of fantastic elders and mentors.

After coming out to folks in ACT UP, I came out to my family and other students at my high school. And then I got involved in calling for better sex education for the student population. I have ACT UP to thank for that.

ACT UP Milwaukee meetings happened on Wednesdays in a community room in a Catholic church. The fact it took place in a church was surprising—to think that a space which has historically been so anti-gay provided space for this group of folks to get together. The meeting would open by asking if there were any police or law enforcers there, saying very explicitly that they should not be there. It's an old wives' tale that if you ask somebody if they're a cop that they have to tell you, but we still did it anyway.

We were a diverse group of individuals coming together to combat HIV/AIDS—that was important. We weren't just gay men, and we weren't just for white folks living in large and/or coastal cities. We were working for Black folks, Latine folks, people who were working-class, people who were unhoused, people who used injectable drugs. We were for folks who at the time may have seroconverted because no one had been paying attention to the blood supply.

All of us mattered. Everyone.

With ACT UP, I went to my first Pride event. I did my first die-in. I remember being in the hallway by the school cafeteria using the pay phone to call the drug company Burroughs Wellcome to zap their phone line as part of an ACT UP action in the middle of the school day!

While I was doing all of this, I was on the student council at my school. I wanted to change the way that sex education was happening, because I knew that the teaching we were currently getting wasn't good enough. Kids weren't being taught about AIDS. They weren't being taught about how to protect themselves from HIV or other STI transmissions.

Working with other ACT UP members and with the help of the Milwaukee AIDS Project, I said, "Look, I need resources to persuade the school board that this matters. Give me educational materials. I don't know what I'm doing."

Speaking at the school board was terrifying as an awkward eighteen-year-old kid. But I believed in what I was doing. I still do. We should make it normal to talk about sexual health, about pregnancy, about menstruation, about HIV, about STIs. We should be talking about sexual pleasure and what feels good! We should be talking about loving people, about how to be open and honest.

You need to understand that what I was asking for was huge. Imagine being a student and trying to get the school to change *any* part of a curriculum. Maybe you only have one math class a week. You and your friends are like, "Hey! We need more math education!" You go to the principal and the board of governors and say, "We need to expand math class! Math is prominent in our lives but people just aren't getting it! The math you taught us when we were first-years doesn't prepare us for the math we experience as seniors!"

Taking that initiative, of course, your peers are going to have mixed reactions. Folks who are pro-math are going to have your back, but others are like, "You only want to do this because you're promoting your pro-math agenda."

You make the proposal.

You talk to the adults.

But the adults just say, "No way! We can't do that! It's going to cost too much money, and we don't believe in math education like that. Hey, maybe math should be reserved for when you're married and we shouldn't teach anyone it at all!"

That's what we were up against. But it wasn't math, it was sexual health.

We weren't asking for protractors and rulers and calculators, we were asking for free condoms, free dental dams, freely available information about HIV/AIDS.

We did a bunch of petitions of the student body before we presented our argument at the school board. We could make our case that 75 percent of the graduating class agreed that sex education was substandard.

In the early 1990s, people just weren't ready for queer high school students at all. Some folks acted like I must have AIDS because I was queer, but others appreciated the underlying message: We deserved good sex education, we deserved good health education, especially as we transitioned to young adulthood.

The response to my proposal was intense. I got death threats sent to me. People calling me a faggot, telling me that I was going to die, burn in hell.

But miraculously, the school board voted in favor of our proposal.

There was a major caveat, though: They committed to improving sexual health education in the school and to making condoms available at school, but only if you went and asked for them at the nurse's office.

It was a start, and it was a win. But it still wasn't enough.

Hilariously, I was rewarded for being such a troublemaker and for making so many folks in the community mad. At the end of the year, the school gave me a Student Spirit award! I was called up in senior assembly to receive it.

I even invited my friends from ACT UP and one of my best not-yet-out-as-queer guy friends to my senior prom! Rather than going to prom ourselves, we stood outside and handed out condoms and safer sex information to all the high school students. They were all in tuxedos, and we were in Doc Martens and rolled-up jeans and leather jackets. We looked like tough-ass queers! Afterwards, we all went dancing at one of the all-ages nights at a club called Mad Planet. So we still got to go dancing but in a much less formal and much more queer way.

That was thirty years ago. These days, I still go past my old school sometimes when I use the pool. Nowadays, there are big posters in the window which say *All students are valuable* and display the trans rights flag. That's crazy to me. It's beautiful to see the transformation. Change has to start somewhere. It certainly wasn't all done by me, but I'm proud that I played a small part in making that change happen.

Our community said: *This is important, we're going to support our students, and that means supporting students' sexual health.*

# Fighting Words: Larry Kramer vs. Anthony Fauci

Any activist faces a fundamental question when working to get the government to change: They can fight the system, calling it out from the outside, making enough noise to force it to change. Or they can work within the system, using diplomacy and personal collateral to convince other people within the system to improve it.

In the case of AIDS activism at the height of the epidemic, the stakes couldn't have been higher: People were dying, and the government that controlled the medical options was working far too slowly. If treating HIV/AIDS patients wasn't made a priority, and if funding wasn't given to finding a successful treatment (if not an outright cure), then hundreds of thousands of Americans were going to die. Activists were desperate for the government to take AIDS as seriously as possible, preventing new infections through education, speeding up access to new treatments, and forbidding pharmaceutical companies to sit on drugs as they waited to maximize profits. But how to best push the government to deliver an ethical amount of resources and push Big Pharma to get drugs into the bodies of the people who needed them?

On the scream-and-shout side was Larry Kramer, the activist who had helped found both Gay Men's Health Crisis and ACT UP. With good reason, he did not trust the government to save the lives of the dying. In fact, Kramer told as many people as possible that the government was doing the opposite, using the plague to wipe out gay men. The only way to fight this, he felt, was to fight it vocally and relentlessly. He didn't mind being an asshole. To him, being an asshole was a strategic choice to help save lives.

> I discovered that anger got you further than being nice.... I was better TV than someone who was nice....
>
> I don't consider myself an artist. I consider myself a very opinionated man who uses words as fighting tools.

On the work-within side was Dr. Anthony Fauci. In 2020, Fauci led the CDC response to COVID-19, but thirty-five years earlier, he was entrenched in the governmental response to HIV/AIDS, becoming the director of the National Institute of Allergy and Infectious Diseases (NIAID), part of the National Institutes of Health. In a later interview, he remembered the years from 1981 to 1985 in this way:

> My entire existence with my colleagues was 12 hours a day taking care of desperately ill young men, and seeing them die no matter what you did for them.... And in order to be able to accept that and continue going, you had to suppress it.

To Kramer, Fauci represented everything that was wrong about the government's response to HIV/AIDS. In May 1988, Kramer addressed Fauci in a column in *The Village Voice*.

> I have been screaming at the National Institutes of Health since I first visited your Animal House of Horrors in 1984. I called you monsters then and I called you idiots in my play, *The Normal Heart*, and now I call you murderers.
>
> You are responsible for supervising all government-funded AIDS treatment research programs. In the name of right, you make decisions that cost the lives of others. I call that murder.
>
> At hearings on April 29 before Representative Ted Weiss and his House Subcommittee on Human Resources, after almost eight years of the worst epidemic in modern history, perhaps to be the worst in all history, you were pummeled into admitting publicly what some of us have been claiming since you took over three years ago.

You admitted that you are an incompetent idiot.

Over the past four years, $374 million has been allocated for AIDS treatment research. You were in charge of spending much of that money.

It doesn't take a genius to set up a nationwide network of testing sites, commence a small number of moderately sized treatment efficacy tests on a population desperate to participate in them, import any and all interesting drugs (now numbering approximately 110) from around the world for inclusion in these tests at these sites, and swiftly get into circulation anything that *remotely* passes muster. Yet, after three years, you have established only a system of waste, chaos, and uselessness.

It doesn't take a genius to announce that you have elected to personally supervise the study of a broad range of new drugs. Yet, two years later, you are forced to admit you've barely begun.

It doesn't take a genius to request, as you did, 126 new staff persons, receive only 11, *and then keep your mouth shut about it.*

It takes an incompetent idiot.

After imploring, "YOU FUCKING SON OF A BITCH OF A DUMB IDIOT, YOU HAVE HAD $374 MILLION AND YOU EXPECT US TO BUY THIS GARBAGE BAG OF EXCUSES!" Kramer invoked the efforts of gay activism.

The gay community has been on your ass for three years. For 36 agonizing months, you refused to go public with what was happening (correction: not happening), and because you wouldn't speak up until you were asked pointedly by a congressional committee, we lie down and die and our bodies pile up higher and higher in hospitals and homes and hospices and streets and doorways.

Meanwhile, drugs we have been *begging* that you test remain untested. The list of promising untested drugs is now so endless and the pipeline so clogged with NIH and FDA bureaucratic lies that there is no Roto-Rooter service in All God's Christendom that will ever muck it out....

The gay community has, *for five years,* told the NIH which drugs to test because we know and hear first what is working on some of us somewhere. You couldn't care less about what we say. You won't answer our phone calls or letters, or listen to anyone in our stricken community. What tragic pomposity!

"THERE ARE MORE AIDS VICTIMS DEAD BECAUSE YOU DIDN'T TEST DRUGS ON THEM THAN BECAUSE YOU DID," Kramer went on to write.

ACT UP was formed over a year ago to get experimental drugs into the bodies of patients. For one year ACT UP has tried every kind of protest known to man (short of putting bombs in your toilet or flames up your institute) to get some movement in this area. One year later, ACT UP is still screaming for the same drugs they begged and implored you and your world to release. One year of screaming, protesting, crying, cajoling, lobbying, threatening, imprecating, marching, testifying, hoping, wishing, praying has brought nothing. You don't listen. No one listens. No one has ears. Or hearts.

Kramer, a Jew, likened the Reagan administration to Nazi Germany, with Fauci playing his role.

I don't know (though it wouldn't surprise me) if you kept quiet intentionally. I don't know (though it wouldn't surprise me) if you were ordered to keep quiet by Higher Ups Somewhere. You are a good lieutenant, like Adolph Eichmann.

Kramer tried to include at least one thread of hope in his despair, closing his letter:

You may (God help us all) be the best that will be given us. You may, like John Ehrlichman, once accused, seek redemption and forgiveness by rethinking, retooling, and, like Avis, trying harder. Even more miraculous, those Supreme Murderers in the White House might tomorrow acknowledge that families simply everywhere have gay sons and daughters.

But I fear these are only pipe dreams and you'll continue to carry on with your spare equipment. The cries of genocide from this Cassandra will continue to remain unheard. And my noble but enfeebled community of the weak, and dying, and the dead will continue to grow and grow—until we are diminished.

A month later, on June 26, 1988, when Fauci was being honored by a charity that was raising funds to fight HIV/AIDS, Kramer wrote an open letter to him, which was published in the *San Francisco Examiner.* It began:

Anthony Fauci, you are a murderer and should not be the guest of honor at any event that reflects on the past decade of the AIDS crisis.

The letter said Fauci was a murderer because of the deadly clinical trials the government was undertaking, "piss[ing] away billions of dollars testing dangerous compounds that DO NOTHING to improve the quality of life, to stop opportunistic infections or to extend survival for people with HIV." Kramer blasted Fauci for not focusing on boosting immune response in people with HIV and relying on a testing standard that had been invented by drug companies to maximize their profits.

Few people besides actual murderers and Nazis like to be called murderers and Nazis. It would have been all too easy for Fauci to dismiss Kramer's concerns because of the volume and vitriol of the name-calling. Within the government, Fauci felt he was fighting to get the crisis as much attention and the NIAID as many resources as possible. It would have been natural for him to be defensive or dismissive.

But Kramer had gotten his attention.

Referring to Kramer's San Francisco "open letter," Fauci said in a later interview:

> I was a little bit shocked when that article came out, because I didn't expect that. No one had ever done that to me or any other scientist. It was just unheard of. He was breaking all the ground rules, but I never really took it personally.

While Kramer was calling Fauci a murderer, Fauci started meeting with other members of ACT UP. As activist Peter Staley later wrote about meeting Fauci for the first time in 1989: "Mr. Kramer had labeled him our enemy, but I couldn't shake the feeling that as the head of our government's AIDS research efforts, Dr. Fauci had my life in his hands." Fauci was willing to eat, drink, and (most important) talk with Staley and other activists. Wrote Staley: "We couldn't help but love the guy, but his research program sucked."

Fauci attended an ACT UP meeting in October 1989 and met regularly with some of its leaders. He felt like an advocate for the activists on the inside, telling his scientific colleagues that ACT UP members should be included in discussions about drug trials. Of his colleagues, Fauci said, "I was pushing and pulling these people and screaming, 'Hey, we have to deal with them.' I was in a difficult position because I was trying to convince the establishment that ACT UP had something to offer."

The problem was, Fauci wasn't getting results. At least not fast enough for ACT UP leaders, who were still seeing people with AIDS die at horrifying rates. ACT UP decided a protest was needed.

In May 1990, over a thousand activists stormed the NIH headquarters. They set off rainbow-colored smoke bombs and sounded an air horn every twelve minutes to represent the rate at which people were dying because of HIV/AIDS in America. The activists brandished signs that read *Red Tape Kills US* and *NIH—Negligence, Incompetence and Horror* and *NIH, you can't hide, we charge you with genocide*. A mock graveyard was set up in front of Building 31, where Fauci's office was located, and one protestor hoisted an effigy of Fauci's head on a stick. Activists faced off against police in riot gear; many were arrested. They were demanding faster research, the inclusion of people living with HIV/AIDS in research committees, and more focus on women and people of color with AIDS.

After he was arrested, Peter Staley saw Fauci, who asked him if he was all right. "I'm fine," Staley replied. "Just doing my job. How about you, Tony?"

In the next day's *Washington Post*, Fauci worried that the activists' actions were "interesting theater" but "not helpful" since they would further alienate his scientific colleagues. But over time, Fauci's view changed. He later recalled:

> These guys came in with Mohawk haircuts, multiple earrings, black leather jackets, making a lot of noise. Scientists ran for the hills. They could be preaching the gospel and scientists wouldn't listen to them.
>
> But what they said made really great sense to me. . . .
>
> Fortunately I had a good friend—that was George H. W. Bush. When I explained it to him, he thought it was a good idea.
>
> I learned an important lesson: Be nice to everybody in Washington, even the low-level people, because one day they are going to be high-level people.

It's certainly possible to see a different lesson here: The ACT UP activists didn't get Fauci to listen to them by being "nice." Although their willingness to meet with him and talk with him was just as important as his willingness to meet with them and talk with them, it took a more dramatic, antagonistic statement on ACT UP's part to get results. A month after the demonstration, it was announced that activists, journalists, and people living with HIV/AIDS would be let into the AIDS Clinical Trials Group, and that the trials would include women of color, drug users, and children with AIDS.

As Fauci began to meet regularly with ACT UP members, there was one person conspicuously absent from the meetings: Larry Kramer. This was by design. (Kramer had memorably left his leadership position at Gay Men's Health Crisis because other leaders did not invite him to a meeting with New York City Mayor Ed Koch, whom Kramer loathed unsparingly.) But Kramer's and Fauci's paths ended up crossing... when Kramer was out walking his dog at night in Montreal, which was hosting an AIDS conference.

The two men met not as adversaries, but as two men walking down the street with a dog. Kramer would later call it "a historic meeting" because it led to enough trust being established for Kramer to arrange for Fauci to meet with more activists. Impressed, Fauci started to welcome activists into meetings they had been thrown out of before. As Kramer recounted:

> That was the beginning of a major turning point. Dr. Fauci has become the only true and great hero in all of this, in the government, in the system.... I acknowledge him every chance I can, because we certainly got off to a rocky start.

Fauci remembered meeting Kramer on the street in Montreal, "like two generals in a war on opposite sides coming together for a little bit of a truce.... We found out at the end of that that even though we still disagreed on how to do things, we didn't disagree on what needed to be done."

A true answer to the fight vs. work-on-the-inside question started to form: What if this was a false dichotomy? What if you need both in order to save lives? Kramer could exert hostile pressure from the outside while Fauci exerted friendly persuasion from the inside.

Kramer saw this dynamic pay off when it came to the issue of "fast-tracking." Basically, Fauci successfully changed the rules so that new drugs in clinical trails could get into the bodies of the people who desperately needed them as quickly as possible. This change allowed trials to happen even before conclusive data was in hand.

Kramer said:

> Actually it was his idea, because he sensed that because of the work that we were now proceeding with, we had enough mechanisms in place to allow certain things to go out faster. We had relationships with drug companies; we had a few treatments that needed to be tested and a lot of dying patients who were desperate to test them. What it needed was a government official to make the first move, and that's what Tony Fauci did.

There were, however, limits to the tag-team approach. Even as their friendship developed, Kramer still disagreed with how Fauci worked with his other "friend," the president.

As Fauci recounted, "During the administration of George H. W. Bush, he told me, 'Tony, you should chain yourself to the gates of the White House.' I said, 'Larry, how would that help? I can go talk to President Bush any time. He's a friend.' He said, 'You should still do it.'"

Fauci pointed out to Kramer, "If you chain yourself to the White House fence you will be a hero to Larry Kramer for an hour-and-a-half and then you will never again get into the White House."

Kramer replied, "I concede there were things he couldn't do in the early years, that he needed to get inside, but after that there's no excuse."

By both Kramer's and Fauci's accounts, a deep, long friendship formed between them. It was not without its tension—"He wants to kill me more than I want to kill him," Fauci once observed. In the 1994 edition of his book *Reports from the Holocaust: The Making of an AIDS Activist*, Kramer wrote: "Before I knew [Fauci] personally, it was in no way difficult for me to come after him like a maniacal tiger. As I came to know him over the following years (now that I'm HIV-positive, he's even one of my doctors), even though I'm just as furiously angry at him for what he does and doesn't do, it's become painful for me to call him names.... He's a nice man with a lovely wife and he works seven days a week and rarely sees his kids. I have to remind myself that my idol Hannah Arendt pointed out for us all how nice people can perform so many evil deeds."

In private, they had dinner together, and Fauci helped Kramer when he was diagnosed with liver cancer. In public, they would honor each other . . . but Kramer continued to hold Fauci to task. Because there was always more that needed to be done—once a treatment was found, Kramer felt the government stopped its efforts to find an all-out cure. He also refused to revise history; he still said Fauci had "blood on his hands" from early and continuing AIDS-related deaths. Even as they continued their friendship, Kramer would regularly trash Fauci on TV. In 1993, Kramer chastised him on C-SPAN for selling "bureaucratic bullshit" and for not speaking out as much as he could. "Tony, more than anyone in this world, knows how awful everything is, knows what has to be done and yet he can never say it in public like I can say it in public," Kramer declared.

Fauci recounted another appearance:

> All of a sudden Larry starts trashing me. He says I'm a disgrace. That I'm doing this, and that I'm doing that. And I'm saying to myself, "What's going on with Larry?" He made it look like we were mortal enemies.
>
> About 15 minutes after I got home, the phone rang. It was Larry. He said, "That was really great, wasn't it, Tony? We really did well." I said, "What do you mean we did well?" He answered, "We made our point." I said, "I know, Larry, but you called me a dirty rat in front of 10 million people on *Nightline.*"
>
> He thought that people were losing attention about the importance of HIV. He figured that a good way to get attention was to trash Tony Fauci in front of 10 million people.

In 2018, after Kramer called him "the consummate manipulative bureaucrat who speaks out of too many sides of his mouth," Fauci replied, "Although Larry can be confrontative and combative, I consider him a friend and a hero of the AIDS activist movement." This mix of combativeness—sometimes performative, sometimes genuine—and friendship continued into the 2020s, as Fauci became a national figure on TV once more in the first years of the COVID-19 pandemic and Kramer's health began to fail. Their complicated dynamic stayed intact to the very end. As Fauci recalled in a piece he wrote for *The New York Times* after Kramer's death in 2020, the last interaction they had was this:

> He said with a mischievous smile, "I still think that you should have chained yourself to the White House fence." . . . I am so pleased and grateful that the last words we had the opportunity to say to each other were, "I love you."

What did it take for the activists on the outside of the power structure to make a key player on the inside listen to them? The answer, ultimately, is empathy. That is the connector between agitation and diplomacy. As Fauci told an interviewer after Kramer's death:

> "It's hard to fine-tunedly psychoanalyze yourself. But as a person who's devoted their lives to taking care of people, no matter who they are, what they're doing, what their status in life is, I felt a great deal of empathy for the situation that these mostly gay young men were going through. . . . They were suffering and dying at an extraordinarily frightening rate.
>
> "There was a certain degree to which most of the scientific establishment reflexively pulled back from them and shut them out . . . so rather than being intimidated by the theatrics and the confrontation, what I did was say, '[L]et me put myself in their shoes. What would I do if I were in their shoes, experiencing what they were experiencing? . . .'
>
> "It didn't come easily. It wasn't all over a sudden early night. But over a period of months and then years, gradually, we gained greater respect and confidence in each other," says Fauci. "Because they were dead on right in most of what they were saying. They weren't always right . . . just the way the scientists and the regulatory

establishment got things wrong. When we worked together, then we all got it right."

Asked . . . if he had any regrets, Fauci says: "Certainly nobody's perfect, least of all me. Early on, I could have acted a little bit more quickly in some of their suggestions. . . . [E]ven though I acted more quickly than anybody else [in government], maybe I could have acted even more quickly and embraced some of their more daring approaches."

As Peter Staley said, "Dr. Fauci walked through the fire with us, and his friendships with AIDS activists deepened with time, bound by a shared trauma." But if Fauci walked through the fire, Kramer *brought* the fire—knowing the government would act only when they felt it was in their best interest to act.

Michael Specter wrote in *The New Yorker*:

> Kramer's actions helped revolutionize the American practice of medicine. Twenty-first-century patients no longer treat their doctors as deities. People demand to know about the treatments they will receive. They scour the Internet, ask for statistics on surgical success rates, and if they don't like what they hear they shop around. The Food and Drug Administration no longer considers approving a new drug until it has consulted representatives of groups who would use it.

In the same article, Fauci told Specter, "In American medicine, there are two eras. Before Larry and after Larry. There is no question in my mind that Larry helped change medicine in this country. And he helped change it for the better. When all the screaming and the histrionics are forgotten, that will remain."

Kramer believed that "being gay is a natural normal beautiful variation on being human. Period. End of subject. Therefore, any argument which says differently is an immoral supremacist one. Call it out as such. . . . Be outraged, offended, angry and intolerant of any discussion or any one who describes you as unequal, undeserving or unnatural for being just as you are." From this passionate belief, he and his fellow activists forced Fauci and many others to change. They became, in Fauci's words, "brothers in arms."

# Addressing the Need: Needle Exchange and HIV/AIDS

Making sure that people who inject drugs were able to do so as safely as possible became a mission for many AIDS activists in the 1980s and 1990s. But this mission was beset by challenges and charges from other members of society, who felt that providing drug users with clean needles was tantamount to promoting drug use. In a lethal moral judgment with more than a few echoes of the gross indifference for the health of gay and trans people, politicians and lawmakers held to the line that drug users should be punished, not helped . . . even if it made the AIDS epidemic worse.

One of the most common ways for people to become infected with HIV is for drug users to inject themselves with needles that have already been used by someone who is HIV+. Needles and syringes for injecting drugs are inexpensive to manufacture; they're used legally and safely in medical settings every day all around the world. But they're often hard to get hold of because in many states they're classified as "drug paraphernalia"—which means they're illegal to have without a doctor's prescription. Because of the nature of drug addiction—particularly addiction to "hard drugs" like heroin and opioids that are injected intravenously and cause horrible, dangerous withdrawal systems when stopped abruptly—when access to new needles is cut off, drug users aren't going to stop using until they get clean ones. Instead, they will use old needles. Since HIV is transmitted by blood, and needles are injected directly into blood, the needles are easily contaminated. If you use a contaminated needle and put it into your vein, you're mixing the previous user's blood with your own. For a lot of drug users, especially in the 1980s and 1990s, that meant unknowingly contracting HIV and developing AIDS in the years that followed.

The solution to this problem should be obvious: If the drug users are being killed by using old needles, give them new needles. And then, while you're giving them new needles, provide them with a judgment-free space where you can warn them about the disease, give them condoms so they don't spread it sexually, provide access to HIV testing, and offer resources to help combat their drug use.

Sounds like a good plan, right?

Unfortunately, it's still a controversial one. And in many places, it's still an illegal one.

Luckily, unjust laws rarely stop people from trying to save other people's lives.

If we tried to detail all the things most American politicians got wrong about drug policy in the 1980s, this chapter would become as long as the book itself. But to boil it down to the basics, America's drug policy was both disturbingly and predictably similar to its AIDS policy. Politicians and their supporters from the self-proclaimed "moral majority" prioritized shame and stigma over compassion and service. They imposed a narrative of personal choice over a difficult situation involving disease; like gay and trans people who became infected through sex, intravenous drug users were alleged to have brought it on themselves and deemed undeserving of the government's care—even as the government spent billions of dollars on medical care for people whose cigarette use led to lung cancer and other forms of cancer. In the eyes of the Reagan administration (as well as plenty of other Republicans and Democrats), drug users were bad people doing bad things within their control, just as gay and trans people with AIDS had become sick because of their own actions—not because of an underlying illness that didn't give a shit who they were. The Reagan administration's antidrug slogan "Just Say No" is predicated on the idea that people who are addicted to drugs, who face severe physical and psychological blowback if they fight that addiction, can freely and without consequence say no anytime they want.

This has never been true. The reality of drug use and drug addiction is complicated, especially when it comes to the extremely addictive drugs that people inject into their veins. These drugs can have a powerful allure, even if the consequences are ultimately devastating. When your body adjusts to the presence of the drug in your bloodstream, it builds a tolerance to it. That tolerance means you need more of the drug to achieve the same effect. This spiral is chemical and biological, not solely a matter of choice.

Because the government refused to stop blaming the victims, it was willing to let them die. When activists and medical professionals asked for clean needles to be given to drug users (often in exchange for used needles) to prevent them from injecting themselves with HIV, the national government and many state governments . . . just said no. Especially when the primary populations at risk were poor, BIPOC, and/or queer.

Critics of needle-exchange programs claim that they will only encourage more drug use, get in the way of drug-prevention efforts, increase crime, increase the presence of discarded needles, and ultimately not deter the spread of HIV. While there wasn't much data about this at the start of the AIDS epidemic, by now there is plenty of data—and all these arguments have turned out to be wrong. According to the CDC, participants in syringe-exchange programs are five times more likely to enter drug-treatment programs and three and a half times more likely to stop injecting drugs. Other research demonstrates that 90 percent of all syringes that are distributed are returned, meaning that neighborhoods aren't flooded with used needles when new ones are distributed.

According to a 2021 article in the *American Journal of Preventive Medicine*, "Research over the past 3 decades has provided compelling evidence on the effectiveness, safety, and cost effectiveness of SSPs [syringe services programs] in preventing HIV infection among PWID [people who inject drugs]." SSPs also help reduce additional health risks for intravenous drug users, such as viral hepatitis, life-threatening bacterial and fungal infections, and overdose deaths, and benefit the larger community by increasing the safe disposal of used syringes and the number of people seeking treatment. Finally, the article concludes, "SSPs have not been shown to increase drug use or crime."

Many politicians remained impervious to this data. They stuck to their story.

So if the government wasn't doing the right thing . . . who was?

From the age of fourteen to the age of nineteen, Jon C. Parker was a heroin addict, convicted over twenty times for drug-related crimes, breaking into so many pharmacies that he was known as "the Rexall king" (after the pharmacy chain of that name). He later went into recovery and became an academic. After thirteen years of sobriety, he saw the toll AIDS was taking on drug users and decided to act. In 1987, he began to buy needles in places where it was legal to buy them and then go up and down the Northeast to cities from Boston to Philadelphia, distributing them in places where needle exchange was illegal. By 1989 he was known as "the Johnny Appleseed of needles," distributing over 50,000 needles and founding the National AIDS Brigade to hit the streets and do the work, raising AIDS awareness and advocating for drug counseling while giving users safe needles and syringes. It cost him everything—according to the *Chicago Tribune*, "Parker buys the needles he distributes with his own money. He pays for the gas for his van and the rent on two storefront offices. Because of those expenses, he is several months behind in the rent on his apartment, and has shut-off notices for the gas, phone and water."

As Parker told *The New York Times*, "I'm trying to save lives. I'm trying to stop AIDS. We don't condone drugs, but we're trying to keep people AIDS-free till they get into drug treatment. . . . Thank God, when I was shooting up, AIDS was not around."

For this work, Parker was arrested in Boston.

His defense against the charges was a "defense of necessity," meaning that he admitted to, in the words of his lawyer, "committing a smaller wrong to prevent a greater evil."

Judge Sally A. Kelly acquitted him, saying Parker had acted "solely with the purpose of limiting the spread of AIDS."

The National AIDS Brigade marched on, shrugging stigma to the side to save people's lives.

In 1988, it was against the law in California to possess syringes without a prescription. A group of volunteers began a group called Prevention Point, handing out needles, bleach, cotton, alcohol wipes, condoms, and referrals to drug-treatment programs and social services. They had to keep their efforts hidden—at times, a baby carriage was used as the camouflage to deliver new needles to drug users. But they got results. A study in 1992 of their efforts showed that the percentage of people who reported sharing needles went from 66 percent to 36 percent and the number of HIV cases for people who inject drugs dropped by 50 percent.

In March 1992, San Francisco's mayor, Frank Jordan, declared a public health emergency and committed $138,000 to Prevention Point. It didn't matter that their actions were still technically illegal in the state; the city knew what needed to be done.

Decades later, other cities and other states still haven't gotten the message.

Needle exchange still faces resistance, even during the opioid epidemic, which has introduced a new wave of HIV transmission. Even in states or counties where possession of syringes without a prescription has been decriminalized, in most states, people working for syringe services programs can still face arrest for any drug residue that remains on the "dirty" needles exchanged for new needles.

In 2015, there was a remarkable HIV outbreak in rural Scott County in Indiana. In the town of Austin, Indiana, 235 people out of a total population of 4,100 were infected in "the worst drug-fueled outbreak ever to hit rural America."

In response, Indiana's governor, future Vice President Mike Pence, approved the first needle exchange in the state's history, over three decades after its first documented case of HIV. He said, "I will tell you that I do not support needle exchange as anti-drug policy. But this is a public health emergency." (It is worth noting that this "emergency" was only declared after an outbreak in a rural, massively white area of the state, and not in an urban area with primarily BIPOC residents.)

The needle exchange was startlingly effective. Five years after the outbreak began, three-quarters of the people who'd been infected were under regular treatment and had an undetectable, untransmittable HIV status. And there was only *one* new reported case of HIV through intravenous drug use in all of 2020. In March 2021, NPR noted that "the county's One-Stop Shop in Austin, Ind., provides testing for HIV, hepatitis C or sexually transmitted infections. There's food and the people who work there can connect users with health insurance, housing and recovery opportunities. It serves around 170 people a month."

But that didn't stop the Scott County commissioners from voting 2–1 to end the program.

Why?

In a Facebook post he later deleted, one of the commissioners, Randy Julian, called it "a welfare program for addicts." The same old ugly biases showing their face again.

If anything, the fight against needle-exchange programs, like the inability to sufficiently fund a cure for HIV/AIDS, shows how tenacious these biases can be. Congress has yet to allow taxpayer dollars to be spent on funding syringe services, adhering to laws introduced by Republicans in 1990, at the height of the AIDS crisis. (The ban was briefly lifted during the Obama administration but reinstated when Republicans took back control of Congress two years later.) This even though the CDC estimates that syringe programs can reduce the contraction of HIV and hepatitis C by *50 percent* without added medication-assisted treatment to address opioid-use disorder, and by *67 percent* with the added treatment.

Why do people let this happen? Because they are still stuck on the idea that injecting drugs is something "bad people" do, and that they can "just say no" at any time. Just as gay and trans people died and still die because their illness is blamed on their identity. There is a lesson here, one that echoes Surgeon General Koop's earlier words: When it comes to disease, there should be no room for moral judgment. There should only be room for the people who show compassion and work to keep everyone safe from a disease (or many diseases) that none of them asked for.

# Tina Valentin Aguirre

*When named a Latino Heritage Month honoree by the Instituto Familiar de la Raza, longtime queer activist Tina Valentin Aguirre said, "I like to model fearlessness. Some of us have it in us to jump in when we don't know what's going to happen but we know our work is needed." This is the story of how Tina jumped in.*

> Like it or not, AIDS is now an issue of concern to the Latino community. Several organizations have started up in the wake of the epidemic to provide information and education to Latinos who know little about the virus. While the disease has been primarily associated with the white/gay community, the Instituto Latino AIDS Project in San Francisco is one of the newly formed Latino groups focusing on the controversial issue. It has emerged with an agenda which calls for urgency, prevention, and education regarding the lethal virus.

Tina Valentin Aguirre was a student at Stanford University when they wrote these words in a 1988 issue of *Estos Tiempos,* a publication for Latine students. Tina grew up in a working-class family in San Diego. They were always the odd one out—wearing makeup at school, finding a genderqueer identity from a young age. After moving to the Bay Area for college, Tina started to notice a lack of awareness around AIDS in their community, especially when a friend was suspected to have AIDS. Tina thought that many in the queer Latine community saw AIDS as just a problem for white gay men—not them.

At Stanford, I experienced lots of alienation, isolation. I grew up poor and being Latino, it was an alienating experience to live at Stanford. Lots of princes, rich people, people who did not know how to do the basics of self-care. They didn't even know how to change a roll of toilet paper.

I started writing about AIDS because one of my peers at Stanford, a journalist, a gay Chicano man, was rumored to have gotten AIDS. It was '86, '87.

We knew that lots of us were coming to San Francisco and were having sex and were vulnerable. I was getting tested. I spoke to health care providers who weren't talking to each other because they were in competition with each other. I asked questions without filters—questions about queer and trans people.

Quickly, I learned about many systemic problems. Most of these problems came down to the fact that we as queer and trans people weren't leading the efforts to protect our communities against HIV/AIDS. So I wrote an article. In essence, it pointed to great dysfunction and argued that this dysfunction was going to lead to lots more deaths in my community.

After the article appeared in *Estos Tiempos,* Tina connected with like-minded queer people who belonged to the Latine community in San Francisco, forty miles northwest of Stanford. Stanford might have been geographically nearby, but San Francisco was a whole different world. Stanford was stuffy and academic. San Francisco was a bohemian city overflowing with sex, drugs, parties, and progressive politics. Rents were still cheap. After the hippie movement of the 1960s inspired an influx into the city, San Francisco had gained a reputation as a destination for waifs and strays, hippies and artists. This migration into the city helped to make its enduring bohemian spirit, but it created problems that city planners and community organizers had to grapple with. HIV/AIDS was fast becoming one of those problems among the city's population, particularly those who injected drugs and/or sold sex in the city's sleaziest districts, and across the city's LGBTQ+ population.

For Tina, like so many young queer people, San Francisco held the promise of home. The city was loud, lively, and full of people who looked like Tina and felt like Tina. People who wanted to have the same conversations. People who wanted to change the world. The increasing threat of AIDS was a fundamental feature of those conversations. Finding ways to prevent further cases of AIDS became the main way to change the world.

> I got a chance to come to San Francisco. I painted a mural with an artist, a hippie, who was really open about everything. She asked me, did I know about Esta Noche, a gay Latino bar in San Francisco?
>
> I went to Esta Noche. That first night, I promptly met some people who were part of a response to AIDS in a gay Latino context. I said, "Oh, well I wrote this article." They were like, "We need writers in the movement! You need to meet some people." They introduced me to people. Other activists.
>
> I was really happy about making the connections. I went back to Stanford. I plugged into the National Latino Lesbian and Gay Organization that was just being created at the time. It became a national organization. I was a youth activist there. Part of our demands were that we get programs to protect us as young people.

Still barely out of their teens, Tina was aware of the treacherous circumstances that meant that many young queer kids in the Bay Area were coming into contact with HIV without realizing it.

> Unfortunately, youth have always been extra susceptible to HIV. And in San Francisco, like lots of meccas, survival sex and also just power dynamics often get lost in the stories we tell about how this happened and what occurred. Think about the need for connection. The need to learn from older adults. Without AIDS, that could be

a positive thing, but with AIDS, it became a very dangerous thing. Once you add in all the poverty and inequities, it created a situation which led to many young people being exposed to HIV and succumbing to HIV.

For Tina, finding a sense of belonging in the Latine queer community in San Francisco was a survival strategy. And this survival was joyful.

> I met my first boyfriend at Esta Noche. He was there the first night I went, and he was there when I went back again.
>
> We started dating. I ended up leaving Stanford, coming to San Francisco. I didn't know until the day I was in the U-Haul driving my stuff down that he was HIV+. When he told me, it was after a long period of me trying to get him tested. He'd say, "I've never gotten tested, I'm afraid to get tested."
>
> We had safe sex but it was still devastating to get this news right as I was moving to San Francisco. And it informed my development as a person.
>
> I started doing HIV outreach in the streets, passing out condoms and bleach, especially on 16th street, which was a gay Latino corridor.

What was that like?

First of all, it was a lot. But as a Mexican American, death is a part of my culture. I understood that death is just a part of my life. It always was, and it always will be.

And coming to San Francisco, finding community—it was tremendous. Just walking down the street you'd find community and meet people.

For me, I was always looking at individual, peer, community level, and then city, national, international levels of how issues impact us. I just think that way. And it turned out that perspective was needed. So when I got to the city and started to bring up these questions, I got lots of feedback—from everybody. People on the street, people in organizations, people who have great distrust for public health.

Along the way, I connected with some leftists. I learned how groups like the Brown Berets, the Black Panthers, United Farm Workers, organized during the civil rights movement to create health care systems which were peer based. The original systems were so racist that they would've died if that had not happened.

So as AIDS came about, one of those people was Pat Norman—a Black lesbian activist. She created the Institute for Community Health Outreach. To undo the fear and stigma of AIDS, we had to share information. She established a curriculum to teach people using radical leftist community organizing principles. Like, go out on the street. Have engaging conversations. Listen to people. Make sure that you're succinct. Be able to stop people. You're able to engage very quickly. Use whatever you have. I have some charm. I have the ability to stop people and I've always used that in this kind of work. And then you pivot quickly to serious things—things that people don't often talk about. Sex. And risk. But in a fun way.

It was a training. Lots of us activists got trained as AIDS test counselors, and then took this training. In 1989, I worked at a liquor store by day. But by night, I was a journalist, and I was organizing with people. And then I was doing HIV outreach. The training made us ready to enter HIV prevention programs as staff.

And that meant:

*We became our own experts.*

First, we just started out with a table of condoms to hand out and bleach for drug users to clean used needles. We'd just stand there and stop people. 16th and Mission Street is a neighborhood where a lot of injection-drug users went to buy drugs. On the strip, there were sex workers picking up johns. Plus, just people going to the bars. There were lots of bars. So it was very easy. And fun—I want you to know the whole thing was amazingly fun. And cruise-y!

There were lots of artistic people, lots of projects happening. There was this *rush*—an impetus for people who were dying, or people who were witnessing the death, people who were older, to hurry up and come together.

They recognized that something was happening. We needed to come together. The full extent was not clear. There was bias. People of color groups thought, "Oh, we're not white, we're not getting AIDS at the same rate, it's really a white disease."

But I knew that it was coming. And so some of us were doing that work.

It was awesome.

I would go to the panadería down the street from where we were. I knew one of the twins who worked there, and his brother was gay and closeted. When the brother was at the register, and I'd been getting my burrito or whatever after giving out condoms on the street, he'd be like, "Hey, can you hand me some condoms?" I'd pay for the burrito and put some condoms under the cash.

And then word gets out. That you're trustworthy. That people will share their details with you. You're not going to spread them. Instead, you're just there, consistently. And if people needed help, they started to know: They could trust me and others like me.

So it was fun.

San Francisco in the late 1980s was very vibrant and happening. But it also was different for people of color with AIDS—it did hit us later—the waves hit us later.

Tina was focused on reaching people who were left out of mainstream conversations to stop the spread of HIV/AIDS. Identity is a slippery thing. Tina knew this firsthand through their experience growing up as genderqueer in San Diego.

> My experience was always different because I've always been genderqueer. In high school, I was using makeup. It shocked people. They'd be like, "Why do you have makeup on?" And I'd say, "Because it's Tuesday?" I'm not gonna sit here and talk about why I have makeup on. I just do.

And when Tina got to San Francisco, they saw how differences within the queer community made it harder to protect people from HIV. Gay men were treated as a single group, despite the fact that many gay men shared friendships, relationships, and desires with other LGBTQ+ people, and with men who remained in the closet because of homophobia. But Tina also saw how the community rallied together.

> When I came to the queer community in San Francisco, the splits in the community were by gender. This split got reenforced by AIDS, because of risk. The narrative is out there that lesbians helped gay men, and that's true. However, it's much more complicated. There were radical leftist separate feminists, and then trans people, and drag, and genderqueer people like me. We were all on the outskirts and we found each other.

As Tina handed out condoms on street corners and built relationships with local sex workers and with closeted men, they realized how important it was that people understood that AIDS wasn't a disease affecting just white gay men.

> What I learned is that it's all complicated. Sex is complicated. Desire's complicated. And risk categories are useful, but they're not borders. We're not made any more safe by those borders or by those categories. It actually puts some of us at more risk if we're not considered, and if we don't consider the porousness of sexuality. That was a part of what I brought to wherever I went.

\* \* \*

You can't talk to Tina about their youth in San Francisco without talking about the mother they found there. For many queer people at that time, in that place, chosen family was about staying off the streets. The queer kids who'd arrive in San Francisco in search of freedom had often been disowned and misunderstood by their biological families. At Esta Noche, Tina found a new family of other Latine queers—trans women and drag queens. Tina was never a sex worker, but some of their sisters were. They'd all party at the bars, support each other's drag shows, and some of their sisters would hustle—exchanging sex for cash with interested men. They'd discuss their relationship to their gender, taking notes on whether they wanted to start hormones, get gender-affirming surgery, and, really, what it meant to them to be a woman and to be queer.

> On 16th Street, I first met a whole bunch of sisters. They were drag performers, some of them. We would talk, we would track each other: Are you going to get hormones? Are you going to have any surgery? After their shows, they would come out to smoke cigarettes and maybe find johns. Some of us were sex workers, some of us were just sluts ... who did not make any money at all! That's me!
>
> Anyway, we would connect, and talk. We all loved each other. Then they would do fundraisers for people when they were sick. They liked my journalism, my community activism, I liked what they did.
>
> We became family. We supported each other. We were all young! I was way too young to be going to that bar. But I did! And they did too.

This family was led by Teresita La Campesina. Her name started as a drag persona, but it's inseparable from the rest of her life. Teresita was a Mexican American trans woman who'd been part of the scene in San Francisco since the early 1970s. She became well known as a drag superstar who sang her own songs with a huge operatic voice, rather than lip-syncing. She was beloved as a mother, offering LGBTQ+ kids shelter, safety, and solidarity.

> She didn't have a lot of shame. Societal expectations and family stuff. She was quick to share that a lot of that is destructive to us as queer and trans people, sissies—people who don't fit the norms. She would say, "You as a straight family parent unit cannot deal with your queer children. Send them to me. We'll be fine."
>
> For me, the concept of chosen family was solidified through her.
>
> We all just called her Mother.

As a queer elder and a role model, Teresita helped Tina understand their own unfolding relationship to their gender in their early twenties.

> She really helped me to understand that it's okay. It's nobody's business where we are at, if we ever get certain procedures or some things done.
>
> Some of her sisters, my aunties, had had vaginoplasty. Let's say they had "everything" done. They'd look at us and say, "Oh you're not actually transexual!" That was the word they used at the time. They meant "You're not actually a woman." We'd just say, "Fuck you, we get more men than you. Whatever you want to say, girl!"

Teresita was born in 1940 to Mexican parents in Los Angeles. She was their twenty-first child. By the age of fifteen, she was made homeless by her family for being queer. She made a living singing with mariachi bands across the city and singing Spanish songs on the radio under the name Margarita. As a young person, she was regularly stopped by the police for "masquerading"—dressing in women's clothing—a problem for trans people at that time. Teresita was under attack by city police and oppressive laws simply for being herself. By the 1970s, she had made her way to San Francisco, seeking the same refuge that the city offered so many young queer people by the 1960s.

In San Francisco, she worked the notorious streets of the Tenderloin district. When Tina joined Teresita's chosen family, Teresita was still selling sex on the city streets. Tina often worried about Teresita coming into danger as she tried to make money, but Teresita was used to the risks that came with who she was.

> One time I was driving on the freeway and I saw her off the side of the road and I was like, "Oh my God, my mother!" so I got off the freeway, came back, stopped, and got her. I was like, "Oh my God, why are you here? Do you need help? What's going on?" But she just was like, "I'm trying to make money!" She didn't like competition, so she'd wait by the freeway and get truck drivers who knew she would be there. They'd stop and she would make money.
>
> Teresita was a fabulous person. A star amongst us. With great talent.

For trans women, sex work has historically been one of the few available sources of income, because ignorance, transphobia, and inequality make it harder for trans people to work in "normal" jobs. But sex work can bring danger, too. In the early 1990s, that meant not only violence but also increasing your chances of contracting HIV, even though sex workers and their customers were more mindful of the need for condoms by that time. By Tina's account, Teresita was a fabulous performer and a loving drag mother who provided the care that so many vulnerable young queer people sorely needed. Her life as a sex worker—the choices she had to make, the things she did to get money for food and shelter—didn't negate that.

Teresita found out she was HIV+ in the early 1990s. She would travel to Nevada to work as a sex worker at the casinos, until she was wanted by police for soliciting as an HIV+ person, since HIV had already been criminalized to an unjust degree (to be explained further in the next chapter). She was public about her status during her performances at nightclubs around San Francisco, even as her health went up and down over the final decade of her life. She wouldn't let the crowds forget that the person whose beautiful voice they were enjoying was a person living with AIDS—living against the odds, living for today. Teresita's diagnosis made her even more enthusiastic to support Tina's work in HIV outreach. Teresita spoke at international AIDS conferences about her experiences and campaigned in San Francisco to encourage LGBTQ+ people to vote during an important mayoral election in 1999.

As a young person in the early 1990s, Tina was already close to burnout after taking on a leadership role in AIDS activism in their early twenties.

> By 1990, I was already plugged into the Latino Coalition of AIDS, working across activism and advocacy. I was born in 1968, so I was young. Shockingly young! And thrust into a position of leadership out of necessity because many of the people who were the leaders were already starting to get sick.
>
> I helped build a coalition with the Gay Men of Color Consortium that included the American Indian AIDS Institute, the Black Coalition on AIDS, the Gay Asian Pacific Alliance, the Community HIV Program. The coalition helped on a city level with the Ryan White Act. We needed to look at the massive amounts of funding that were not getting distributed to us as communities. I became a direct services provider, worked as a case manager and then a health educator for the Center for Positive Care. And in 1991, I worked with a gay Latino homeless group as a case manager.
>
> I was starting to experience great loss in the community. By 1992, I was already experiencing burnout. A lot of my friends were dying. Friends I'd only met five years before. It was really awful. A lot of them were young. Some were not. I decided to step back. I needed time for myself.

Tina started to make documentaries about their experiences in San Francisco. The city was rapidly changing around them, gentrifying, and so many of the city's most colorful figures had died because of AIDS. Making art was a form of therapy for Tina.

> There were writing groups, movie-making groups. It was a means for us to deal with grief and self-esteem issues so that we could actually

stay HIV-negative, or try to stay healthy. We used culture as part of the plan, part of the medicine.

Tina's relationship with Teresita became fraught in the year before Teresita's AIDS-related death, shortly before Tina returned to Stanford to recommence the undergraduate degree she had paused fifteen years previously to work in HIV outreach.

> Her death was around 2000. Before I went back to school, there was a lot of loss that I experienced, including her. We ended up not talking right before she died. She grew up poor, she never left poverty. And there were some people that thought that because I made movies I had lots of money, or maybe because I went to Stanford, I had lots of money, even though I'd dropped out. I never had lots of money.
> 
> I became her manager in some ways, I'd organize shoots. I would help her negotiate her fees and I'd bring her equipment. She was bad talent though, because she didn't like to rehearse, and she didn't like musicians. Ultimately I realized that I couldn't be her manager after all. If I were to actually manage her, she would need to get a discipline which she never wanted. It was impossible.
> 
> The saddest thing is that her voice started to give out. That was the worst.

Teresita died, and Tina went back to Stanford.

> I did end up going back to Stanford to finish my bachelor's. I'd stopped out my sophomore year. I was just like, "I'll come back to it when I want to."
> 
> And I did finish—in the early 2000s, I got my bachelor's. It was interesting going back to Stanford as a thirty-three-year-old who'd had all this experience, who'd seen everything I'd seen, who was an adult.
> 
> People would ask me, What are you going to do now?

I'd say: basically the same thing I was doing. Nonprofits, fundraising, arts work, journalism.

Today, Tina is a central figure in San Francisco's queer community—a storyteller and protector of the legacy of queer Latine people in the city. Tina was elected as the first manager of the Castro LGBTQ Cultural District and has served on the board of the city's GLBT Historical Society. Tina produced a film about Teresita, *Wanted Alive: Teresita La Campesina,* which remains a powerful testimony to Teresita's vitality.

When you experience unimaginable pain—when you witness unimaginable levels of grief—art, community, and storytelling are ways to keep the light on against the odds. Tina's remarks today about young people and HIV are much the same as they were in the mid-1980s, when Tina was a teenager writing articles about AIDS for the student magazine and dreaming of San Francisco.

> I'm HIV-negative. I wasn't always confident that I was HIV-negative. I definitely didn't think that I was going to stay HIV-negative. After the AIDS cocktails came out, I was able to start to put that behind in me. It really was about grief.
>
> AIDS definitely informed my development from a young person to an adult. It took quite some time to undo that. For people of my age, we weren't really allowed to date in junior high or high school in ways which were healthy at least, or open. We didn't have the practice. Our twenties, maybe early thirties, were times to screw everything up. HIV is an issue that needs to be focused on, but it won't get solved if we ignore economics, if we ignore self-esteem, if we ignore so many of the other things that lead young people to make decisions that are high-risk.
>
> I grew up with a complete fear of sex. But also still titillated, you know? A teenager with hormones, good luck trying not to think about sex. Having a little bit of sex but not that much, being really careful. And then coming to San Francisco, it was like: Holy crap,

*everything* is here. There were lots of sex clubs, and cruising. You could find sex walking to the corner store to get a loaf of bread.

Welcome to San Francisco!

So I grew up with all of that. I learned about my sexuality, but it took me a long time to actually . . . It took until I was thirty-five to understand what I needed and what I wanted. I want to know it's fun, but I'm not into everything. Not all menu items are options for me. You have to be clear. You have to be smart and funny. And you have to be really good at communication.

It is important to remember the immense fear and misinformation that people with AIDS and their advocates remain up against. Once a lie becomes lodged in the cultural consciousness, it is hard to remove it completely. At the less consequential end of the spectrum, AIDS is still a punch line in a number of jokes about gay people. More seriously, there are still threats that people with AIDS are under that go beyond the medical. At the height of AIDS hysteria, a number of laws were created to criminalize people with AIDS, maliciously insinuating that the ill would use their illness to deliberately spread harm.

Over thirty years later, many of those laws remain on the books.

*What if someone broke into this chamber and started kissing and sticking people, infecting others simply to take their lives?*

# HIV Is Not a Deadly Weapon

"What if someone broke into this chamber and started kissing and sticking people, infecting others simply to take their lives? . . . AIDS is behaviorally driven and we have to have the mechanisms to control it, if necessary."

These were the words of State Representative Alphonse Jackson Jr., a Democratic legislator in Louisiana who in June 1987 sponsored HR 1041, a bill that would allow people with HIV to be arrested and quarantined. Health officials would be able to hold and jail people with HIV without a court hearing or bond as a "danger to public health." In other words, the law would create state-sanctioned internment camps for people already struggling to get good medical care. It was a chilling prospect—a literal manifestation of the conservative US Senator Jesse Helms's exhortation that "we're going to have to quarantine if we are really going to contain this disease"—no matter the civil rights implications. In 1987, with no successful treatment for AIDS available, quarantine would mean that people with AIDS would have to spend the rest of their lives imprisoned. In the absence of a remedy, the only release would be death.

The bill had been requested by Louisiana's Department of Health and Human Resources. It passed the lower chamber of the state legislature 62–27.

When asked at a news conference if he supported the bill, Louisiana Governor Edwin W. Edwards said, "No. This is America, man! I'm not going to sign anything that allows anybody—even a member of the news media—to be jailed without due process."

After Edwards announced that he would veto the bill, Jackson tabled it. America was spared its first legal internment of people with AIDS.

Other laws against people with HIV/AIDS were soon enacted—not just in Louisiana but across the country. While these laws were ostensibly aimed at people who might wield their illness as a weapon, they ended up ensnaring many innocent people whose only crime was being HIV+.

In the same month that the arrest-and-quarantine legislation was killed, the Louisiana House passed a bill that made it a crime for someone HIV+ to "intentionally expose" another person to the virus—the first state legislature to do so. HIV+ people who did not disclose their status to sexual partners could be sentenced to ten years at hard labor in prison, fined up to $5,000, or both. (Initially the bill's sponsor, Representative Kernan Hand, wanted intentional transmission of HIV/AIDS to be treated as a second-degree murder charge, which would have meant a sentence of life in prison without the possibility of parole.)

Gary Clements of the American Civil Liberties Union of Louisiana said, "We are going back to the Middle Ages. It is impossible to prove intent in this bill."

Clements and other critics pointed out that the bill had the effect of encouraging people to *avoid* being tested for HIV, making the health crisis worse, not better. Because if people didn't know their status, then they couldn't be found guilty of withholding it.

A month after it was introduced and passed by the House, Governor Edwards signed the bill into state law. Many other states followed with their own forms of this legislation. Eventually, more than two-thirds of the states in America would have laws criminalizing the transmission of HIV. Many of these laws—drafted in the late 1980s or early 1990s, before successful treatment of HIV/AIDS and before much was definitively known about transmission—stand to this day. According to the CDC, as of 2022, thirty-five states still had laws that criminalized HIV exposure.

In 1993, Louisiana's law was amended to cover exposure through any other means or contact besides sexual contact. Among these other means or contact? Spitting, biting, stabbing with an AIDS-contaminated object, or throwing blood or other bodily substances. None of these actions are at all likely to spread HIV. Even though the science has been clear on this for decades now, eleven states still criminalize it.

You would think that, with the rise of effective treatments and the ability of HIV+ people to live with the virus as undetectable and untransmittable, these laws would have been repealed or greatly modified. But that is not what has happened. It was not until 2018 that Louisiana took out the parts of their law that involved "other means or contact"—acknowledging decades too late that things like spitting could not transmit HIV. But the law about having to disclose your HIV status to anyone you come into sexual contact with, as well as to any police or medical officer you might be "exposing"—that remains the law, even if your HIV status is undetectable.

Robert Suttle knows all too well how unfair these laws can be. He was working as an assistant clerk at the Second Circuit Court of Appeal in Shreveport, Louisiana, in 2008 when police showed up and arrested him in front of his coworkers. The charge? Intentional exposure to HIV. The accuser? One of his exes.

Suttle is a Black, gay, HIV+ man. As he remembered it, when he first met his ex at a New Year's party, he disclosed his HIV status. But the ex remembered differently, and after their relationship was over, he went to the police. It was one man's word against the other's; even though Suttle had not actually transmitted the virus to his ex, it was still a crime that he *could have*. Suttle, worried about what might happen if the case went to trial (especially as a Black, gay, HIV+ man in Louisiana) and wanting to get it behind him, pleaded guilty. Instead of receiving the two years' probation he expected, he had to serve six months at hard labor in prison . . . and was then added to the state's registry of sex offenders. Later, when he moved to New York state, he was forced to register as a sex offender there, even though New York does not have a similar law criminalizing intentional exposure to HIV.

After his imprisonment, Suttle became an activist, fighting against the laws that derailed his life. As he told the website AIDSVu:

> These stories are real people's lives. They may sound like something that happened a long time ago, but there is still more to be said about it. You might not see it on our faces, but some of us are still struggling with the consequences of these convictions every day when we try to manage relationships with our families and friends, secure employment, access housing, or continue our education.
>
> We are trying to get our lives back on track and it's difficult to push forward when you have a felony or conviction on your record. Most importantly, we are trying to remember who we are after our unjust treatment in the criminal justice system. We can only hope that this egregious experience changes us for the better, but sometimes you may find yourself feeling incapable of living a full life. I want people to know about these realities and problems that we constantly face because of HIV criminalization.

According to the Williams Institute at UCLA School of Law, which tracks the criminalization of HIV/AIDS, thousands of people have been prosecuted for "HIV crimes" in the United States—and "the vast majority of arrests, prosecutions, and convictions are pursuant to state laws that do not require actual transmission of HIV, the intent to transmit, or even conduct that can transmit HIV." In addition, being convicted of an HIV crime can lead to a long sentence "and create lifelong collateral consequences from a felony conviction."

There is also an inherent bias in these arrests, which disproportionately affect Black people and are used to give sex workers harsher sentences. In Louisiana, 91 percent of the people arrested for HIV crimes are Black men, even though only 44 percent of people living with HIV in the state are Black men—an example of the inequity in the way the law is applied. There are some states where there are movements to repeal or revise these laws to reflect the fact that HIV is no longer a "deadly weapon" and that if you are untransmittable, disclosure is not necessary to keep your partner safe. But few legislatures are making this a priority issue. In the meantime, people with HIV live in legal limbo.

Just as very few owners of knives ever use a knife as an intentional weapon, there are very few cases on record where an HIV+ person has deliberately transmitted the virus with an intent to harm or kill. Still, the myth of HIV as a deadly weapon persists, in no small part to demonize and disenfranchise queer and BIPOC people. Had people with COVID-19 been arrested for spreading it to the people they came in contact with, there would have been justifiable outrage. We now need that same kind of outrage on behalf of people with HIV so these laws can reflect science, once and for all.

## TIMELINE

# 1987–1991

### March 1987

On March 19, 1987, the FDA approves AZT (azidothymidine) as the first drug to treat AIDS. While most drugs take eight to ten years to be tested for federal approval on such a scale, AZT's approval takes twenty months. Still, for the more than 33,000 Americans who've been diagnosed up to this point, it is far too slow, and for more than half of them, it's already too late.

AZT was not invented to fight AIDS. It was, in fact, a failed cancer drug from the 1960s, derived from herring sperm (and later synthetically created). When AIDS hit in the 1980s, Burroughs Wellcome, like many other pharmaceutical companies, tested a variety of drugs they had on the shelf, to see if anything would work against the disease. One of the things the scientists at Burroughs Wellcome tested was Compound S, a re-creation of the original AZT. When they put it in a dish with animal cells infected with HIV, it stopped the virus from replicating. (AZT works by preventing HIV from creating more versions of itself within cells.)

Burroughs Wellcome sent its findings to the FDA and the National Cancer Institute, and the approval process began in a speedy way. Eventually, a test was done on human AIDS patients—a test that is still controversial, because it was a standard scientific study with half the patients getting the medicine and half getting the placebo. When it became clear that the patients on the placebo were dying far faster than the patients on the medication, the study was halted, and all the patients were given the drug. And even before the FDA's approval, a further 5,000 patients were given the drug to test.

While the announcement of the FDA's approval is greeted by some with hope, doctors are careful to point out that it isn't a cure or even a proven long-term treatment for AIDS—it might prolong life, but it won't rid the body of the disease. It also has many horrendous side effects, including severe intestinal problems, damage to the immune system, and nausea. And, in some patients, it actually increases the presence of the virus, for reasons doctors can't identify. For the next few years, people with AIDS will debate whether it is better to take this, the only available treatment, even if it proves to be just as toxic as the virus.

And then there's the price. A year's supply of AZT costs as much as $12,000 in 1987. (To put it in some perspective, the median family income in 1987 is $30,853.) Especially cruel is the fact that the 5,000 patients who were put on AZT as a trial are now expected to pay for it if they want to continue.

The activism against pharmaceutical companies to lower the price of AIDS treatment is discussed elsewhere in this book. And ultimately the scientists were both right and wrong about AZT—it was helpful in fighting HIV . . . but it only became effectively helpful on a long-term basis once other drugs were added to the regimen.

## May 1987

The Reagan administration's Public Health Service proposes adding HIV to its list of "dangerous infectious diseases," requiring anyone who wants to get permanent residence in the United States to have a negative HIV test. Within months, not only is this proposal enacted, but *all* HIV+ travelers—whether they are coming to visit family, get medical treatment, do business, or simply go on a vacation—are banned from entering the United States.

While there is an exception for married heterosexual couples, there are no exceptions made for gay couples (who are unable to get legally married). As a result of the HIV travel ban, relationships are disrupted, families are unable to reunite, and treatment by US doctors is effectively limited to US residents. All international AIDS conferences move outside the United States in protest, especially after a Dutch scientist, Hans Paul Verhoef, is banned from entering the country to speak at an AIDS conference in San Francisco because of his status.

The ban remains in place for twenty-two years.

Upon its repeal in 2009, President Barack Obama says, "Now, we talk about reducing the stigma of the disease, yet we've treated a visitor living with it as a threat. . . . If we want to be the global leader in combatting HIV/AIDS, we need to act like it."

## October 1987

"This subject matter is so obscene, so revolting, it is difficult for me to stand here and talk about it," Senator Jesse Helms tells the Senate. "I may throw up."

The "subject matter" is a safe-sex comic book distributed by Gay Men's Health Crisis to try to prevent the spread of AIDS. Even though no public funds were used to create the comic book, Helms uses it as the central reason he is amending a federal spending bill at the last minute.

The amendment's purpose is listed in the *Congressional Record* as:

> To prohibit the use of any funds provided under this Act to the Centers for Disease Control from being used to provide AIDS education, information, or prevention materials and activities that promote, encourage, and condone homosexual sexual activities or the intravenous use of illegal drugs.

When the Senate votes, only two senators vote against it: Lowell Weicker (Republican of Connecticut) and Daniel Patrick Moynihan (Democrat of New York). Senator Edward Kennedy (Democrat of Massachusetts) calls the amendment "a foolish exercise"—and then votes for it anyway, along with ninety-five of his colleagues.

Even if senators agree that it's absurd to think you can prevent the spread of AIDS if you don't talk about "homosexual sexual activities," with a big election year coming up, they don't want their opponents to be able to say they are pro-homosexuality. Their political futures matter more to them than medical imperatives.

Weicker insists that "education is the only tool we have at hand which is effective," while Helms says, "I just want the American taxpayer's dollars to be spent in a moral way"—proving once again that the definition of "morality" is very much in the eye of the beholder.

## November 1987

When Debra Fraser-Howze was the director of youth and social welfare at the New York Urban League, she was used to seeing cases of teen pregnancy that came from a lack of access to condoms. When one of her colleagues told her about a young father in her office who had tested positive for HIV, she knew it was a different problem with a similar cause: lack of information about safer sex and lack of access to things like condoms that could limit exposure to the virus.

In 1987, Fraser-Howze sends out a call to Black leaders across the city, saying that a coordinated response is necessary. They come together and in November found the National Black Leadership Commission on AIDS.

In a later interview for the New York City AIDS Memorial, Fraser-Howze says, "The community did not want to own it, and at the same time they were being impacted in ways that were unimaginable. . . . They all saw it as a white gay male epidemic and it was very hard to break through that stigma and noise."

## November 1987

Randy Shilts's book *And the Band Played On,* one of the most noteworthy works about the AIDS crisis published in the decade, is released. Shilts, a reporter based in San Francisco, tries to weave together a history of the new disease, grounding the scientific story within the greater story of institutional indifference and ineptitude. Although some of his reporting—such as his portrait of a Canadian flight attendant who introduced AIDS to North America as "Patient Zero"—proves inaccurate over the course of time, the book remains an important time capsule depicting what was known when it was written. At that time, the book and the subsequent miniseries based on the book introduced many readers and viewers to the complexity of AIDS history. Said David M. Smith of the National Gay and Lesbian Task Force, "He broke through society's denial and was absolutely critical to communicating the reality of AIDS."

Shilts was tested for HIV while writing the book but asked his doctor to hold off on telling him the results. On the day he wrote the final page, he learned he was HIV+. He lived for almost seven more years, and died in 1994 at the age of forty-two.

"Any good reporter could have done this story," Shilts told an interviewer when *And the Band Played On* was published, "but I think the reason I did it, and no one else did, is because I am gay. It was happening to people I cared about and loved." And in a later interview done after he revealed his HIV status, he said, "Every gay writer who tests positive ends up being an AIDS activist. I wanted to keep on being a reporter."

Ultimately, he was both.

## February 1989

Princess Diana attracts a large amount of interest from the American press on her first official overseas visit as a member of the British royal family without her husband, Prince Charles. As she tours New York City, crowds of admirers flock to see her, creating traffic jams and what the tabloids called "Di-mania." While she attends a lavish cocktail party and a gala dinner filled with the city's rich and famous, it is the less glamorous side of her itinerary that makes the trip so remarkable. Diana, long a supporter of people with AIDS, makes a point to travel to Harlem Hospital in Manhattan to visit its pediatric AIDS unit. With a full retinue of reporters and photographers in tow, Diana meets with the doctors, nurses, and other health care workers who keep the ward running. She talks to the patients, laughing and smiling. The press snaps photos of Diana as she scoops the children up into her arms, holding them in an embrace. The power of these photographs really can't be overestimated: The fear and stigma of AIDS remain enormous, and here's the future queen of England hugging and spending time with children affected by a condition that makes them pariahs. She looks relaxed and happy.

A reporter notes a moment when the princess holds out her finger for an eleven-month-old to grip: "As the boy looked up at her through big brown eyes, Gayle Alston, a nurse who works at the hospital, told him, 'I have brought her here specially to meet you.' Diana smiled but tears formed in her eyes."

*She's not afraid.* That's what the photos say to the millions of people around the world who see them in the papers and on TV the following day. *You don't need to be afraid. These children deserve support. They deserve recognition. They deserve dignity. They deserve to be held with love and kindness, just like any other child—just like anyone affected by AIDS.*

Diana understands the value of her celebrity. She knows that the newspapers and TV cameras follow her wherever she goes, and that her influence is far-reaching. She is well aware that most politicians, on either side of the Atlantic, have little interest in being photographed with people affected by AIDS. Her decision to align herself with people with AIDS plays a notable role in shifting public perception of the crisis—it helps to dismantle people's misplaced fears about the risk of contracting HIV through casual contact, and to demonstrate compassion in a time of fear.

## March 1989

Photographer Robert Mapplethorpe dies on March 9, 1989, at the age of forty-two, the latest of so many countercultural, subversive artists to be felled by AIDS. In particular, the New York art scene, centered in the lower reaches of Manhattan, has been decimated by the disease. We could just as well highlight May 6, 1982 (Hibiscus, age thirty-two), August 6, 1983 (Klaus Nomi, age thirty-nine), May 28, 1987 (Charles Ludlam, age forty-four), November 26, 1987 (Peter Hujar, age fifty-three), November 10, 1989 (Cookie Mueller, age forty), February 16, 1990 (Keith Haring, age thirty-one), March 10, 1990 (Tseng Kwong Chi, age thirty-nine), December 7, 1990 (Reinaldo Arenas, age forty-seven), July 22, 1992 (David Wojnarowicz, age thirty-seven), June 29, 1994 (Assotto Saint, age thirty-six), January 9, 1996 (Felix Gonzalez-Torres, age thirty-eight) . . . all fixtures of the New York City queer scene, and they are only representative of the many, many more who did not have the chance to leave as large a mark or create as big a lasting body of work.

## October 1989

After a meeting about people of color and AIDS called by the Office of Minority Health in the Department of Health and Human Services, a number of Asian and Pacific Islander (API) activists decide to form a new group, APICHA (Asian and Pacific Islander Coalition on HIV/AIDS), to offer support and a voice to those in their community. Along with Native American people with AIDS, API people with AIDS were largely overlooked in the discourse about the plague; even at conferences devoted to "minority" groups with AIDS, they were viewed as a minority within the minority.

Besides setting up workshops and working within the API community, APICHA partnered with Native American advocates to change the policies of the Centers for Disease Control. Until late 1989, the CDC lumped these groups together in the category of "Other" when tracking data on diseases. After meeting with the activists from these groups, the CDC agrees that "Asian/Pacific Islander" and "Alaskan Natives and American Indians" deserve to be their own categories. This leads to greater visibility for the impact of HIV/AIDS on these groups and further activism to make sure their voices are heard and needs are met.

## November 1989

> Good afternoon. My name is Ralph Hernandez. I am a Viet Nam vet. I am homeless, and I am living with AIDS. When I went to Nam, the government told me I was putting my life at risk for my country. I believed what they told me. And because I believed in my country, I became disabled and finally I got AIDS. Now that I am sick, my country doesn't want to do anything for me.

So begins Ralph Hernandez's testimony on November 2, 1989, to the National Commission on AIDS. Hernandez is a member of Anger into Direct Action (AIDA), a group formed in New York City by a number of homeless and formerly homeless people living with HIV/AIDS. They work with ACT UP and the Coalition for the Homeless to make vulnerable people aware of HIV and rally for greater awareness of the unique set of problems that homelessness and AIDS present.

The plights of HIV/AIDS and homelessness are intertwined. No safe place of shelter. No roof over your head. Park benches. Subway trains. By the late 1980s, activists in New York have realized they are dealing with an epidemic within an epidemic: homelessness and AIDS. Then as now, people experience homelessness for any number of reasons. Something goes wrong, and before you realize it, there is nowhere to go. It isn't unusual for queer kids to be rejected by their families and find themselves sleeping on the piers. People who use drugs can find themselves addicted to them, and as addiction takes control, they run out of money, out of options, cut adrift. It's a fact that everyone deserves safety, everyone deserves shelter, and you need both to heal. In the case of people living with HIV, homelessness only exacerbates their vulnerability, because homeless people are among the most vulnerable people in society.

It wasn't unusual in the 1980s for someone to be made homeless simply because they had HIV. People living with AIDS faced being unfairly and unlawfully evicted from their homes—it wasn't until the Fair Housing Amendments Act of 1988 that housing discrimination against people with disabilities, including people with HIV or AIDS, was prohibited—and even then, enforcement was far from complete. In cities both large and small, the rise of homelessness for people with HIV/AIDS put even more pressure on the limited services and charities that were trying to help the homeless population.

In November 1988, another AIDA member, Denise Walker, saw an advertisement for a research trial at a hospital in Harlem. You had to have a history of drug use and you had to consent to getting an HIV test, but if you met those criteria, they'd give you ten dollars. Her HIV test came back positive.

Two weeks after her diagnosis, something terrible happened:

> We lost our apartment where we were squatters for two years. The managers of the building knew we were there because we requested a lease and were told to wait for a court date. Finally, when we did get to court, we were thrown out of the place. We were willing to pay rent there but that was not to be. So we became members of that new, exclusive society, "the homeless."

Denise and her husband sought help through official channels but found themselves getting moved from shelter to shelter and hotel to hotel. City officials refused to provide them with steady housing, saying their health didn't meet the necessary criteria, despite Denise's multiple hospitalizations and poor health.

On November 28, Denise testifies to the New York City Council Select Committee on Homelessness and the Committee on Health about where the Division of AIDS Services (DAS) and the Medical Assistance Program (MAP) placed her:

> The place where they placed us took some getting used to. The kitchen and bathroom were out in the hall, you couldn't put your pot on the stove and go in your room because someone would go in it. The people in the room next door were constantly fighting or playing

their television at ear-splitting levels. The place was overrun with drugs. My husband and I separated for a few days and I went back to MAP to be rehoused and guess what? They placed me back in the SRO [single room occupancy hotel] that was supposedly no longer being used and, ironically, in the same room. We lost our belongings downtown, and are starting all over again.

Does MAP/DAS have any real policies or are they doing as they want? The way they can move you around or deny a person doesn't seem fair. I am ill and the stress is that last thing I need them to inflict on me. There has to be a better and easier way for people like myself to receive some assistance with less aggravation. I was told they had filed for my SSI [Supplemental Security Income, administered by the Social Security Administration]. I haven't heard anything yet. When I ask where to go, they give me all the misinformation possible. I think I will have to do it myself.

Ralph Hernandez served in the Vietnam War until he was honorably discharged after becoming disabled in the line of duty. When he came back to the United States, he brought another disability home with him: drug addiction. By the mid-1980s, his life was coming undone after years of trying to balance his job and family with his need to shoot up heroin. He lost his wife, his children, his apartment, and his job. The streets became his only option.

In front of the National Commission on AIDS, he testifies:

In 1987, I started getting sores on my skin and my physical appearance started deteriorating. I left my wife and started shooting up more and more. I felt too weak to go to work. Soon I lost my apartment and then my job. I tried to get into the VA hospital but they wouldn't see me because I was homeless. They wouldn't even let me into the detox program. They told me to just stop shooting....

I went to the Washington Heights Shelter. When I took my clothes off in the shower, the other homeless people kicked the shit out of me. Then they called the guards and the guards threw me out. I went to another shelter but I was afraid to stay there. So I started living in the tunnels under Grand Central Station. Even there I had to hide so no one would see the condition I was in.

Hernandez speaks of the stigma he felt, and of being emboldened by AIDA to fight against it:

I wish you knew how I feel when I go on the subway and see people move away from me. It's a fucked up feeling.

I served my country in time of crisis. Now that I'm in crisis, where is my country?

I am not the only one who has experienced this. There are thousands of homeless men and women with AIDS struggling to survive....

We are tired of being beaten up by other homeless people, who think they can protect themselves from AIDS by hurting us. We are tired of not being allowed in your shelters, of having to hide our illness to get in to them, and we are tired of being treated like dogs when you find out we are sick. We are tired of living in the streets and dirty hotels.

We demand housing for people with AIDS now. We demand adequate services for homeless people with AIDS now. We demand medical care and treatment for homeless people with AIDS now. We demand the right to live our lives with dignity. And we are turning our Anger into Direct Action.

ACT UP!
FIGHT BACK!
FIGHT AIDS!

By speaking about their experiences in public hearings, members of Anger into Direct Action refused to be shamed or silenced. Instead, they demanded change on behalf of the many others left on the streets by HIV/AIDS.

## July 1990

Congress passes the Americans with Disabilities Act (ADA), which gives federal civil rights protections to people with disabilities and guarantees equal opportunity for individuals with disabilities in public accommodation, employment, transportation, state and local government services, and telecommunications. People with HIV/AIDS are included as a category of individuals whose impairments prevent them from leading normal lives and doing normal activities, requiring employers, public businesses, and governments at all levels to make accommodations for those who are ill.

This groundbreaking law is still in effect, the bedrock for challenging discrimination against those with HIV/AIDS. The US government website gives the following examples of what is no longer allowed—all of which were all too plausible in 1990:

- An automobile manufacturing company has a blanket policy of refusing to hire anyone with HIV or AIDS.
- An airline extends an offer to a job applicant and then rescinds the offer after the employer discovers (during the post-offer physical) that the applicant has HIV.
- A university fires a physical education instructor after learning that the instructor's boyfriend has AIDS.
- A retail store generally rotates all sales associates between the sales floor (where they can earn commissions) and the stockroom (where they process merchandise) except for the sales associate who is rumored to have HIV, who is never rotated to the floor.
- A company contracts with an insurance company that has a cap on health insurance benefits provided to employees for HIV-related complications, but not on other health insurance benefits.
- A dentist categorically refuses to treat all persons with HIV or AIDS.
- A moving company refuses to move the belongings of a person who has AIDS, or refuses to move the belongings of a person whose neighbor has AIDS.

- A health club charges extra fees to persons who have HIV, prohibits members with HIV to use the steam room or sauna, or limits the hours during which members with HIV can use the club's facilities.
- A day-care center categorically refuses admission to children with HIV or the children of mothers with HIV.
- A funeral home refuses to provide funeral services for a person who dies from AIDS-related complications.
- A building owner refuses to lease space to a not-for-profit organization that provides services to persons with HIV or AIDS.
- A cosmetology school refuses to enroll a student once they learn that she has HIV.
- An overnight summer camp where children sleep in group cabins requires a camper with HIV to sleep in the camp infirmary.
- A pharmacy requires customers to stand in line to be served. A person with AIDS finds it too tiring to stand in line. It would be a reasonable modification of the pharmacy's procedures to allow the person to announce her presence and/or take a number and then sit down until her prescription is filled. It may also be a reasonable modification for the pharmacy to provide curbside service.
- A restaurant refuses to admit an individual with AIDS: This violates the ADA because HIV cannot be transmitted through the casual contact that occurs in a restaurant setting.
- A gynecologist refuses to treat a woman with HIV: Health care providers are required to treat all persons as if they have HIV or other blood-borne pathogens, and must use universal precautions (gloves, masks, and/or gowns where appropriate, etc.) to protect themselves from the transmission of infectious diseases. Failure to treat a person who discloses that she has HIV out of a fear of contracting HIV is a violation of the ADA, because so long as the physician utilizes universal precautions, it is generally safe to treat persons with HIV or AIDS.

As with all laws, the key to justice is enforcement, and often the burden is on the discriminated-against to call out the discrimination.

But at least now there is federal recourse, and an acknowledgment that people struggling with HIV and AIDS deserve the same level of accommodation as others who find they are living in a world that has not been designed for their health and needs.

## November 1990

The Housing Opportunities for Persons with AIDS (HOPWA) Act is passed as part of the Cranston-Gonzalez National Affordable Housing Act of 1990. The act gives communities resources and financial aid to provide housing assistance and support services for low-income people living with HIV and AIDS.

## March 1991

In the spring of 1991, a group of artists connected to the organization Visual AIDS meets up for a conversation. They want to create an easy symbol for people to show solidarity with people affected by HIV/AIDS. They settle on the idea of a ribbon, because ribbons are easy to make. They decide the ribbon should be red, because red is an attention-grabbing color. It is the color of blood, the color of love, and the color of anger.

The Red Ribbon Project is born.

The instructions are simple: *Cut the red ribbon to a six-inch length, then fold at the top into an inverted V shape. Use a safety pin to attach to clothing.* People get together to make ribbons by the hundreds and thousands, ready to be handed out for a charity donation on street corners. In New York City, Visual AIDS works with a shelter for homeless women, paying them a weekly fee for preparing ribbons, which has the added bonus of making a vulnerable population more aware of HIV/AIDS than they might be otherwise.

The red ribbon becomes widely known in June 1991, when Visual AIDS teams up with Broadway Cares and Equity Fights AIDS. These organizations support HIV+ people who work in the entertainment industries. Together, they make sure that as many people as possible at the forty-fifth Tony Awards wear a red ribbon, turning a mainstream televised awards ceremony into a sign of solidarity with everyone fighting HIV/AIDS. This sets the standard for many years of awards shows to come, with celebrities wearing red ribbons on the red carpet.

But it's not just celebrities.

*Make a donation, pin a red ribbon to your jacket.* Everyone who walks by you will know that you stand in solidarity with people affected by HIV/AIDS. Most people don't like being asked to think about HIV/AIDS. The red ribbon makes them think about it anyway.

The red ribbon (or "AIDS ribbon") is never copyrighted. This is deliberate: The artists who create it want to maximize its potential impact. In 1988, World AIDS Day was launched by the World Health Organization—making December 1 an annual day of AIDS awareness and reflection, emphasizing AIDS as a problem for the entire world. The red ribbon becomes a powerful symbol to mark this event, and remains so today.

## September 1991

On September 5, 1991, seven activists from the ACT UP offshoot TAG (Treatment Action Group) cover Senator Jesse Helms's house with a huge yellow condom.

Across the condom are these words: *A CONDOM TO STOP UNSAFE POLITICS. HELMS IS DEADLIER THAN A VIRUS.*

TAG leader Peter Staley would later write in *Poz* that they believed humor was one of the best weapons in an activist's arsenal. "If you can get folks laughing at your target's expense, you diminish his power. I wanted the country to have a good laugh at Helms' expense. . . . And I wanted Senator Helms to realize that his free ride was up—if he hit us again, we'd hit back."

The activists had the giant condom made from inflatable material—the same kind that would be used for an inflatable animal outside a car dealership. Funded by gay multimillionaire David Geffen, they choose a day they know Helms won't be at home and (after a practice run at a TAG member's house) make their move. All they need are the giant condom in a large duffel bag that Staley carries, a heavy portable generator, a long extension cord, two ladders, rubber mallets, plastic stakes, a very early portable phone, a small cold-air blower for the ground, and a large blower with a custom-built stand for the roof. Staley and another activist climb onto the roof of Helms's house, unroll the condom, and hook it up to be inflated. It takes seven minutes for the police to arrive . . . and in those seven minutes, reporters get plenty of pictures. (You can see video of the action on YouTube.)

Helms denounces the activists from the Senate floor . . . but he never manages to pass anti-AIDS legislation again.

The TAG activists are brought before the law . . . in the form of a parking ticket, for parking their truck in the wrong direction.

A virus doesn't know or care who you are. To it, you are just a collection of cells. You are not a person—you are a body. Your fame, your wealth, your status, your history—none of it matters.

But it does matter to other people who you are. Especially when it comes to caring about strangers.

Which is why in order for AIDS to be taken seriously as a threat, it had to strike some very famous people. Because of this, it landed on the front pages of newspapers around the world.

*I think sometimes we think, well, only gay people can get it—"It's not going to happen to me." And here I am saying that it can happen to anybody, even me. . . .*

# As the World Watched: Rock Hudson and Magic Johnson

What is the definition of a celebrity?

A celebrity is someone who can make the world pay attention.

And a celebrity who has an otherwise ignored disease?

Well, that celebrity can make the world pay attention to that disease, too. In ways that no ordinary person could ever do.

This is why it's impossible to talk about the history of AIDS without talking about Rock Hudson and Magic Johnson, two people who undeniably brought it to the world's attention.

When backed into a corner, Rock Hudson spoke his truth and, in doing so, changed the way the world perceived AIDS. His activism was voluntary, but only barely so—it wasn't until he was at death's door that he let the world understand who he truly was and what was happening to him.

During the late 1950s and early 1960s, Rock Hudson was one of the biggest stars in Hollywood, topping box-office charts and garnering an Oscar nomination. On-screen, he was the personification of the stereotype of a "man's man"—handsome, rugged, tall, charming. Whether in a light comedy or a heavy drama, he was a compelling romantic lead. Off-screen, gossip magazines found him to be a compelling romantic lead, too, telling their readers all about his loves and drama (much of it manufactured by the studios). Thousands of women a week wrote him fan letters, and he made it clear in interviews (also manufactured) that he adored being adored.

It was the performance of his life.

Hudson was born Roy Scherer and came to Hollywood right after a stint in the navy during World War II. There, a gay agent named Henry Willson spotted him and took him under his wing, changing his name ("Rock" for the Rock of Gibraltar, "Hudson" for the river in New York). As Rock's star rose, his personal life had to be pushed further into the shadows. He had longtime male partners and innumerable gay flings, but if even a whisper about them had hit the press, his career would have been over. So he lied. When one tabloid threatened to out him, a marriage was hastily arranged with Willson's secretary, Phyllis Gates. (And, for good measure, Willson sold out a lesser-known gay actor to the tabloid, so it would still have its lavender-scare headline.) The marriage didn't last, but the secrecy did—even after Hudson went from being a movie star to a TV star to a TV guest star. Post-Stonewall, Hudson still didn't want to jeopardize anything by being truthful. And, in fairness, it was also nobody's business but his own.

In 1984, this all changed. One of Hudson's friends noticed an irritation on Rock's neck. Rock had thought it was a pimple, but his doctor told him it was a KS lesion and that HIV/AIDS was the cause. Hudson continued to work, but it got harder and harder to maintain the secret of his diagnosis as he lost more and more weight and was ravaged by night sweats and other symptoms. He flew to Paris to get an experimental treatment, which worked at preventing the disease from growing worse . . . but only for a short time. When he returned to Paris in July 1985 for another treatment, he collapsed and was rushed to a hospital that did not ordinarily treat AIDS patients. There, he was told by the hospital: *If you do not announce your condition, we will have to.* So a press conference was arranged, and a French friend of Hudson's broke the news to the world:

> Mr. Rock Hudson has acquired immune deficiency syndrome diagnosed over a year ago in the United States. He came to Paris to consult a specialist. Prior to meeting the specialist he became very ill at the Ritz Hotel and his personal business manager Mark Miller advised him from California to enter the American hospital immediately.

Later, Hudson's friends would speculate: If he'd collapsed in Los Angeles and been taken to a hospital more sympathetic to Hollywood cover-ups, the true nature of his disease might have never been known. But once the news was out, Hudson did not shy away from it. He allowed his name to be used to rally people to the cause of finding a cure. And while at first his suffering did not demonstrably change the mind of his old friend Ronald Reagan (who called him in the Paris hospital to wish him well), the Reagan administration *did* increase its spending on AIDS shortly after Hudson's announcement. And friends of Hudson's—most notably Elizabeth Taylor—used his sickness and death to galvanize other celebrities to use their celebrity to put a spotlight on the disease. Said comedian Joan Rivers, "Two years ago, when I hosted a benefit for AIDS, I couldn't get one major star to turn out. I received death threats and hate mail." But now things were different.

Proclaimed *People* magazine, "In the aftermath of Hudson's announcement, AIDS is no longer an underground, underreported disease." As gay author Michael Kearns told the magazine, "Now everybody knows someone who has AIDS."

Hudson's revelation—and his refusal to shy away from it once it was public—made him an instant role model for many gay men, but his emergence as the best-known person to die because of AIDS made him a tragic trailblazer. As Ron Najman, the media director of the National Gay Task Force, pointed out at the time, there was something very wrong with the American health care system when someone as wealthy and connected as Hudson had to fly to Europe for treatment.

Fame and riches couldn't help Rock Hudson—he died on October 2, 1985, a year and a half after his diagnosis. But fame and riches *did* help elevate the profile of AIDS in the public consciousness, setting the stage for a lot of the activism—particularly Hollywood activism—that followed. Celebrities like Elizabeth Taylor and Elton John were galvanized to plunge loudly into the fight, and soon one of the most visible symbols of support for AIDS research was the red ribbon worn at awards ceremonies. (Taylor later told *Vanity Fair* that she decided, "I could take the fame I'd resented and tried to get away from for so many years and use it to do some good. I wanted to retire, but the tabloids wouldn't let me. So I thought, If you're going to screw me over, I'll use you.")

There was, however, a double standard in the elevation of Rock Hudson as Hollywood's most notable AIDS casualty. One of the reasons he was such an effective symbol was that he had appeared so *straight* to millions of moviegoers. When more queer-perceived celebrities like Liberace and Freddie Mercury died, it didn't hit as close to home for straight America as Rock Hudson's death did.

Even if Rock Hudson was seen as the straightest of romantic leads by America, he was still in the queer-perceived world of acting. But the world of sports? Nothing in America is more coded as straight. So to have a genuine sports legend announce he was HIV+? That was a game-changing revelation.

Earvin Johnson Jr. was born in 1959 in Lansing, Michigan, to an assembly-line worker and a school janitor. He devoted himself to basketball at an early age and was only fifteen when a sportswriter dubbed him "Magic"—a nickname that would stick with him for the rest of his life. He went on to play for Michigan State and, in what was then the most-watched college basketball game of all time, took the team to the championships in 1979. Later that year, he joined the NBA, taking his place on the Los Angeles Lakers. There, he became one of the most accomplished, famous basketball players in the sport's history—in the following twelve seasons, he scored over 17,000 points and led the Lakers to the national championships five times. He was an idol, not only on the court but in commercials and on talk shows. Everyone knew him.

The reaction to his press conference on November 7, 1991, was seismic. In front of the whole world, he announced his HIV status, saying, "I think sometimes we think, well, only gay people can get it—'It's not going to happen to me.' And here I am saying that it can happen to anybody, even me, Magic Johnson." He vowed, "Life is going to go on for me, and I'm going to be a happy man. When your back is against the wall, you have to come out swinging. I'm going to go on, going to be there, going to have fun."

According to the Associated Press, "The day after he told the world, people talked and cried and thought about little else." Calls to testing centers doubled that day, and almost overnight an important truth was brought home to many Americans: HIV did not happen only to white gay men, but also to Black men and straight men.

As one Lakers fan who headed to the team's arena after the announcement told *The New York Times,* "I came here because I was shocked when I heard about it. I wanted to actually see if it was true. It's still hard to believe. Magic Johnson, of all people. He's the last person I would expect to be HIV-positive." Anthony Fauci later said it "really jolted people into a much more empathetic view towards people who were living with HIV."

In his announcement, Johnson promised to become a spokesperson for people with HIV/AIDS and also said that he would retire from basketball. Only one of these two things ended up being true.

Within three months, Johnson was back on the court at the NBA's All-Star Game, scoring so well that he was named its MVP. Then, in the summer of 1992, he was part of the USA Dream Team that won gold at the Summer Olympics. Finally, in September 1992, he announced he was rejoining the Lakers, although he ended up not playing in the regular season, in no small part because of pushback from players on other teams who were afraid to play against someone HIV+. After a stint coaching, he officially returned in January 1996, then retired on his own terms after that season was done. He would later find great success in the business world, owning a billion-dollar investment firm as well as shares in the Los Angeles Dodgers and Sparks teams.

Meanwhile, as promised, he became one of the most vocal proponents for people with HIV/AIDS in the world. Not only did he raise millions of dollars for research, but he also continued to spread the message: If I can have this, you can too. Finding a cure was everyone's responsibility, and he was willing to lead the charge—speaking nationally and internationally to raise awareness and fight stigma. He was candid that he was likely to have contracted the virus because he'd had unprotected sex with a number of female partners, and he used that candidness to encourage safer practices in others. At the same time, he did not distance himself at all from the gay and bisexual people who were also fighting the disease. (Still, it cannot be denied that Johnson's straightness was essential to the way he was embraced by the general public; had he also come out as gay, it is highly unlikely at that time that the public's sympathetic reaction and his subsequent positions of authority would have been the same.)

Within days of his announcement, Johnson was asked to join the National Commission on AIDS. Ten months later, he resigned with a letter to President George H. W. Bush that did not hold back. "I cannot in good conscience continue to serve on a commission whose important work is so utterly ignored by your administration," Johnson wrote, weeks before Election Day in 1992. "Mr. President, when we met in January I gave you a letter in which I expressed my hope that you would become more actively involved in the fight against AIDS. No matter how good the team may be, I said, it won't win the championship without the owner fully in the game. I am disappointed that you have dropped the ball, and that your administration is not doing everything that it must to fight this disease."

Johnson's mastery of advocacy didn't just come from the grand scale of celebrity. Instead, he understood that he was most effective on a human level—closing the distance between himself and everyone else, rather than maintaining his elevation. "I did become the kind of spokesman I wanted to be," Johnson said, citing in particular a program he did for kids on Nickelodeon in 1992 called *Conversations with Magic*. During the program, he spoke to kids about HIV and AIDS, including two who were born HIV+. One of them, Hydeia Broadbent, would grow up to be an AIDS activist herself. But in 1992, she was a seven-year-old sobbing out her truth to a sports idol who was more than willing to listen.

"I want people to know that we're just normal people," Hydeia told Magic, rubbing her eyes and starting to cry.

"You don't have to cry," he told her, leaning in and touching her back in consolation and solidarity. "Because we are normal people, okay? We are."

SOURCE MATERIAL

# A Little Magic and a Lot of Faith

by Patricia Eldridge

*Patricia Eldridge was thirty-four years old and her son was ten when she wrote this essay for* Fingernails Across the Chalkboard. *She worked in the HIV/AIDS support ministry at Trinity United Church of Christ in Chicago.*

I could tell the time was coming, the time when I would tell my son my HIV status. Many times over the years, I struggled with whether or not I should tell him I was HIV positive, or what to say. Because I never had peace about the decision, I simply tabled it for another time. In the meantime, however, I did begin to build my foundation. I had always told my son to be careful with people's blood, especially Mommy's. I told him blood was dirty and it could carry germs that could make him sick.

I also talked to him about Magic Johnson. My son loves basketball and he knows all the great players, past and present. Magic has always been one of his favorites. Magic has also always been one of mine, ever since the time of short shorts, long socks, and big afros. I loved Magic. He was my hero. Now he is my hero in another arena as well. I used him as my building block in talking to my son about HIV.

The innocence of a child is so amazing. They don't come with preconceived notions about diseases. They don't have irrational fears and attitudes. They aren't judgmental. When I talked to my son about Magic, he was concerned and sounded sorry to hear that some people had treated him badly because he was HIV positive. I told him how AIDS kills a lot of people, but luckily, we have some medicines that help some people like Magic to stay healthier. Periodically I would find ways to revisit this conversation. I wanted to be sure he knew the facts about HIV. How you get it and how you don't. In addition, we talked about the stigma and the way some people felt about it.

I say I knew the time was approaching because I felt it in my spirit. Over a period of two weeks several people, all of whom did not know each other, asked me out of the blue when I was going to tell my son. I began to think about that question seriously and considered how and what to tell him.

It wasn't 100 percent clear to me until a situation arose that made me realize by not telling my story it was costing people their lives. By not sharing my experience and knowledge I was denying others real lifesaving information they needed. Granted, we all have some basic facts about HIV/AIDS. However until you put a face to it, a familiar face, a healthy face, it is surreal.

During this time, I went with a friend of mine to get tested. She found out the man she was dating was HIV positive. He had not told her, much like the person who had infected me. I told her my story and encouraged her to get tested. By the Grace of God, she was fine. I was able to see, in an intimate way, how important it was for me to share my experience with others. I knew in order to speak out I had to tell my son first. I didn't want to have someone else to tell my son my status before I did.

*2 Timothy 1:6-7: Hence I remind you to rekindle the gift of God that is within you through the laying on of my hands; for God did not give us the spirit of fear but a spirit of power and love and sound mind.*

I went to the Youth Pastor at my church for counseling. I was an emotional wreck and didn't know how I could do this. God told me to weave a net of support, and that He would not let my son fall. I began by calling everyone who knew my status to tell them I was preparing to tell my son. I asked them if I could count on them to support him. I wanted to see if they could offer him a safe place to come and talk about his feelings and ask questions if needed. Of course, they all said yes.

When I went to speak to the Youth Pastor, I didn't know what to expect. As we talked, I gained a new sense of peace. I came to realize that in telling my son now, he would be able to see my walk of faith. I realized that is what was important to me. I wanted him to understand the faith that has brought me, us, this far. I don't know if I will ever develop AIDS or if AIDS will kill me. But I do know that God has done many miracles in my life and He continues to do so. My Youth Pastor offered to be there when I told my son. I thanked him and considered his offer. I decided that in my situation I wanted to tell my son in a very casual atmosphere.

My son and I talk quite a bit on a regular basis to each other and have a strong relationship. I wanted him to feel comfortable in the space we were in for him to be able to react. I knew he might have lots of questions and would be worried about me dying. He asked me about death when he was younger. I told him no one knows when they are going to die, and we live here on earth until God feels that our job is finished. I was prepared to revisit this conversation.

I sat down on the carpet for a game of cards. After a few rounds, I began the conversation by talking about Magic. After my stuttering a few times, my wise 8-year-old son asked me.

"Mom, what are you trying to say?"

I took a deep breath. "You remember what I told you about Magic Johnson and HIV?"

"Yes." He answered.

"And about how HIV can cause AIDS and many people can die from that?"

"Yes."

"But there are medications people take in order to help keep them healthy like Magic Johnson. Do you remember how I told you some people treat Magic when they found out he had HIV because they were afraid of HIV?"

"Yes."

"I just wanted to tell you that I also have HIV, like Magic."

He sat there thinking about what I had just said before finally asking if he had HIV as well. I told him that he didn't. I explained to him how I had to take medicine while I was pregnant and how God had protected him. "That is why I am always telling you what a miracle you are."

"Oh," he answered and trailed back into thought. After a moment of silence he sat down in my lap, put his arms around my neck in order to give me a big hug and said, "I don't care if you have HIV, because I love you!"

Without these three ingredients: power, love, and a sound mind, I would have never been able to tell my son I was HIV positive. I had been preparing him for a long time, and I had been preparing myself. I have learned to weather the elements, but I wanted to protect him. I wanted him to know the miracles that God has performed in both of our lives. I wanted him to see the goodness of God and that He is real. God spared my son's life when he was born and he saved it when he was baptized. I have seen God's spirit in my son in the bravery he has shown. When I told him I had HIV, he climbed up into my lap, hugged me and told me he didn't care if I had HIV. That was love. When I had a conversation with him later and told him I felt I had been called to speak about HIV, I put forth some hard questions to him. I asked if it would hurt his feelings if people didn't want to play with him, or if they told him I was going to die soon? He answered quite honestly and said yes. That is sound mind. In my fear and natural instinct to want to protect my son, I asked if it was still okay if I went and did speaking engagements on HIV where I would reveal my status. His response? "Yes because they need to know! They need to know not to be scared!" That is power.

A few months later, I took him to a church to see Magic Johnson speak. I asked Magic to tell us how he told his children he was positive and ended up recounting my story. My son got to hug his hero and mine that day. It is a moment I will never forget, neither will he. As a matter of fact, he said he was going to write his autobiography starting at that moment.

## Pedro Zamora and the New Reality

Travel back for a moment to 1994.

You have never seen a young gay man with AIDS on TV before. If you've seen people with HIV at all, it's been on the news, and they've been dying horrible deaths. You're not supposed to make any connection with them—they pass in and out of your life in a matter of minutes. Yes, there have been TV movies and after-school specials about AIDS, but in those, the HIV+ people (almost all white, almost all men) have been played by actors. Healthy actors. It's not the same as reality. It doesn't have the same impact.

Then along comes season three of *The Real World*.

In 1994, "reality TV" is still a new concept, and *The Real World* is leading the way. The concept is simple: Force six or seven (mostly attractive) young people to live in a house together, and film the explosions that occur. It's more addictive than any soap opera. And it also happens to be a perfect platform for a young activist.

Enter: Pedro Zamora.

Pedro was born in Cuba in 1972. His family of nine lived in poverty; his father was not a fan of the Cuban government.

At age eight, Pedro, with his parents and one of his sisters, made a perilous journey to Miami, part of a mass exodus fleeing the Castro regime. Because these emigrants fled from Mariel Harbor in Cuba, they were known as "Marielitos," arriving in Florida with little to nothing. In Pedro's case, his parents left behind five of his brothers and sisters in order to make the journey.

When he was thirteen, Pedro's mother died of skin cancer. She would never know her son was gay. Pedro himself had an idea by that time of who he was and what he liked, and as he got older, he began to act on his identity. By the time he was in high school, at the top of his class, he'd had many sexual partners, often older than him. Even though he knew what AIDS was, he hadn't made any connection between his own identity and his risk of becoming HIV+. He thought it was only sex workers and drug users who got AIDS, not honors students like him.

As a high school senior, Pedro decided to donate blood as part of a Red Cross drive—mostly, he later said, so he could get out of class. It was by then standard procedure for all blood to be screened for HIV ... and Pedro was notified a few days later that his tests had come back as "reactive." He tested again and discovered he was HIV+. He wondered if he'd live long enough to graduate.

Instead of trying to keep his status a secret, Pedro told his family, who were supportive, and joined a local HIV/AIDS organization. Inspired by the people there, he decided to become an AIDS educator and soon was educating far beyond his home state. He went to schools across the country, went on popular talk shows like *Oprah*, and in 1993 testified before Congress.

> There is not one second of my day that I am not aware that I am HIV-positive. I don't want to forget that I have AIDS, and I don't want you to forget that I have AIDS. You have to understand AIDS is part of my life. It's my reality. It's who I am.
> —Pedro Zamora, congressional testimony, July 12, 1993

He would go from school to school, telling students who weren't getting any sex education the truth about safer sex, getting them to listen because he admitted to them that he had contracted AIDS from unsafe sex and was likely to die before he was thirty. They often listened, but touring around the country was taking its toll on Pedro. (Remember, there were still no good treatments for HIV/AIDS in 1994.) His roommate at the time suggested that he audition for a slot on *The Real World*.

That way he could educate all of America without having to visit all of America. He decided to do it, and out of over 25,000 applicants, he was chosen for the San Francisco edition.

Viewers who tuned in to the first episode of the third season had no idea what they were in for. They were about to meet a Cuban American HIV+ gay man who wanted to get his message across to as many people as he could before he died.

> MTV is pushing the limits by bringing in a gay person and especially a person with AIDS, which is part of why I did it. . . . Even growing up, I never had anybody on TV like, "Oh, he's a gay man like me. I can relate to him."
> —Pedro Zamora to *Entertainment Tonight,* June 1994

What was it like, for a young gay man coming into his own sexuality, to watch Pedro on *The Real World* in 1994, as episodes rolled out week by week?

For many Americans, it was astonishing to see someone with AIDS who was so full of life, who seemed so much like a friend you'd want to have. He was handsome and sexy, but that wasn't the sole source of attraction. He was also smart and vulnerable and dedicated to speaking his truth. In a house full of self-centered twentysomething people, he had clearly centered himself on a much larger calling. He struggled with his health, and viewers got to see his doctor's visits, even when there was bad news. But as important as his status was, the show was much more interested in the relationships that he formed.

At the start, viewers sensed there was going to be trouble with Rachel, who was conservative and Catholic. But Pedro didn't treat her as a potential enemy, and instead approached her as a potential friend, explaining to her that she wouldn't "catch AIDS" just from being in his presence, explaining to her not only how his disease worked but also how his life and his heart worked. Like most viewers, she was won over.

The antagonist turned out to be Puck, a straight, white, obnoxious bike messenger who liked to be disliked by everyone. He especially seemed keen on being homophobic toward Pedro. As a viewer, you'd start to worry every time they were in a room together. Pedro worried too, and about halfway through the season, he told the other house members that he was probably going to have to leave, because Puck's attacks were taking their toll, using up energy that Pedro didn't have to spare.

Then the most incredible thing happened: The other house members got together and decided to kick Puck out of the house. Puck was clearly the show's breakout star, its biggest personality. Would MTV really let that happen? And was it possible that all these other straight people would take Pedro's side over Puck's, without Pedro even having to ask?

Remarkably, Puck was voted off, on a show where you weren't supposed to be able to vote someone off. And MTV allowed it.

Then there was Sean. Sean Sasser, whom Pedro had met in DC at a big gay march in 1993. They started dating while Pedro was on the show, and it became very serious, very fast.

> It was hard for me sexually beyond the physical level. Emotionally it was just not there. I'm still dealing with it. Sean is the first person who I've been able to break through with. When I look at him, I feel an equal level of power. From our second date, I felt no barriers. I felt understanding. I felt safe. I was able to be vulnerable with him, because, for the first time, someone was vulnerable with me.
> —Pedro Zamora, *Poz* magazine, August 1, 1994

Not only was this a gay love story told in real time, but it was between two BIPOC gay men, who were allowed to kiss and flirt and be worried in front of our eyes. On the second-to-last episode, they had a marriage ceremony, even though it was illegal at the time. It was the first same-sex wedding ever broadcast on TV.

A happy reason to cry.

Followed by less happy reasons to cry.

The *Real World* season concluded with Pedro and Sean together, and the other house members vowing to be with Pedro as friends for life, especially Judd and Pam (who would later get married themselves).

After the filming ended in June of 1994, Pedro aimed to resume his travels as an AIDS educator. But soon he was too sick to travel, with Judd often taking his place. Pedro was admitted to St. Vincent's Hospital in New York, where it was discovered that he had toxoplasmosis (a parasitic brain infection) and also a viral inflammation of the brain. Episode after episode continued to air, with viewers not knowing how close to death Pedro had since become.

He died on November 11, 1994, a few hours after the season finale aired. He was twenty-two.

President Clinton summed it up nicely for many of us when, in remarks for Pedro's memorial service, he said, "No one in America can say they've never known someone who's living with AIDS."

> As gay young people, we are marginalized. As young people who are HIV-positive and have AIDS, we are totally written off.
> —Pedro Zamora

> We will never know how many lives he saved as he struggled to deal with his own illness, but they will be his lasting contribution to all of us.
> —Governor Lawton Chiles of Florida

> My greatest challenge in life has been to become an entire person. We fragment people, especially minorities, because we assume it's easier to deal with specific problems if we compartmentalize behavior. Well, I could deal with the fact that I was gay. I could deal with my being a Latino man in America. I could deal with having been sexually abused as a kid. And I could deal with having HIV and

AIDS. But I couldn't deal with them together at the same time. And you have to if you ever want to become a whole person.

Go seeking services and you'll see the compartmentalization in action. But if you can't deal with my having been sexually abused then it's going to be impossible to deal with and understand my HIV because—guess what?—they are connected. And if I'm struggling to be a whole person, and I'm fairly well-informed, how hard must it be for others? No wonder we're also struggling to be a whole community. We're not and won't be until we accept the diversity that is going on.
—Pedro Zamora, *Poz* magazine, August 1, 1994

My life is being threatened every day. I'm dealing with AIDS, so I know I can deal with anything.
—Pedro Zamora, at the end of the *Poz* magazine interview, weeks before he entered the hospital for the final time

At the age of seventeen, Pedro was given what he knew was a death sentence. And what did he decide to do with his one wild and precious life? He decided to get his truth out to as many people as possible, in any way possible. There is a poignant moment in the *Poz* interview when he says, "When I started doing AIDS education, I made myself a promise that there would be a point where I was going to quit and focus on me and take care of myself and do what I really want to do. I think I'm now at that point, and I've discovered that I really don't know what I want to do." The disease took the answer away from him, because soon he was in St. Vincent's Hospital, battling the brain infections that would cost him his life. But in many ways, the disease also gave him an answer, because his impact went far beyond his living years. He died too soon, but his honesty and his willingness to use reality TV to spread the reality of living with AIDS made many other people appreciate their own wild and precious lives a little more.

## What We Lost

I [David] think about them as the missing pieces of the generation before mine, and I think about them all the time.

It is impossible to tally what all the lives cut short would have added to our world if they'd been able to last longer. And because AIDS impacted the creative community so greatly, it's impossible to know what novels went unwritten, what canvases went unpainted, what dances went unchoreographed, what songs went unsung, what stories went untold, in any form. Just when queer people, especially gay men, were liberated to tell their stories in the years after Stonewall, so many of their lives were silenced.

This is why I want to pause here. Because while it is important to discuss and acknowledge Rock Hudson, Freddie Mercury, Eazy-E, Keith Haring, Rudolf Nureyev, Pedro Zamora, Fela Kuti, Robert Mapplethorpe, Marlon Riggs, Paul Monette, and others who attained greatness in their fields before AIDS ended their lives, it is also important to discuss and acknowledge the tens of thousands (if not hundreds of thousands) of other creators who weren't allowed to leave as much of a mark. I have always felt my job is to catch as many of them as I can—to read, listen to, and watch as many of their works as I can, and then to pass word of those works on. As an author, I am often asked who my forebears are, who my mentors were. The reality is, in the world of queer YA literature, where most of my work resides, I didn't have many predecessors, especially out gay male predecessors. This isn't just because of the closet, or because the notion of writing a queer YA novel was so unheard of. The reality is that in the 1980s and 1990s, gay male writers had many other things to face, many other urgent stories to tell if they had the strength or time to tell them. Writing a YA novel was not a priority. Surviving was a priority.

In a collection entitled *Loss Within Loss,* in which writers talk about friends who died and the work they will never be able to create, the novelist Benjamin Taylor observes:

> This subtraction of wit, grace, brains, and beauty from our midst has now become unbearable to contemplate. How is it we haven't, in compassionate horror, pulled the earth up over us? How is it we who are spared have gone on creating, laughing, renewing ourselves with love? Is the appetite for life simply too great, greater than our accumulated griefs? And what, for their part, do the lost travelers under the hill think of us? Do they applaud our flinty resilience? When they come back to us in dreams—at least in mine—it is usually to say that, yes, they do.

These are our ghosts. We must take care of them.

Every year from 1991 to 1997, *Entertainment Weekly* magazine would run a list of people in the entertainment industry who had died because of AIDS. The lists were long and wide, with familiar names beside those of people who'd stayed steadfastly behind the scenes. It was a brutal toll, bringing home how queer creators are so central to the arts of our times, and how devastating it is to the arts when we are wiped out on such a grand scale.

I would love nothing more than to stitch together all those lists and go through them name by name with you, to convey the scope of what was lost, in all fields, on all levels. But that is probably a different book—and you can find the lists online, to look at in your own time, with your own thoughts. What I'm going to do is take one of the names from 1992 and tell you a little about him. He isn't any more representative of the list than anyone else would be—he just happens to be a performer I got to see for one brief, shining moment, and whose voice continues to run through my life.

\* \* \*

It is here that I must digress for a moment and confess to you my irrational, remarkable love for the musical *Chess*. For those of you who aren't familiar (and I would have assumed most of you weren't, until a new Broadway revival was announced), *Chess* is about an American chess player, a Russian chess player, and the woman who is in love with the former but falls for the latter during a big Cold War chess match. The Russian defects. The woman's affections defect. But it isn't so easy to start dating against a backdrop of geopolitical warfare. The music, by the guys from ABBA, is fantastic. The story, however, only occasionally makes sense, which is why the composers and lyricist have been tinkering with it for over thirty years to get it right. The key here is that at the end of the first act, the Russian chess player is given a song, "Anthem," in which he sings about his inner conflict as he leaves his precious home behind in order to reach for freedom and love. It's an astonishing song; when performed well, it is one of the most powerful things I have seen on a stage.

On Broadway, *Chess* ran for only sixty-eight performances. I saw one of those performances.

The important thing here is: The Russian chess player was played by an actor named David Carroll, and his rendition of "Anthem" still gives me chills.

It was not his first Broadway show. He'd played minor parts in major shows and major parts in minor shows before. But this was his breakthrough, and he gave it his all. Even though the show was a flop, he earned a Tony nomination. Because this was the pre-internet era, all I knew about him then was what it said in *Playbill* about his previous credits.

Two years later, Carroll was in a much more successful musical, *Grand Hotel*. He received rave reviews and scored another Tony nomination. But after only a few months, he had to leave the show, only to come back six months later. Even in a legendarily liberal place like Broadway, the reasons were kept a secret. But it's easy enough to read between the lines when you read interviews with Carroll from that time, like the quotes in this "Goings On About Town" piece from *The New Yorker*:

> On December 3, Mr. Carroll will check back into "Grand Hotel," after a six-month absence from his role as the Baron Felix Von Gaigern. He won't be the same impoverished aristocrat, however. For one thing, the mustache he previously sported for the part will be gone. "It got me pneumonia," he joked to us pluckily the other day, referring to the illness that caused him to bow out of the show last spring....
> 
> Is Mr. Carroll back in touch yet with the physical rigors of "Grand Hotel"? "It's funny," he replies. "So much has been made of the Baron's derring-do, of his death-defying leap into space. But climbing the set's monkey bars is nothing like having to hit a high A at the end of a song every night."

Or the next week, in a *TheaterWeek* interview:

> Carroll's sudden illness caused concern in the theatrical community. "It was strange timing," he says, "nothing that I planned on." But he prefers not to discuss it. "I think it's pretty boring when people talk about their health. Let's talk about my career, shall we?"

One of Carroll's costars, the Tony winner Michael Jeter, was also HIV+. In 1998, Jeter would tell *Poz* magazine, "The irony was, I was playing a man who was dying, and the star of the show, David Carroll, really was dying." Jeter only found out that Carroll had AIDS when he saw a bottle of AZT in Carroll's hotel room when they were doing their out-of-town tryout in Boston. "I saw the bottle and just burst into tears," he said. "David made me vow not to tell a soul. And I didn't."

To me, the incredible thing is that Carroll returned to *Grand Hotel* and, by all accounts, found wells of energy to perform a dance-and-song-heavy role night after night. *Death-defying,* in his words. It wore him down, though. Because of contractual disputes, it took two years for the *Grand Hotel* cast album to be recorded. Even though he was very sick, Carroll insisted he was up to the task. He went in and collapsed during his first song. He died that day in the recording studio. He was forty-one years old.

It would be nice to be able to take the cheery route and say, *Well, at least he died doing what he loved.* But really—what an awful way to die. How cruel to be so close to what you once could do, and then to not be able to do it. That is the story of those who were lost in those early years of AIDS: to have a sense of your talent, a sense of your potential, and then to watch as the forces in your body extinguish it all.

The only solace I can get—and it's a deeply imperfect solace—is that there was no way we could have known in 1992 the multiplicity of ways that art could live on. Even if we've lost all the songs David Carroll never got to sing, we at least have a hold of more songs than we might have expected to keep, and we can watch them on YouTube or stream them online. As I've written this, I've put on grainy footage of *Chess,* less grainy footage of Carroll in *Grand Hotel,* during the Macy's Thanksgiving Day Parade, and on *The Phil Donahue Show.* There's even a clip of him acting on *Another World,* a soap opera. It isn't much, and for every performance captured there are dozens that are gone. But it's something. It can continue the conversation I'm having with this particular ghost.

Art lives on, but it always, always needs help living on. This won't make up for the art the artists never got to create. It won't mean that we'll get to know these artists as people, or bring them back in the same way their loved ones' memories bring them back. It is not enough to see their names on a roll call of the dead. Let's talk about what they made, shall we?

It sounds almost too simple, but I have to believe it's true: The way to prevent those who were lost from being completely lost is to go out and find them. For me, this means listening to the Broadway cast album of *Chess.* And flipping through books of Peter Hujar's photos.

And reading Essex Hemphill's poetry. And breaking out my videotapes to watch a series I loved called *A Year in the Life,* which lasted only a year itself, where Sarah Jessica Parker's husband was played by another David, David Oliver, who died five years later at the age of thirty.

And so on, and so on.

It's impossible to remember them all. But there are enough of us to try.

# Deaths in the Neighborhood

For gay men in America, San Francisco was supposed to be the promised land—the place where you could live and love freely, where people came from far and wide to be part of an actual gay *community.* When AIDS hit, it hit hard, decimating the foundation of the community as it took life after life after life.

The *Bay Area Reporter* was the local paper of the San Francisco queer community. And so every week, when a new issue came out, people would open its pages warily, knowing it was likely that they'd find someone they knew in the obituary section, which was forthrightly called DEATHS. It could be a friend or neighbor they hadn't seen in a while. It could be someone they'd dated or hooked up with. It could be a DJ from a club they went to, a waiter from a local restaurant, a volunteer at a local clinic, or someone behind the scenes—a cook, a city planner, a mechanic—they'd never met. The obituaries were the way to keep track of who was still around and who was gone.

To read these obituaries is to get glimpses into the lives these men lived—what they did, how they acted, the people they loved, the people who loved them back. It is not an entirely representative sample—in order to have your obituary in the paper, you had to have someone who loved you enough to encapsulate your life and share it with the neighborhood. Most other newspapers avoided mentioning AIDS in their obituaries. Families were too ashamed to name the cause of death and editors weren't keen to print it. The *Bay Area Reporter* obituaries are notable for their honesty as well as their affection.

These are obituaries from a single month—January 1990, the start of a new decade. Individually and collectively, they give you a sense of what was lost.

## Booker Tyrone Benjamin
### Aug. 24, 1953 - Nov. 23, 1989

Tyrone, as he was known by his family and many friends, passed away peacefully, Thanksgiving Day at San Francisco Kaiser Hospital after a long and painful battle with K.S.

Despite being bedridden the last three months of his life with unrelenting pain, he never lost his tremendous love and zest for life. He frequently told his lover, "Joe, it's gonna be alright."

Those who knew him well would say it was like Tyrone to die on one of his country's most important holidays.

Tyrone was a native of San Francisco. He graduated from Balboa High School in 1971 and attended San Francisco City College. He worked for several years in the service of the city he loved so dearly. He last worked for the S.F. City and County Assessor's office where he made many friends.

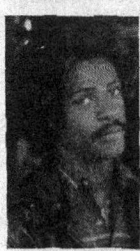

He will be remembered by many for his honesty and out of the closet lifestyle.

Tyrone was a man with artistic and creative ability for fashion design. His fashion designs were seen in many of San Francisco's early Gay Day parades.

He was a man who cared little for the politics and bullshit of life. His interests were family, friends, parties, good times, fashion, loving, caring, giving, cartoons and teddy bears.

Left to cherish his memory are his lover of three years, Joe; his father, Booker; four brothers, Ernie, David, Jonathan and Joseph, all of the Bay Area, and a host of other relatives and eternal friends.

"Biddy," you are missed. ▼

## Cody Jon Vurgason
### Dec. 17, 1959 - Dec. 24, 1989

Cody moved to San Francisco in July 1984 and soon became involved with Shanti project.

He was named site coordinator and was critically involved in the major undertaking of finding new quarters, remodeling and moving Shanti to 525 Howard St.

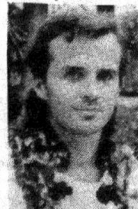

He was proud to be a friend of Jim Geary and Jess Randall, and helped in the vital role Shanti played by training volunteers, while giving his love and support to all who needed it.

Cody then worked as a home nurse for VNA Hospice before joining the staff of Operation Concern in 1987 as a counselor, working there until fall 1989 when he became too ill to continue.

During this period he was enrolled in the graduate nursing program at San Francisco State University, working toward his master's degree.

He loved the outdoors, and was especially comfortable at Wildwood where he often served as staff nurse for PWA weekend retreats.

He ended his 27-month battle with AIDS gently in the early morning hours, cuddling his favorite teddy bear, surrounded by his lover, David Fagundes, his wonderful parents, Tom and Frances Vurgason, and his beloved best friend, Danny Johnson.

This special, beautiful man is also survived by his sister, Vickie, and brothers Scott, Alex, Gary and Tom. He will live forever in all their hearts and in the hearts of his many friends who loved him. So long, Codycakes, we'll always love you.

Memorial service and party pending. Call 861-3637 or 648-8847 for details. ▼

## Bill Henderson "William Bear"
### Dec. 10, 1951 - Nov. 8, 1989

Bear died in his home Nov. 8, two and a half years after he was diagnosed with AIDS. He was born and raised in Kansas (he sometimes called himself Prudence of the Plains). He earned a B.A. in English from Phillips University in Enid, Okla., and a master in theatre arts from Fort Hays State College in Hays, Kansas.

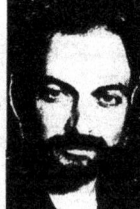

In 1973 he moved to the Bay Area, spending most of that time in San Francisco. In the early '80s he served as a guest instructor at San Francisco State University in the Theatre Arts Department.

An accomplished performer, he was a veteran of more than 30 productions, counting among his favorite roles Littlechap in *Stop the World, I Want to Get Off*, Lucky in *Dames at Sea*, and the Red Queen in *Alice*. In the late 1970s, he toured in the scandalous *Let My People Come*. Perhaps his most notable role was in the highly successful 1984-85 production of *Side by Side by Sondheim* at the Plush Room.

Bear was a wild amalgamation of warmth, irascibility, generosity, sardonic humor, hedonism, sanity and courage. His talent and friendship will be missed by all those who knew and loved him. ▼

## J.D.
### Jan. 10, 1958 - Dec. 1, 1989

All I have to say is: Goodbye and I'll love you forever.  —Kurtie ▼

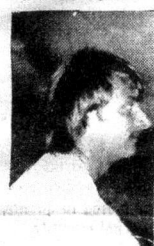

## Jay Adrian

On Dec. 18 Jay quietly and peacefully left this Earth, as his lover Burt was holding his hand.

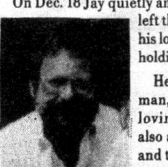

He was a gentle man, sweet and loving. He was also a hell-raiser, and that was also part of his charm. He'll be missed by many, for a long, long time.

His ashes will be scattered in his beloved Texas, by his daughter Markita.

Goodbye for now, Captain Midnight... we'll meet again. ▼

## Henry Freeland Osborn
### Aug. 1, 1953 - Jan. 3, 1990

Henry Osborn died peacefully in his sleep on Jan. 3, after a brief struggle with AIDS. His lover, Anthony, was with him at the time of his death.

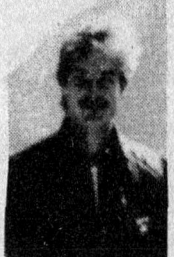

Henry (a proud Leo) was a native of Nashville who never lost his charming Tennessee accent. Henry's first love was playing the piano. His crowning achievement was winning a Tennessee statewide piano competition at the age of 17, which earned him a four-year scholarship to Vanderbilt University and the Peabody Conservatory of Music.

Henry moved to San Francisco in 1979 and always felt at home here. He worked as an accountant and as a piano teacher. He received his B.A. from St. Mary's College in Moraga, Calif. in 1985.

Henry loved classical and gospel music, street fairs, the Russian River, weekends at Harbin Hot Springs, and "play space." Most of all, he loved the many people whose lives he touched. His winning smile, sense of the nuance, kindness, compassion, and love will be missed by his family and friends.

Henry is survived by his lover, Anthony; his father, Alstein Osborn, a retired Baptist minister whom Henry loved and respected throughout his life; his Aunt Ovella; his lifelong friend Nita Hulsey of Nashville; and a host of other eternal friends.

Services are tentatively planned for Saturday, Jan. 13. Call 647-3472 for details. ▼

## Randy Tyler
### May 7, 1957 - Nov. 28, 1989

The San Francisco community was diminished greatly by the announcement of Randy's passing. Artistry, creative-genius, in the mix, Mr. D.J., don't stop the music.

Randy's turntables spun fire and grace for years at Buzzby's, the Endup, Bench and Bar, and numerous events that were favored by the leather-Levi crowd.

He leaves behind a mom and sister in Indiana where he was buried Dec. 2, and numerous friends, brothers and music lovers.

Is it not a coincidence that the Endup is closing? For years on Sunday morning with his grin, there he was dishing up the best hip-shaking, boot-bopping funk anyone could find, in front of enormous crowds.

To those of us who knew and loved Randy, his entrance onto another stage shouldn't sadden us, he would want us to dance, dance, dance, dance dance!

Your friend since November 1975 — Michael-Howard Roberts. ▼

## Larry Long
### Sept. 18, 1946 - Dec. 13, 1989

Larry passed away peacefully of AIDS complications on the morning of Dec. 13 at the Peter Claver Home in San Francisco. He is survived by his sister of Richmond, Va., and mother and brother of Lexington, Ky.

Larry moved to San Francisco from Lexington in 1977 and immediately established himself as a community personality. His unusual wit and his "down home" sense of humor will be fondly remembered.

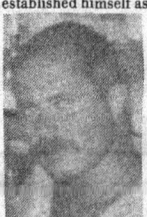

During the past year Larry mellowed considerably, thus achieving a greater sense of peace and happiness. He would like to be remembered as "A good ole wagon that done broke down."

A memorial service will be planned in the near future at the Peter Claver Home. Contact Marta for further information at 563-9228. ▼

## Sava Ranisavljevic
### June 19, 1947-Oct. 17, 1989

The day Sava was born in Zemun, Yugoslavia, his father announced the fact by breaking all the windows in the neighborhood; the day he died, Mother Nature was a bit more destructive with the quake of '89.

Born in Yugoslavia and raised in Germany, Sava immigrated to the U.S. at the age of 15. Sava made quick work of his schooling, graduating as valedictorian of his high school class and then going on to complete his B.A. at Northeastern Illinois University and Masters at Northwestern in four years. 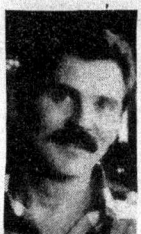 Sava was naturalized in 1968 and served in the U.S. Army before returning to Northwestern to get his doctorate in Spanish and Portuguese. He taught Spanish at Stanford and since 1980 held various positions with the San Francisco Community College District. He was a founding member of the Bay Area Gay Academic Union and the Gay and Lesbian Educational Services Committee.

Sava passed away quietly within a half hour of the quake surrounded by his mother, Katharina of Millbrae; sister Sofija and niece Michele of Chicago; and Chuck, his companion of seven years. He is also survived by a niece, Sue Ann, and grandnephew, Jacob of Chicago, and numerous friends and colleagues in the U.S. and Europe. Special thanks to those friends, colleagues and staff at Davies who gave encouragement, medical and spiritual support over the past year: Patrick, Charles, Leora, Barbara Ann, Stephen, Ron, Mary, Carol, Terrie, Beth, *Dorene*, Cheryl, *Randy*, *Mitch*, Patsy, Yvonne, Nancy, Michael, Jeff, Morris, Phillip, Brian, Janet, Frances, Hillary, and so many more, too numerous to list.

A wake was held Oct. 19 at Sullivan Mortuary and interment at the Serbian Cemetery took place on Oct. 20. Donations were asked to be sent to Shanti or the San Francisco AIDS Foundation.

Sava will be remembered as a lover of people, cultures, languages and education; *possessed with a sharp wit, ready advice and love of entertaining.* A gathering to celebrate Sava's life will be held Jan. 20 at his home, 7-9 p.m. For information call 333-8072. ▼

## Domingo A. Giffuni
### April 29, 1961-Dec. 31, 1989

Domingo died of AIDS related complications at his family home in Caracas, Venezuela, surrounded by his cherished parents, his five loving brothers and a supportive extended family.

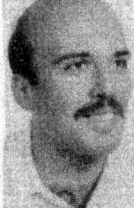

Having lived in San Francisco for the past nine years, it was his ultimate wish to be with his family again. He mustered up all his energy and determination to make it home for the last three weeks of his life.

Domingo was diagnosed with AIDS 18 months ago, one month after losing his beloved companion, Roger. He then gave up his plans for medical school and, finding his strength in these tragedies, devoted his energies to the Names Project, the Wedge Speakers Program in public schools, the Latino AIDS Project, the AIDS Hotline, ACT UP and contributed his time to many other projects and events including giving a series of lectures to AIDS care professionals in Venezuela.

Domingo worked to exhaustion on the projects he supported.

All of us who were privileged to have him in our lives will remember Domingo as the most honest and dependable of friends, a sweetheart who was truly adored. ▼

## Richard Joel Robison
### Jan. 30, 1940-Jan. 13, 1990

Richard Joel Robison, 49, died at his San Francisco home on Jan. 13. His companion Gary Lee Nelson and his mother Joan Kelley Robak of Oakland were with him at the time of death.

Robison was best known as founder and operator of Off The Wall Gallery on Haight Street. Working with other local merchants to develop business and promote public safety, Robison advocated that police presence and other city services be provided at the same level as other San Francisco commercial areas. 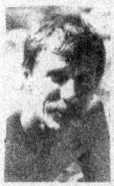 He worked with fellow merchants to establish services and create business opportunities in the Haight Street corridor. Robison sold the gallery and retired in 1986.

In the 1960s and 1970s, Robison was involved with businesses and service organizations which supported the San Francisco gay community. He was involved with the Society for Individual Rights and, *referring to a popular Sutter Street gay bar of the day,* he was known as one of the first "Rendezvous Dolls."

"Richard was proud of his membership in CRIR/Log Cabin Club and his involvement with San Francisco's gay service organizations," said Nelson.

Robison was a charter member of the San Francisco Castro Lions Club, the first predominantly gay club to be chartered by an international service association, Lions Club International. In addition to actively supporting his local Castro Lions Club, Robison was a member of the Russian River Lions Club. Because of his monetary gifts, he was both a Life Member and a Helen Keller Fellow of the Lions Eye Foundation of California/Nevada. This foundation provides major vision care services for indigent patients.

Having been actively involved with gay alcoholic support groups since beginning his own recovery program, Robison looked forward to celebrating his 20th anniversary of living sober later this year. In 1975, he participated in the formation of Acceptance House which provides a supportive environment for gay alcoholics who are starting a recovery program. Among his many friends in the United States and abroad, Robison included the "friends of Bill W.," referring to the founder of Alcoholics Anonymous.

In addition to his companion and his mother, Robison is survived by many aunts, uncles, cousins, friends, and his four cherished cats, Hudson, Sister, Norman and Alex.

Visitation was yesterday at Arthur J. Sullivan, 2254 Market St. Friends may gather there today at 12:30 p.m. and then proceed to Cypress Lawn Cemetery for a *graveside service at 1:30 p.m.*

Robison asked that memorials be made to Coming Home Hospice or to any Lions Club charity. ▼

## Mark S. Ryan
### Sept. 7, 1957-Jan. 1, 1990

Mark Ryan gently died on New Year's Day.

Mark was renowned as one of the best disc jockeys in San Francisco, having spun hits at the I-Beam Tea Dances for many years. Mark was involved in many political and community affairs, but he was most active in the fellowship of Alcoholics Anonymous. As he intended it, his last musical engagement was as DJ at the fabulous Living Sober New Year's Eve Dance in 1988. The recovering community deeply mourns Mark's death.

After leaving the I-Beam at the peak of his career, Mark worked as the volunteer coordinator at the National Council on Alcoholism. Most recently, he worked as a training specialist for the UCSF AIDS Health Project.

*On New Year's Eve* Mark attended the black tie wedding of his sister Laura, to Jamey Sachoy, at his family's summer home in Mattapoisett, Mass., where he was surrounded by family and friends. He died just after dawn the next day, in the company of his lover, Mike Hall.

A memorial service will be held at 11 a.m. on Jan. 20, at St. Ignatius (at USF). Mike requests that donations be made to the Shanti Project or Alcoholics Anonymous, in lieu of flowers. ▼

### Brian Jackson
### Aug. 19, 1954 - Dec. 9, 1989

Brian died of complications from AIDS on Dec. 9, in Jackson, Miss., in the presence of his mother, Virginia, and cousin Mavis.

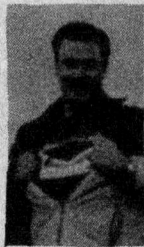

Brian was born in Kodiak, Alaska, where his parents were stationed in the military. He studied fine arts and interior design at the University of New Mexico before moving to San Francisco in 1978.

In San Francisco, Brian taught square dancing through the Foggy City Squares. He recalled this as being one of the most rewarding experiences of his life. He was also involved in several gay bowling leagues through the years.

During his last couple years in San Francisco he worked for Breuner's department store doing display work.

In 1986 Brian served as vice president of the San Francisco Hiking Club during which time he led several club outings and an excursion to the Farallon Islands. He hosted the social hours at the club's monthly meetings and always added his special flair.

Brian loved parties and festivities— the glitzier and flashier, the better. He thrived on getting to know people and experiencing new things. His warm Southern manners and sharp sense of humor could bring a smile to anyone's face.

Many of his friends remember him by his other name—Trudy Yoors. Trudy was always the life of the party. Yet there was also a very complex, serious side of Brian that he protected carefully.

Brian is survived by his mother, Virginia, brother Carle, sister-in-law Melanie and many friends. His ashes will be scattered near Albuquerque, N.M., an area he had a special affection for.

A celebration of Brian's life will be held Jan. 14. Call 285-7710 for details. Contributions may be made in Brian's memory to Project Inform, or to Sandifer House, P.O. Box 8342, Jackson, Miss. 39284. ▼

### Marvin Dale Mabb
### Dec. 31, 1955 - Dec. 24, 1989

Marvin Mabb conquered in death his brave battle for nearly two years with AIDS—with his lover at his side—at Coming Home Hospice on Christmas Eve morning.

Born in Denver, Colo., Marvin lived in St. Louis, Mo., and graduated from high school in Azusa. He served in the U.S. Air Force in Germany from 1970 to 1974 after which he attended the University of Missouri, the European Bible Seminary in Germany, and the Gradwohl School of Laboratory Technique in St. Louis.

After his education, Marvin lived in New Orleans from 1981 to 1985, Seattle from 1985 to 1987, and finally found his permanent home moving with his lover and life-partner to San Francisco in 1987.

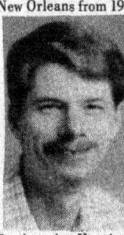

Marvin went on disability from his much loved employer, Pacific Presbyterian Hospital, in October 1987. His life before disability and after has been filled with his loves of studying German, which he spoke, read and wrote fluently, playing his organ and guitar, and studying Unitarian writers. Much of his time was spent meditating on various AIDS publications and therapies.

A kind and extremely gentle man, Marvin is sorely missed and survived by his lover, Chuck Wright, his father, Dean Mabb of Cottage Hills, Ill., his mother, Mary Beller of Pueblo, Colo., his sister, Joan Marshall of San Jose, and his aunt, Katherine Krieg of St. Louis. Marvin also leaves five brothers: Samuel, Rodney, Randolph, Jonathan and David Mabb.

Marvin's interment at Holy Cross Cemetery on Thursday Dec. 28 will be followed by a memorial gathering on Saturday, Jan. 13, at 10 a.m. at the First Unitarian Church Chapel at 1187 Franklin St. ▼

### Bill Lemen
### July 5, 1948 - Dec. 18, 1989

Bill died in his sleep at his home near Lake Tahoe on Dec. 18. He was blessed with good health most of the 29 months he was battling AIDS. He became ill Dec. 16 as the result of a reaction to Compound Q.

Bill was a native of Sacramento and he lived most of his life there. He found satisfaction working with people. His jobs included helping children who had cystic fibrosis and eating disorders at Stanford Childrens Hospital, and counseling troubled youth with the California Youth Authority. Bill spent the last decade of his career helping people buy and sell real estate in Sacramento.

During his life Bill developed many special relationships with people because he understood unconditional love. Bill is survived by his companion of nine months Joe Swain of South Lake Tahoe, former lovers Tom Sachs and Jerry O'Brien of Sacramento, and best friend Craig Chester of Sacramento.

He was preceded in death by former lover David Reeder.

Bill also leaves his parents, Frank and Lois of Sacramento; his brothers, Dick of Pacific Palisades, and Jack of Merced; and his sisters, Virginia Richards of Diablo and Jane Brearly of Auburn.

A memorial service was held at St. Paul's Episcopal Church on Dec. 21. Donations in Bill's memory can be made to the Bill Lemen Memorial Fund established by the South Lake Tahoe AIDS Task Force. The fund will be used to plant a grove of trees in Bill's memory. ▼

## John Victor Mazzei
### June 17, 1956 - Dec. 22, 1989

Relief from a long struggle with AIDS came to Victor Mazzei on Dec. 22. With him when he passed on were his lover, Tom, his father, Gene, and friends, Ryland, Renee, Paul and Tony, surrounding him, as he had always surrounded others with his love and loyalty.

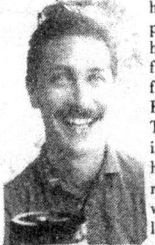

Victor was born in Albuquerque, raised in San Diego, and spent many happy years in the Bay Area. In 1978 he received his BA in Business from UC Berkeley, then worked several years at IBM in San Francisco.

Wizard in the kitchen, connoisseur of the art world, and lover of the environment, Vic charmed our lives with his sharp mind, great sense of humor and smile. We will miss this self-proclaimed "eternal optimist," who, in impossible settings, at any hour, always found a parking place!

To hear Rachmaninoff, now, is to hear you. Every act with style. Every gesture with grace. Well done, Vic! We love you.

Contributions in Vic's memory can be made to Project Open Hand. ▼

## Frank Polello

Frank L. Polello (Frankie) made his peaceful crossover on Nov. 22 at the Maitri Hospice. Frankie's love for life and living, his incredible ability to make each day fresh and new will be with us forever.

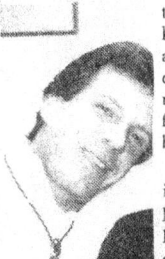

Frank was born in Spokane, WA, March 23, 1954. He loved his parents very much, who he is now finally with once again.

Frankie's happiest memories were when he was a dancer with the Silver Spurs Dance Troupe. Undeniably, Frankie's faith and courage in his fight against AIDS was his best show ever.

Frankie's wish was for memorials to go to Project Open Hand and the Maitri Hospice. Memorial services pending. We miss you, Frankie, and thank you for sharing your life. ▼

## Robert Lee Ferrell, Jr.
### May 27, 1947 - Dec. 30, 1989

Bob Ferrell passed away on Dec. 30 in the arms of his lover of 9½ years, Dennis Rhodes, and surrounded by his sister and dearest friends. Bob fought a courageous and inspiring two year battle with AIDS. He believed that death, no matter how young and unfairly it strikes, is what gives life its meaning and urgency. And the quality of life lived is ever so much more important than the quantity.

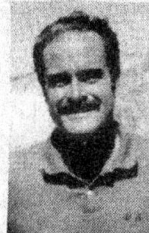

Born in North Carolina, Bob became a San Francisco resident in 1978. He had worked for Development Associates and at the time of his death was on leave from Bank of America where he held a management position.

Enough cannot be said about this wonderfully intelligent and charismatic man. He made a difference in his life and in the lives of many others. He lived life fully and will be truly missed, but will live on in the lives he touched.

Thank you, sweetheart, for helping me learn to love and believe in myself, for 9½ wonderful years, and for loving me. I love you.

I want to live, I want to grow./ I want to see, I want to know./ I want to share what I can give./ I want to be, I want to live. ▼

## Carl M. Marshall
### Feb. 6, 1948 - Jan. 4, 1990

Carl passed peacefully and with dignity into the light at his home in Hercules in the company of his friends.

He was a computer software designer who lived and worked around the Bay Area since the early '70s.

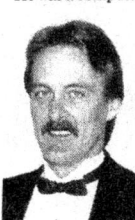

The last weeks of his life here were made difficult by a debilitating stroke that left him unable to communicate his thoughts.

He was, however, able to leave us with these words: "A friend is someone who leaves you with all of your freedom intact but obliges you to be fully what you are."

Carl will be missed by all who knew and loved him. ▼

### Ronald "Rony" Fox
**March 6, 1954-Jan. 13, 1990**

Rony Fox died peacefully and gently on Jan. 13 of renal failure and complications from AIDS at Hospice by the Bay's Hodge House Hospice, San Francisco. With him when he passed on was his loving family.

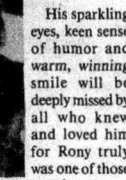

His sparkling eyes, keen sense of humor and warm, winning smile will be deeply missed by all who knew and loved him for Rony truly was one of those rare individuals who won hearts.

Born in Corpus Christi, Texas, Rony grew up and was educated in San Jose. While he also lived in Minneapolis, Houston and Los Angeles for extended periods of time, Rony considered the San Francisco Bay Area his home and always returned to either San Jose or San Francisco to live, work and play. In 1973, Rony enlisted in the U.S. Air Force and served as one of those handsome-men-in-blue, stationed mostly in Montana, until 1975.

While he was employed in the insurance industry and as a nurse's aid for brief periods of time, his real love was working as a bartender or as a chef in gay businesses, where he was always popular with both staff and customers.

Rony also had a deep passion for pool, contract bridge, gourmet cooking, science fiction and the San Francisco Giants.

One of Rony's proudest moments in the last year was taking part in the 20th Anniversary of Stonewall by participating in the Gay Freedom Day Parade with the Garden-Sullivan Hospital Staff and Volunteer contingent. Even his wheelchair could not keep him from making the long trek from the Castro to the Civic Center to display his pride in who and what he was.

Rony is survived by his mother, Rena Reed; his stepfather, Don Quigley; his sisters, Cindy, Stephanie, and Sharrie; an aunt, Gerry Davidson; two nieces and a nephew; and his good friend and hospice volunteer, Gary J. Palm of Garden-Sullivan Hospital. A memorial gathering was held in his honor Wednesday, Jan. 17 at Hodge House Hospice.

Rony's family wishes to thank the many doctors, nurses, hospice volunteers and other staff persons at Kaiser Hospital, Mother Theresa's Missionary Sisters, Garden-Sullivan Hospital and Hodge House for the wonderful care, treatment and love which they gave Rony during the past year. These persons made the last year of his life a happy, joyous and full one.

We will miss you, dear son, brother and friend, but our lives are richer because you have touched us with your presence and love. You have won our hearts forever. ▼

### Charles E. Henderson, Jr.
**Oct. 31, 1955-Jan. 13, 1990**

Charles "Chaz" passed away in his home in Detroit, Mich. His family was

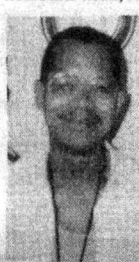

with him when he joined his deceased lover, Paul, and numerous friends who have passed before him. Charles lived in San Francisco for many years and was last employed by a law firm in which our start date was the same day. Charles, through his wit and charm, became my best friend.

Charles loved shopping, stuffed animals, music, the opera, good food, movies and the company of friends. He left behind many friends in the Bay Area: Syl and Maurice, Cindy, Craig, Richard and Jim, Rosie, Alice, Rudy, Kendra and Carolyn, Shirley, Barbara, Jack, Marian, myself (Steve Brown) and too many others to mention. He touched a lot of hearts and we are all better people to have known him.

His memorial service was held on Jan. 17 in Detroit. His cousin, Janet (an opera singer), sang at his service.

Contributions can be made to the Shanti Project in his name. ▼

### Murray "Jim" Buchheim
**1951-Dec. 27, 1989**

Murray Buchheim, affectionately known as "Jim," who made his home in San Francisco more than 20 years ago died from an overdose in his sleep. He was 39 years old.

Jim complemented the San Francisco gay community with his extremely handsome "Harrison Ford" looks and his outrageous personality. During his life, Jim associated with many famous people, including Roy Cohn, and made the most out of his good looks. Jim also traveled extensively

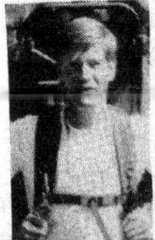

throughout the U.S. as well as Europe and the Pacific. He did a tour of duty for the USMC. He loved the outdoors, hiking and white water rafting.

Until his death, Jim made the Polk Street bars his second home, always in the Motherlode, Polk Gulch, Kimo's or any other party spot.

Jim was caught up in a deep depression since his testing positive for HIV. He isolated himself sometimes for weeks where nobody was able to contact him.

Jim is survived by his long time best friend, Warren, of Irving, Texas, an aunt and uncle from San Diego, and only a handful of trusted friends.

Jim was cremated and his ashes were scattered in the San Francisco Bay. Anyone wishing to talk about Jim's life can call Rod at 775-1754.

Jim, I know you were in deep pain, but now you are free to fly with the angels who came and rescued you from this hard life us gay people sometimes live in. I will miss you, dear friend, and will think of you always. ▼

## Reginald Jay Jones
### Aug. 26, 1949-Jan. 10, 1990

Reginald Jay Jones, playwright, gardener, and bon vivant rolled up his carpet recently, after an extensive battle with AIDS and its primary therapies.

Reggie attended the opera, meetings of the California Horticultural Society, and local playwrights' workshops. He wrote several articles for the *B.A.R.*, introduced the expression "the Sappho strut" to contemporary usage, danced tap, sang the songs of Noel Coward at Fanny's and 544 Natoma, and presented solo and staged readings of his works which dealt with the black experience in our society.

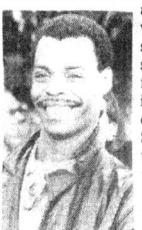

His charm, grace and insightful wit are already missed.

His sister Jennifer's love and assistance was boundless.

He wished no services. ▼

## Stephen Michael Stegman
### Aug. 4, 1946-Jan. 20, 1990

Stephen passed away early in the morning of Jan. 20 with Bruce, his lover of four and a half years, at his side.

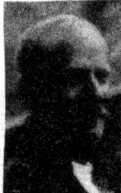

He will be most fondly remembered for his dry wit and engaging sense of humor. He always sought to keep us entertained. If things became too quiet or dull, he would always stir up some trouble.

Most people knew Stephen as the owner of Statements, on Castro Street. It became famous during the late '70s and early '80s.

Stephen grew up in New Jersey and graduated from Western Kentucky University with a degree in art. After teaching art, he worked in wholesale liquor distribution in New York City. He was an active participant on Fire Island in the mid-1970s, and is remembered there for his famous "Orange Party."

Stephen's body has been returned to New Jersey for burial. He is survived by his mother, Ruth, his sister, Ellen, his lover, Bruce, and his cat, Mork.

Stephen's friends will understand that he never stopped doing what he loved the most. The fall that led to his death occurred while shopping.

Stephen, my whole life has been shaped by the love you gave. Thank you for sharing your energy with me.

Memorial contributions should be made to the AIDS Emergency Fund. ▼

## Rene Antonio Zepeda
### Feb. 22, 1951-Jan. 15, 1990

On Jan. 15 at twilight, Rene Antonio Zepeda died as he had lived, sharing love, life and joy, at peace with undaunted honesty. He was alone with his weiner dogs, Doris and Fred. His loving sister Dianna had been with him during his last month, giving her time, love and compassion to her little brother.

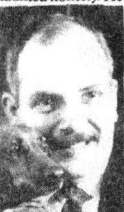

During his short illness, he shared the passing and rejuvenation of his spirit with many friends who came from all parts of the country, illuminating their lives with his compassion.

He made mistakes throughout his life, but always faced them bravely and responsibly.

With a razor wit and a contagious laugh, he radiated happiness to those around him. It was his special talent.

Just before his passing, he was baptized by the Rev. Cecil Williams into Glide Memorial Church, where he found a wonderful home within the people of the church.

It is selfish to say that we will miss him, but we will. And yet, knowing that he is part of the great eternity we will all become, somehow lights the darkness.

Shine on, sweetheart. Buen suenos.

Donations in Rene's name may be made to the AIDS support group, Glide Memorial Church. ▼

# Ed Wolf

*San Francisco General Hospital's Ward 5B was the first hospital ward in the country dedicated to patients with AIDS. Ed Wolf was a nurse on Ward 5B, and here he talks about his personal history and how it led him to be on the front line of the AIDS crisis.*

It was 1969 and I was a college student in Florida.

My roommate ran in: "Oh my God! You're not going to believe what's happened in New York! Some gay people got pissed off with the cops. They set a cop car on fire! They threw rocks!"

I realized there was a community somewhere for people like me.

The minute I graduated, I moved to New York. I found an apartment. I got a job in a factory, working as a typist. (My mother had always said to me, "Take typing classes. No matter where you go, no matter where you end up, you can always get a job if you're a typist.") I wrote back to my circle of friends in Florida, and one by one, they moved to the city and we started our lives. It was the early 1970s! We'd go out dancing. The discotheque was new, and freeing, and unifying. We all felt like we were at the start of something beautiful. I never made it to the sex clubs, but my friends did. I was terrible at having casual sex—I need to get to know someone first! When it got to midnight, I'd leave my friends at the discotheque and go home. I think that might have saved my life. Nearly all of those friends from Florida died early on, horribly, of AIDS. The virus was already out there infecting people. We just didn't realize it yet. We were sitting ducks. We had no idea what was coming.

Life in New York seemed wonderful at first. But by the mid-1970s it got the three D's. It was *dirty*. It was *dangerous*. And it was *depressing*.

Nearly every single woman I knew had been attacked or raped, and it felt like my gay friends were just getting one STI after another. In the end, I moved to San Francisco. San Francisco's like Rome or London or Paris—one of those cities that conjures up wonderful feelings. It was great. But I still had the same problems I'd had with the gay community in New York. I never seemed to fit in. Every image of a gay man was always a macho guy, standing on the corner with a cigarette—a cowboy hat, a leather jacket. I was always the tallest, skinniest person wherever I went. I had terrible buck teeth. I didn't fit in. You never saw any photographs of a gay man who looked like me.

It was probably 1982 when I first heard about AIDS. I was at the big movie theater on the Castro. In those days, you could still smoke inside the theater, and my friend and I wanted to smoke some pot. I went out to the drugstore on the corner to buy some rolling papers, and I noticed all these Polaroid photos. The photos showed all these big red splotches on someone's body. Their mouth. Their arm. The backs of their legs. There was a caption underneath which said: *GAY CANCER: BE CAREFUL OUT THERE.* That moment was when I first became aware that something bad was happening.

It was the summer of 1983 when I started working with people with AIDS. At that point, nearly all of the AIDS cases in San Francisco were among members of the gay community. When I answered an advert in the local paper calling for volunteers, I thought to myself, *Some of these men in need are the men I can't fit in with. But maybe I can help them.* The direction of my whole life changed that day. It was called the Shanti Project; they trained me to help people with HIV/AIDS.

My first client had just been discharged from the AIDS ward at the hospital. I was extremely nervous when I first went to his apartment. What's he going to look like? How sick is he going to be?

He opened the door and said, "Hi, I'm Ed."

And I said, "Oh, I'm Ed, too."

Working with Ed helped me to realize there wasn't anything wrong with me. It was a lightning bolt: *I'm perfect! I'm fine!* Sex didn't come easily to me. I didn't know how to cruise. I always wanted to talk to people and connect with them before I could start to think about having sex with them. That used to embarrass me; like I couldn't behave like a "real" gay man behaves. But my desire to get to know people turned out to be an incredible skill when it came to helping people with AIDS. It wasn't a deficit after all.

Not long after, Ed died. Back then, people died very quickly, because there was no HIV test. The only way you knew you were HIV+ was if you already had symptoms of AIDS.

In 1986, I quit my job as a typist and started working full-time on the AIDS ward. When it first opened in 1983, Ward 5B was a seven-bed unit. By the time I arrived, there were so many people with AIDS coming into the hospital that it moved across the hall onto 5A, a twenty-bed unit. The ward was a terrifying place. All these people, most of them barely thirty years old, dying very young and very terrible deaths. These days, people don't understand all the diseases that untreated AIDS causes. They don't realize what it does to the human body. It could be horrific. But I had made my commitment to seeing these people through.

It was a terrible and beautiful place to work. Beautiful because I was part of a movement of people who showed up to help when the rest of the country didn't care. But terrible because many of these people—the early AIDS volunteers and AIDS activists and AIDS spokespeople—would discover they had AIDS as well. It was stunning to be around such spectacular individuals, literally dying while on airplanes to Washington, DC, because they were determined to lobby for the cause. The efforts they went to were heroic.

Sometimes it was the little things. There was a man who made teddy bears. The teddy bears were beautiful; they had moving parts and so much character. He'd bring them in as gifts to all the patients. But one day, he got sick too. He stayed on the unit, this time as a patient. A patient brought him one of his own teddy bears. Not long after, he died.

The nurses were in a hurry to clean the room and get it ready for the next patient (it seemed like there was always another patient arriving). But his little teddy bear was just sitting on top of the trash can, looking at me. I grabbed him. I still have him all these years later. There was another man who'd visit the ward. He'd bake the most extraordinary, elaborate cookies for the patients. But he got sick. He died too.

And then there was Rita Rockett. She was a phenomenon. In her normal life, she was a travel agent. An everyday, heterosexual, married, white woman. One Easter Sunday, she came to the unit to make lunch for all the patients. She was such a hit that it became a regular thing, and on Sundays she'd turn up with a whole bevy of leather guys who helped her cook all the food and serve it up. She was a tap dancer; she'd dance on the ward. She was such an anomaly; most straight people were repulsed by gay men with AIDS. A straight woman who'd put on a French maid's outfit and bunny ears to cook food and tap-dance for gay men who were dying of AIDS? And at one point she was pregnant while she was doing this! She was very powerful, very unusual.

No matter where you work, things are going to happen which are inadvertently humorous. One day, one of the patients said they saw a mouse in their room. Now, the ward was on the fifth floor of a hospital. The idea that a mouse could have somehow gotten up there was absurd. But talk of the mouse travels, and other patients start claiming they've seen it too. We have to call up the maintenance guy who's very hunky, and everyone's checking him out, but the mouse never appears.

There were humorous times. But mostly? It was like being in the army.

Sick people are surrounded by people telling them what to do. *You need to take this medication. You need to get to this appointment. You need to eat more. You need to get out of that bed.* But a lot of my job was about helping them in a more holistic way. Sometimes it was my job to sit and watch TV with them. Sometimes it was to hold their hand. Maybe it was to help them write a letter. People who are very sick—people who are dying—are the experts on their own lives. Not the doctor. Not the nurse. Not the physical therapist. Certainly not me. They know what they need. They know what works for them. You have to respect that.

We had nothing. Nobody cared. We had to do it ourselves. The stigma and the homophobia that goes hand in hand with AIDS lands clearly on the laps of the straight people in leadership at that time. There was no real HIV funding from the government until 1985 when Rock Hudson died, and that was only because Ronald and Nancy Reagan were friends with him. Even then, it wasn't much money compared to the gravity of the situation. It seemed like nobody in power wanted to treat AIDS as the crisis it already was. AIDS funding only reached an acceptable level when Ryan White died in 1990. He was so young, so white, so "innocent"—*he didn't bring it on himself the way those fags did.* When the general public began to care about Ryan White, only then did funding for AIDS research start to improve. I'm still angry about that. The fact it took that poor kid to get people to care. We will never know how many people could have been saved if the consensus had galvanized sooner.

It was easy to think there'd never be effective treatment, because we just didn't matter to anyone in power. *It's just the fags, their lives don't matter, they've brought it on themselves.* By the late 1980s, we were seeing a lot more straight people on the ward. Some of these people were drug users or ex-drug users. Sometimes drug use led to sex, and that was how the infection happened. Sometimes people contracted HIV from sharing the equipment they were using to get high. It's just another form of penetration; penetrating someone with a needle, exchanging fluids. AIDS tore apart the gay community, but it didn't stop there.

The local gay paper used to run obituaries of all the people who had died of AIDS in the area that week. On Thanksgiving 1989, the paper printed all the photographs of everyone who had died that year. Hundreds and hundreds of people. As I pored through the photos, I couldn't believe how many of them were of people I'd gotten to know at the hospital. Something inside me shifted.

I realized, *Okay, enough. This is too much. I need to do something else now.*

But I stayed connected to HIV/AIDS services. I moved into counseling and testing; it became my job to let people know their HIV test results. Then I moved into training other people to work in HIV/AIDS services, and then I worked overseas in South America and Africa. The direction of my whole life changed, simply because that day in 1983 I decided maybe I could do something to help.

## Floyd Sklaver

*Floyd Sklaver is an AIDS elder who lived in New York City at the height of the epidemic. Here he tells his story.*

It's been such a long time now that my memory plays tricks on me. I'm pretty sure I read that first article when it was published in *The New York Times*. The one which said gay men were getting sick with some sort of strange cancer. Then one day, my upstairs neighbor spoke to me. "You should start using condoms if you're sleeping around. There's this thing going around. We think it's sexually transmitted." It seemed kind of unfair and ironic that something as fun as sex could be so dangerous.

I'm pretty sure I contracted HIV in 1984. When I was diagnosed, I told the guy I was seeing at the time, and he immediately cut off all contact with me. After that experience, I learned to only tell my closest friends. Then I met Marc. I was working for a Broadway show and Marc was a gofer for one of the producers. He walked into my office one day and I just thought he was so cute.

I decided to tell him I was HIV+ on our first date. *If he can't handle this, then this isn't going to go anywhere.* We went to the Halloween parade in Greenwich Village. We stood there together wearing masks and watching all the people in scary costumes go by. Back in those days it was a very ragtag affair; there weren't any corporate sponsors and the whole parade was probably only ten blocks long. We were on MacDougal Street. He was wearing this long, expensive, black overcoat that he couldn't afford. It was a cold day. When I told him I had HIV, he just wrapped his coat around me and pulled me into an enormous embrace.

After the parade was done, we got Chinese food. I ordered kung pao chicken, Marc ordered fried rice, and when I asked for chopsticks, he did too. But he'd never eaten with chopsticks before. When they cleared his plate, he'd made such a mess. I thought that was the cutest thing in the world.

I remember laughing. I remember feeling like I could trust him.

We've been together ever since.

I didn't want HIV to appear on my health record. I avoided telling doctors I had HIV. I didn't want to lose my insurance. I was afraid of anybody finding out. People were losing their jobs. People were losing their homes. Back then, health care workers were still wearing hazmat suits to push food towards people with AIDS in the hospital. Your loved ones weren't even allowed to visit you as you were dying.

So Marc and I lived our life together as if a disaster was about to happen. We set up our finances so that everything was held in both of our names. I saved up as much money as I could because I knew that if I got sick and couldn't work, it would take at least a year and a half for me to die.

New York had been a place of freedom for me in the late 1970s, ever since I started getting the train into the city from college. It was exciting. It made me feel irrepressible. *If it feels good, do it.* And it did feel good.

But the bars shut down. The bathhouses closed. The men disappeared. We became afraid of sex. I knew men who were abandoned by their partners when they were diagnosed with AIDS. The AIDS crisis drove the gay community apart. It made gay people afraid of each other. You'd see a young man on the street whose face looked old and shrunken and you'd turn away. Young men in the prime of their lives, suddenly looking skeletal. You knew something was wrong. It was heartbreaking. And it terrified me because I was waiting for it to happen to me too.

One day I ran into a guy I'd dated. Now he had Kaposi's sarcoma lesions on his face. He'd lost a lot of weight. He still had his enormous smile. He still bopped around like he used to. But he was sick. All these reflections around me. Gay men started to try to gain muscle. You didn't want to be perceived as wasting away. If you bulked up, it implied you couldn't have AIDS.

It's hard to convey the extent of the loss. Broadway lost a generation of directors and choreographers. We lost a generation of mentors. There were no greats to learn from. The greats all died. I began to feel like if I stayed in New York, I was going to die too. I needed to get out.

So Marc and I moved to Oregon. In 1994, I finally started to get sick. My vision was failing, I was fatigued; it was getting harder and harder to work. I knew it was happening. I knew I needed help. I was scared of being helpless, scared of being in pain. I didn't have a doctor. A friend gave me the name of a doctor who was supposed to be excellent. I called the doctor's office. Ten years of fear boiled up in that phone call. I asked for an appointment. But the nurse on the phone said the doctor wasn't taking any new patients.

I couldn't help it. I started to cry. "Look," I said, "I don't know what to do. Can you recommend somebody else? Can you help me?"

She called me back fifteen minutes later and said, "The doctor will see you."

I found out later she'd gone into his office and said to him, "I have a new patient and I want you to take him on." Thank God, he agreed.

But there was still no hope until late 1995. No hope meant no future.

The doctor tells you, "Something is coming down the pipeline. Drugs that work. Hold on a couple more months."

December. January. February. March. You hold on.

My T-cell count was low. I had full-blown AIDS. I didn't have any visible lesions, thankfully, but I was wasting away. I'd go in every couple of weeks and I'd ask him when the treatment was going to be available.

"It's coming."

"It's coming."

And then the first antiretroviral medication became available at last. It was like Lazarus coming back from the dead. I went from not being able to get out of bed one morning to full strength within a couple of weeks. It was a rigid regimen. There were three different medications. You took two of them twice a day, one of them three times a day. You had to time your food. Some of the pills you had to take on an empty stomach; others you had to take right after eating. I bought a Casio wristwatch that had five alarms on it. The alarms were always buzzing to remind me. I stayed on those drugs for years and I never missed a single dose.

The funny thing is, I was lucky. I'm a white middle-class man. I had insurance that paid for it. Not everyone was so fortunate. Having HIV sucks. I'm not going to lie about that. I wish this hadn't happened. But it did. I like to think I've made the best of it, made the best of my life, done the best that I could.

I was never an activist. I wish I'd been more courageous. I have friends who did the bravest and most marvelous things. I've made a number of mistakes in my life, and all of them revolved around fear. Fear became a survival strategy. But today, I feel a responsibility as a longtime survivor. I wasn't courageous when I was younger, but I can be courageous now by talking about what happened.

So don't be afraid like I was. Find your voice. Go for greatness. Young people still contract HIV today. I want to wrap them in my arms the same way Marc wrapped me in his arms that Halloween on our first date. I want to say, "I don't know what's going to happen. But I know you're going to be okay."

## Blood Sisters

In matters of life and death, sometimes the best thing you can offer is your blood.

In 1983, in response to the HIV outbreak, all gay men were prohibited from donating blood for those who needed it—a prohibition that would last forty years.

Lesbians, however, were not prohibited from donating blood.

Many stepped in to fill the gap.

This is an important point to understand in a book about the AIDS epidemic: Even though they were one of the lowest-risk groups in the population, many lesbians were galvanized to help in the fight against AIDS. They were caregivers, marchers, advocates, fundraisers, and witnesses. They gave time, they gave energy, they gave support. And, in many cases, they gave blood.

The San Diego Blood Sisters held their first blood drive on July 16, 1983. Nearly 200 women showed up to donate.

The Blood Sisters were an offshoot of the Women's Caucus of the San Diego Democratic Club. After more than half of the men in the Democratic Club's leadership fell ill from HIV/AIDS, the women knew they had to do something.

As Barbara Vick, one of the founding Blood Sisters, later told *Diva* magazine, "There was a powerlessness everybody felt, but the lesbian community seemed immune to the disease. I don't want to say there was guilt, but you look at counterparts bearing this burden for no reason. At that time, women had less to give economically, but blood is such a basic thing."

Said Wendy Sue Biegeleisen, another founding Blood Sister, "We could not sit by and watch everyone we love die and do nothing."

"Women came out of the woodwork; women that didn't want to have anything to do with men—even gay men," fellow Blood Sister Peggy Heathers said in an interview with the Women's Museum of California. "It was an incredible experience to see the caring and the support."

It might be assumed that gay men and lesbians were natural allies, but their relationship prior to the epidemic was often fraught. Recalled one gay man in California about the early 1980s, "Suddenly, the hospitals were full of lesbians who were volunteering. . . . I remember being so moved by them because gay men hadn't been too kind to lesbians. We'd call them 'fish' and make fun of the butch dykes in the bars—and yet, there they were."

The Blood Sisters made sure the blood they donated didn't go into the general blood supply but instead to a private account that could be exclusively directed to people with HIV/AIDS who needed transfusions. As Vick later told the Lambda Archives of San Diego, "Groups like the Blood Sisters were about more than just fighting AIDS; they were about fighting prejudice, uniting a community, and showing the authorities that blood really is thicker than water."

The San Diego Blood Sisters inspired many other groups of queer women across the country to start their own blood drives, often hosted by queer religious congregations. Even though the women donating blood were not in an at-risk category, they were still met with resistance in some places. In 1985, at a time when there was a critical shortage of 6,000 units of blood in Los Angeles and Orange Counties, the American Red Cross pulled the plug on a lesbian-sponsored blood drive at the Gay and Lesbian Community Center in Garden Grove. The reason given? The Red Cross was afraid the general public would think they were letting gay men donate blood because of where the drive was being held. Said Dr. Benjamin Spindler, the American Red Cross chapter's medical director of blood services, "We declined to go to the gay community center (to collect blood donations) because of the confusion our other regular donors might have."

"Apparently, the need for blood in Orange County must not be as great as stated when you permit prejudice and fears to cancel a blood drive," the community center's chairman, Stuart Smith, replied.

The Blood Sisters were not deterred, however. In San Diego, they continued to hold blood drives and then became a pivotal part of the establishment of an ACT UP chapter in that city, broadening their efforts to include the distribution of clean needles and loud advocacy for better treatment for all people with AIDS, on top of the voluntary caregiving already being done to make up for the lapses of the medical establishment and biological families that refused to be there.

Blood here is a truth, and it is also a metaphor. And while it's easy to focus on the blood in the name, the "sisters" is equally important. What groups of queer women like the Blood Sisters did not only sent a message to the establishment, but also sent a message to the people fighting against HIV/AIDS: *You are not alone. There is something in our queerness that equals kinship, that equals family. We will fight for you now, and when we have triumphed, we will fight together for more.*

Which is, four decades later, what has largely come to pass.

# John D'Amico

*One of the few people openly living with HIV to be elected to public office, John D'Amico served two terms as the mayor of West Hollywood and on its city council from 2011 to 2022.*

My connection to HIV/AIDS is straightforward. I'm part of the cohort of gay men who got infected in the 1980s. I tested positive for HIV in 1988. I was twenty-four years old.

I used to have a motorcycle. I'd ride my motorcycle home from work—I worked in this super-fancy restaurant in Los Angeles. One time when I got home, there was a guy laying on my front lawn. He was super hot. I asked him if he was okay, because it was one-thirty in the morning. He said, "Yeah, I'm just a little stoned." We struck up a conversation. I was a young kid, working in a restaurant, riding around the city on my motorcycle. A hot guy was a hot guy. We ended up having sex.

He told me his name was John D'Amico. I was like, "That's so weird! We have exactly the same name!" I was young. Today, older and wiser, I figure he didn't really have the same name as mine. He was just fucking with me—literally. He gave me his phone number, but when I rang, I was told there was nobody living there with that name. So that was the end of it. In a theatrical way, it feels kind of like I infected myself—this mysterious man saying he had my exact name.

I got sick. I started having night sweats. I felt really bad. I didn't have any health insurance. I went to the free clinic, and they suggested I take an HIV test. I picked up my results before going into work. I was sitting in the parking lot trying to process what I'd just been told, and I just thought, *Well, I guess I better go to work.* It's hard to explain how little information we had. It was 1988. You couldn't Google it. You could barely even find accurate information about HIV/AIDS at the public library.

I first heard about HIV in 1982, although it wasn't called that then. I was still in Hawaii, in Honolulu, which was where I grew up. There was a time in America when Americans believed what newscasters were telling them. Tom Brokaw was the voice of whatever was happening in the world. I remember his report on a mysterious new illness appearing among "homosexuals." I remember feeling so agitated. Like, why is he talking about homosexuals when I'm right next to my mother? She's going to know it's about me! She might talk to me about it! I was more concerned about Tom Brokaw saying the word "homosexual" than the report about a deadly illness affecting gay men in other parts of the country.

At eighteen, I moved to California for college. I was a young, dumb kid. I rode a motorcycle, I smoked, I drank, I did some drugs. By the mid-1980s, AIDS was harder to ignore, but it seemed like something older gay guys got. Not young guys like me. *Condoms, sure, whatever, but I don't really need to worry about it.* The first person I met who was living with HIV was named Scott. He was a little older than me. He was from a famous Chicago family—the archetypal gay son who moved to Hollywood in the 1970s and made a lot of money. He died in 1989. It made me so mad at his memorial because AIDS wasn't mentioned. It seemed so messed up. They hid the fact he had AIDS to protect his family.

Becoming HIV-positive made me think about what I wanted to get out of my life. I decided to go to graduate school so I could get health insurance. I figured I'd finally be able to move forward with my goals, and stop living one day to the next in Los Angeles. I was optimistic. That's important. I was grateful to have the opportunity to get my life together. So many of the HIV-positive people in my life talk about their diagnosis having a similar effect. By the late 1980s, we knew having HIV didn't necessarily mean immediately dying. Finding out you were positive meant saying to yourself: "I guess it's time for me to get my shit together."

After my graduate degree, I knew I needed to work in HIV because I needed to be as near as possible to up-to-date information. I got a job running a team of researchers who were interviewing young men aged fifteen to twenty-two years old about HIV. Five of us would go out to venues across Los Angeles County where young gay men would go out. Sometimes it was Griffith Park, sometimes it was Vaseline Alley, sometimes it was a disco or a nightclub or a rave. Over the course of the night we'd interview young men passing by. We were collecting data about their sex lives to help us understand the direction and prevalence of HIV in this community. How often did they have sex? Who did they have sex with? Do they have sex for money or food or lodging or drugs? And what part of the county did they grow up in? What was their cultural background, their ethnicity, their race?

After that, we'd give them an HIV test.

The HIV test was totally anonymous. We'd send them an anonymous notecard to remind them to come and pick up their results. Confidentiality was important for two reasons. Getting an HIV test was shrouded in secrecy because of ignorance and fear about AIDS. And many of the young men we were testing wouldn't want the people they lived with to know they were having sex with men or going to gay bars. Especially the young kids who were often still living with their families and most often still in the closet.

But another reason the test was confidential was because communities of color and ethnic immigrant communities and the gay community were all concerned about inadvertently creating a registry of people who were HIV+. The fear was that someday, two elections from now, it could be turned into a list and used against us by politicians. There'd been a ballot to segregate HIV+ people in California. The ballot failed, thankfully. But as time went by and a cure was still nowhere to be found, there were concerns about whether such a plan might be revived.

I remember having such empathy for the boys who were under eighteen. You could sense that many of them were so lonely. They were coming into the city and going to gay bars because they wanted to be included. It's complicated being young. You have raging hormones. The dividing line between being a child and being an adult is a single birthday. Some of the kids were homeless, but most of the kids we spoke to were middle-class kids who'd drive into the city from the suburbs in pursuit of fun and adventure. Hang out, meet someone, hook up at the bar, take the bus home when their friends left without them. The older I got, the more I realized how young I'd been when I became HIV-positive. I wanted to protect as many young people as possible.

The results of the study showed us what turned out to be correct: Young men were in general at risk of contracting HIV, but people of color, especially young Black men, were at a really intense risk. About 10 percent of the young men we tested turned out to be HIV+; that's a very high percentage. The epidemic in Los Angeles County pretty much panned out how the data suggested. HIV moved into communities of color in South and East LA and plateaued in the white gay neighborhoods.

A big reason why HIV plateaued in West Hollywood was because it had already ravaged most of that community. West Hollywood has a population of about 35,000. Over the course of the 1980s and 1990s, about 10,000 people died from AIDS there—maybe 2,000 or 1,000 people every eighteen months. It was an unbearably intense time for the city. You'd go to the gym and there'd be guys with catheters hanging out of their chests in the shower. Living out loud with HIV was part of the narrative of the city at the time. AIDS was everywhere.

We all have a clock ticking in our lives. Sometimes I ask myself: Have I been cheating death for more than thirty years now? I was never meant to make it past thirty. I didn't start taking medication until 1992. I never had AIDS. I never had fewer than 200 T-cells and I never had an opportunistic infection. I have no explanation for it. I have no understanding of how seventy people in my life died of AIDS, but I didn't. Not to mention my friends who've lived just as long as I have. I don't know why they're alive and their friends are not. There are no logical answers.

AIDS is an age-old story. Who survived the bubonic plague in the medieval ages and who died? Who survived the Vietnam War and who didn't? No one knows why some people survive and some people die. All the people who died can't tell us what the answer is. The survivors have to deal with the ambiguity of going on living.

I have younger friends who can't name a single person in their lives who died from AIDS. But *seventy* of my friends died from this horrible disease in ten years. Look at your life and imagine so many of the people in it disappearing. Forever. Sometimes it doesn't feel any different from if they just moved away. Like everyone just moved out of town and didn't give me an address to write. Some of my best friends. Some of my acquaintances. You'd hear that someone else had died and it would be like, "Oh, I knew Paul. Bill's downstairs neighbor, right?" He was not going to change my life. He was not going to cure cancer. But I knew him. He died of AIDS.

When my friends were dying, I tried to help them be comfortable. I was smart enough to know I couldn't actually change the course of their sickness, but I needed to feel like I could help in their final days. I used to bring my friend Bill hot peppers. I don't even know why, I just wanted him to have more spice in his life. My friend Tony, I used to spend so much time just sitting with him. I needed him to know he wasn't alone. I'm glad I was able to be present with my friends who were dying. I'm glad I spent my time as a young person being of service to my friends who were dying, because it taught me a lesson for life: You have to show up. Because eventually the people you love will be dead and you won't be able to show up anymore.

I still treasure those times, even though they were so horrible. It helped me to grow up, to stop being such a knuckleheaded kid. I still get angry when I think about a lot of the parents. They found out their kid was gay and had AIDS at the same time. I had so many friends who weren't out to their parents. And the parents would just throw them away. They wouldn't have anything to do with their sons. But then they'd turn up at the end and march out with whatever was left, all the art.

It went on and on. The deaths didn't seem to end until 1997. Once antiretroviral medication became available, deaths fell off a cliff. California had a program called ADAP, the AIDS Drugs Assistance Program, which meant anyone could get access to antiretroviral medication. HIV became a completely different disease. It became about health care management, not palliative care.

I'm the last person to suggest that the younger generation should learn something from me. They don't need me. Go invent the world you want to live in. I don't know what that world is. You do. Go invent it. But if there's anything that older LGBT people can do for younger LGBT people, it's to try to create a safer environment for the next generation. Every person, every community, every generation is going to face a complex crisis. AIDS was ours. Being optimistic is a very useful survival strategy. It kept me sane in the darkest times. Today, HIV is a manageable condition—in fact, it's a completely manageable condition. But young people still need to understand that they don't want it. You don't want to be HIV+. You don't want it at all.

**SOURCE MATERIAL**

## Parachute

### by Tim Dlugos

*Tim Dlugos was a poet active in the 1970s Lower East Side literary scene in Manhattan. After being diagnosed with HIV, he studied at Yale Divinity School to become an Episcopalian priest. He died in 1990 at the age of forty.*

The Bergman image of a game
of chess with Death,
though not in a dreamscape
black-and-white as melancholy
films clanking with symbols,
but in a garden in Provence
with goldfish in the fountain
and enormous palms whose topmost
fronds cut into the eternal
blue of sky above the Roman
ruins and the dusty streets
where any door may lead to life's
most perfect meal: that is what
I think of when I remember
I have AIDS. But when
I think of how AIDS kills
my friends, especially
the ones whose paths
through life have least
prepared them to resist
the monster, I think of

an insatiable and prowling beast
with razor teeth and a persistent
stink that sticks to every
living branch or flower
its rank fur brushes
as it stalks its prey.
I think of that disgusting
animal eating my beautiful friends,
innocent as baby deer. Dwight:
so delicate and vain, his spindly
arms and legs pinned down with needles,
pain of tubes and needles, his narrow
chest inflated by machine, his mind
lost in the seven-minute gap
between the respirator's failure
and the time the nurses noticed
something wrong. I wrapped
my limbs around that fragile body
for the first time seven years
ago, in a cheap hotel by the piers,
where every bit of his extravagant
wardrobe—snakeskin boots, skin-tight
pedal pushers in a leopard print,
aviator's scarves, and an electric-
green capacious leather jacket—
lay wrapped in a corner of
his room in a yellow parachute.
It's hard enough to find a parachute
in New York City, I remember thinking,
but finding one the right shade
of canary is the accomplishment
of the sort of citizen with whom
I wish to populate my life.

Dwight the dancer, Dwight the fashion
illustrator and the fashion plate,
Dwight the child, the borderline
transvestite, Dwight the frightened,
infuriating me because an anti-AZT
diatribe by some eccentric
in a rag convinced him not to take
the pills with which he might
still be alive, Dwight
on the runway, Dwight on the phone
suggesting we could still have sex
if we wore "raincoats," Dwight
screwing a girl from Massapequa
in the ladies' room at Danceteria
(he wore more makeup and had better
jewelry than she did), Dwight planning
the trip to London or Berlin where he
would be discovered and his life
transformed. Dwight erased,
evicted from his own young body.
Dwight dead. At Bellevue, I wrapped
my arms around his second skin
of gauze and scars and tubing,
brushed my hand against
his plats, and said goodbye.
I hope I'm not the one
who loosed the devouring animal
that massacred you, gentle boy.
You didn't have a clue
to how you might stave off
the beast. I feel so confident
most days that I can stay
alive, survive and thrive

with AIDS. But when I see
Dwight smile and hear his fey
delighted voice inside my head,
I know AIDS is no chess game
but a hunt, and there is no
way of escaping the bloody
horror of the kill, no way
to bail out, no bright
parachute beside my bed.

## TESTIMONY

# Robert Levithan

### (How Do You Feel?)

In the days when T-cells were our only indicator of immune system health, I remember coming home one day from an appointment with Trevor Hawkins, my MD. My T-cell count was down a hundred points or so. Not in a dangerous place, but moving in that direction.

I came into my house on Armenta Road, and Patrick Brown, the photographer who was renting my extra bedroom that summer, greeted me and asked what was up:

I was upset: "My T-cells are down."

"How do you feel?" Patrick asked.

"Good, but my T-cells dropped."

"How do you feel?"

"Good. I'm freaked about my T-cells...."

"How do you feel?"

This may have gone on even longer, but finally he reached me.

I feel good! The numbers do not change my state of being unless I give them that power!

Thank you, Patrick. I have applied this lesson many times to situations where information was scaring me but had little relevance to the actual present circumstances.

### (Andrew)

I wasn't supposed to be at home on Tuesday evening at 7, but I had strayed from my plans. The phone rang. Michael's numbed voice on the answering machine stated the facts: "Andrew passed at 4:15 this afternoon. You can call me at the house or come by."

I arrived at the once elegant, mansard-roofed and ridiculously adobed house on Reid Street by 7:15. I let myself in at Andrew's door. At the top of the stairs I was met by the smell of burning candles and a subtle smell which I am beginning to recognize as peaceful death.

Michael was alone. The family had cleared out. Andrew's mother, whom he had not seen in years, had arrived somewhat unexpectedly two hours before his death. Now, she was gone for good. Michael and I hugged. Dry-eyed, I ventured from the kitchen into the only other room—the bedroom.

There he lay, a miniature Rasputin; delicately dressed in a wine-colored vest, jeans, black velvet slippers, and a hat that covered KS lesions, patchy scalp, and set off his nubby beard.

He was quiet; he was still; he was surprisingly Andrew.

I sent dear exhausted Michael out for a dinner break and sat alone with Andrew's body—the room aglow with holy candles and bunches of red and white and purple and pink flowers.

I prayed for Andrew. I prayed for myself. I let go of the need to <u>do</u> anything.

Later Denise came by. What a relief her fervent tears were—to hold her and feel her grief, to talk with her about Andrew.

I had heard about the night from hell before: That Sunday a couple of months ago when Andrew's mind was like a record that keeps skipping and repeating. He got to "do" finding out he had AIDS over and over, every fifteen minutes, for most of the day. Denise said it was horrible—and that it was the one time he let her and Deborah, her partner, truly love him. That night he accepted tenderness.

I had feared that he would never experience that in this lifetime. I was so relieved.

Then Marc arrived and I photographed him and Denise on the bed with Andrew—a tableau of life and love amidst death.

I finally cried when I got ready to leave.

**SOURCE MATERIAL**

# Tiara

## by Mark Doty

*Mark Doty is one of the foremost chroniclers of the AIDS crisis, his work deeply informed by the death of his partner, Wally, in 1994. There are dozens of poems of Doty's we could have included here, and we encourage you to seek out both his poetry and his memoirs, most notably* Fire to Fire: New and Selected Poems *and* Heaven's Coast.

Peter died in a paper tiara
cut from a book of princess paper dolls;
he loved royalty, sashes

and jewels. *I don't know,*
he said, when he woke in the hospice,
*I was watching the Bette Davis film festival*

*on Channel 57 and then—*
At the wake, the tension broke
when someone guessed

the casket closed because
he was *in there in a big wig
and heels,* and someone said,

*You know he's always late,*
*he probably isn't here yet—*
*he's still fixing his makeup.*

And someone said he asked for it.
Asked for it—
when all he did was go down

into the salt tide
of wanting as much as he wanted,
giving himself over so drunk

or stoned it almost didn't matter who,
though they were beautiful,
stampeding into him in the simple,

ravishing music of their hurry.
I think heaven is perfect stasis
poised over the realms of desire,

where dreaming and waking men lie
on the grass while wet horses
roam among them, huge fragments

of the music we die into
in the body's paradise.
Sometimes we wake not knowing

how we came to lie here,
or who has crowned us with these temporary,
precious stones. And given

the world's perfectly turned shoulders,
the deep hollows blued by longing,
given the irreplaceable silk

of horses rippling in orchards,
fruit thundering and chiming down,
given the ordinary marvels of form

and gravity, what could he do,
what could any of us ever do
but ask for it?

## SOURCE MATERIAL

# What the Living Do

by Marie Howe

*Marie Howe's 1997 collection* What the Living Do *is haunted by the death of her younger brother, John, from AIDS complications. In the title poem, she tries to find a balance between the lives of the living and the dead.*

Johnny, the kitchen sink has been clogged for days, some utensil
    probably fell down there.
And the Drano won't work but smells dangerous, and the crusty
    dishes have piled up

waiting for the plumber I still haven't called. This is the
    everyday we spoke of.
It's winter again: the sky's a deep, headstrong blue, and the
    sunlight pours through

the open living-room windows because the heat's on too high in
    here and I can't turn it off.
For weeks now, driving, or dropping a bag of groceries in the
    street, the bag breaking,

I've been thinking: This is what the living do. And yesterday,
    hurrying along those

wobbly bricks in the Cambridge sidewalk, spilling my coffee
    down my wrist and sleeve,

I thought it again, and again later, when buying a hairbrush:
    This is it.
Parking. Slamming the car door shut in the cold. What you
    called that yearning.

What you finally gave up. We want the spring to come and the
    winter to pass. We want
whoever to call or not call, a letter, a kiss—we want more and
    more and then more of it.

But there are moments, walking, when I catch a glimpse of
    myself in the window glass,
say, the window of the corner video store, and I'm gripped by a
    cherishing so deep

for my own blowing hair, chapped face, and unbuttoned coat
    that I'm speechless:
I am living. I remember you.

# Elizabeth Coleman

*Elizabeth Coleman was a young woman when she learned that her dad was living with AIDS in the late 1980s. Here she tells her and her father's story.*

I loved my dad. He was handsome and kind. He painted all of my bedroom furniture with intricate flowers and fruit. He asked questions. He was genuinely interested in what was happening in my life.

It was hard not to be resentful when he moved out after he and Mom got divorced. I'd just started high school. It was still the 1970s. Dad's departure was shrouded in secrecy, because he was hiding the fact that he was gay and moving in with his new partner, Donald. For my dad's generation, being gay was fraught. He was scared that if people knew about him, he'd lose access to his kids or lose his job. There was a lot of hypocrisy, a lot of lies, but it was all just to keep us safe. That's how my dad saw it back then. His lies were his armor.

When Donald came on the scene, no one explained who he was. When Dad introduced us, I remember thinking, *Who is this strange man and why is he spending so much time with my dad?* We went to see *My Fair Lady* on Broadway. I remember feeling so uncomfortable. Back then, the thought that perhaps Dad was gay didn't even enter my head. I asked Dad if he was seeing anyone, and he invented a girlfriend called Sylvia Springfield. He was always making stuff up like that to throw us off the scent. He'd keep a copy of *Playboy* in the trunk of his car to make people think he was straight!

By the mid-1980s, I was in my twenties. I wasn't a kid anymore. I had gay colleagues by then, and gay friends. One summer, I was boating with

Dad and Donald upstate. I watched how they were with each other, and suddenly it all made sense to me. *Dad's gay. And Donald's his boyfriend.*

One time, my dad asked me if I realized that my boss was a homosexual.

I looked at him and said, "Yes, Dad, I do."

He asked, "How do you feel about that?"

"Dad," I replied carefully, "I'm fine with it. Just like I'm fine about you and Donald. I know about you two. I worked it out."

He asked me to keep it a secret from my mom and my brother and my two sisters. He was still scared of what might happen to him if everybody knew. He wasn't ready. So I carried on keeping his secret for him.

I kept his secret until Donald got sick. In 1988, Dad called. Donald had pneumonia. My siblings and I flew to New York to be with Dad, who was devastated. By that time my brother and sisters had also worked out that he was gay and Donald was his partner. When Donald died, none of us dared to speak about AIDS. Dad didn't want us to know the truth and he sure didn't want us to voice it. We followed his cues. We'd been well trained not to ask certain questions. We all lived in his denial. Denial is sometimes a form of survival. It helps you to keep moving forwards; it protects you from having to confront certain possibilities.

After that, I was living in San Francisco.

Donald had been dead for a year. The 1989 earthquake happened, and Dad told me and my sister he had HIV a few days later. We were driving over the Bay Bridge to bring my sister back to college.

"Donald didn't die of pneumonia," Dad said. "He died of AIDS."

I remembered being at the hospital as Donald died. I remembered knowing deep down that it must have been AIDS that was killing him. I remembered Donald's funeral, how Donald's family ignored Dad, how they acted like he wasn't an important person in Donald's life. Dad was heartbroken. And now, driving over the bridge with my dad as the city recovered from the worst earthquake in almost a century, Dad was talking about himself at last.

"I'm HIV-positive," he said.

I thought to myself: *Donald died of AIDS, and Dad's HIV-positive. So Dad's probably going to die too.* But he didn't want to discuss it. Dad having HIV became one more thing we didn't really talk about.

Eventually, as his health got worse, Dad gave up having two separate lives, his gay life and his life as our father. He asked me and my sister to tell our other siblings that he had HIV and was getting sick. In 1990, I moved to New York to live with Dad in the apartment he'd shared with Donald on the Upper East Side. I started to meet all their friends, the people he'd kept us from. Dad's friends were in ACT UP, they were eccentric artists. One friend was a cabaret singer who split her time between the East Village and Provincetown. I found photos she'd taken of Dad and Donald: strange, beautiful artifacts of the life they'd shared together for fifteen years—a life he'd never let us be part of. It was fun to see his life finally, but it hurt too, because he'd kept it hidden until too late.

In the last year of Dad's life, I no longer felt excluded by him, especially because I was living with him. It felt like I was his teenage daughter again, except this time, he let me see who he really was. It made me happy to know that I was finally getting to see all the parts of my dad's life that he'd tried to keep separate for so, so long. But then Dad went into the hospital for some tests, because he was beginning to show signs of AIDS-related dementia. He'd forget where he was and what he was doing. While he was in the hospital, he got pneumonia, and things went south. He got really sick, really quickly.

I rang my siblings one by one. "Dad's not doing well. You need to get here right away."

My brother rushed over from Chicago. My sisters came from New Orleans and California. Dad was hanging on by the time we were all there together. He asked to speak to us individually in his hospital room. He knew this was it. He knew he was dying. We all got to see him. We all got to tell him how much we loved him. But even then, we didn't have the tools we needed to really and truly speak openly about everything. The silence in our family about Dad's life had just been so constant and so consuming. It was a silence that we'd maintained for him for decades.

Five days after he'd first gone into the hospital, he died.

We had to plan the funeral. We could have gone the same direction as Donald's family and brushed it all under the carpet. No way were we going to do that. We wrote his death announcement for *The New York Times* and said he was survived by us, his four kids, and that donations should be sent to Gay Men's Health Crisis in lieu of flowers. We asked Dad's gay friends to speak at the funeral. Their eulogies for him spoke about his gay life.

We agreed that no one who came to the funeral should be in any doubt that Dad was gay and had died because he had AIDS. We weren't going to mince our words any longer.

The lies, at last, were gone. They were replaced by pain, but that pain was honest, and the honesty felt good and right. I'd had to carry so much tension about my father for such a long time—because of the closet, because of homophobia, and finally, because of AIDS. All this tension finally started to dissolve when we decided to be honest at last about his life, about who he was. There were so many people at the funeral. So many people had seen the announcement in the *Times*. There were people he hadn't seen in twenty-five years, right there with his gay friends. All the parts of his life came together at that moment.

I think about my dad all the time. I think about Donald too, and the life they built together before AIDS ruined it. It still breaks my heart that it was so hard for my dad to share his life with his kids. But when it comes down to it, what matters is that he was deeply loved. He loved us and we loved him.

# Todd Theringer

*Todd Theringer is the chairperson of the National Native American AIDS Prevention Center. His connection to the AIDS crisis began in his youth when his sister was diagnosed, and his mission to improve outcomes for Native Americans affected by HIV/AIDS continues to this day.*

My sister Janice was twenty-seven years old when she died. She lived in the San Jose area and spent time in San Francisco. She had the precarious life all mothers try to prevent their daughters from falling into. She was a victim of sexual trafficking. She struggled with addictions to love and to substances. This was a struggle she inherited from our mother. Addiction doesn't happen randomly; it reflects intergenerational trauma at work.

If you want to understand my sister's trauma, and what happened to her, you have to understand the collective trauma of Native American people. And that trauma goes back across several centuries. Starting in 1870, the US had a policy called "Save the Man, Kill the Indian." The military would go into Native land and tear the children away from their families. The scared children were sent off to boarding schools, but these places weren't designed to produce functional adults. They were more like orphanages, run by religious organizations as businesses, based on a military model. The children were taught to act like white people—made to act like "real Americans." They were only allowed to speak English. If they were caught speaking their Indigenous language, they were punished. Abuse of every type you can imagine was rife in these institutions.

When they turned eighteen, the kids got released, but no system was in place to support them. They had nowhere to go. If they were lucky, they had a record of where they'd been taken from or they could remember their tribe. If they had the resources to travel back to their community, they'd arrive to discover that their families no longer lived there. Similarly, children in the foster care system still experience similar cycles of alienation today.

Our grandmother Mary was one of these children. She came out of this abusive system at the age of eighteen unable to read, with no idea how to live a normal life. During her lifetime, she had thirteen children, including our mother, and those children grew up in extreme poverty, surviving off of the land on an Ojibwe reservation in Minnesota with alcohol abuse and violence in the community. Our mother and her siblings were taken away from her family in the 1950s, like a lot of Native kids, and put into the foster care system and rehomed by white families. The boarding schools might have closed, but she wasn't protected in the foster care system. She was sexually abused for years, which instilled in her a sense of powerlessness.

She was our mother, but she wasn't ready to be a parent. She fell into alcoholism once she left the foster care system. My sister and I grew up in an alcoholic home, surrounded by predatory adults. You learn that you're powerless when you're a child and one horrible thing after another keeps happening to you. That was my sister's situation, and our mother's situation, and our grandmother's situation. All the harm creates more hurt to the soul; trauma adds a new ring every year like a tree. My sister and I were put into foster care. We were separated and never really saw each other again until we were adults. Even then, our relationship never truly recovered because we were now the ghosts of who we were as children.

When she was thirteen years old, Janice met an older man who lived in the neighborhood. She ran away to be with the first man who told her he loved her. He introduced her to drugs and then he trafficked her for sex. She went missing, but no one bothered to look for her. Soon it was the mid-1980s. Add a virus like HIV into the mix. Tell people HIV only affects gay men even as it's spreading across the country. Growing up, we barely knew what HIV was; it didn't seem relevant to our lives.

When Janice was twenty-two years old, she teared up when she told me she wanted to have a baby. After all her miscarriages, a doctor told her she was unable to have children, thanks to the severe sexual abuse she suffered as a child. I was secretly happy to hear that she couldn't have children. I was sure she would just pass down the family curse of whatever had marked all of us for suffering.

Then, a few years later, she got pregnant. Janice considered it a miracle as she watched her stomach grow. She'd felt left out of life with everyone around her becoming parents; now she would fit in. But the pregnancy made her sick, and no one understood why. The doctors treated her mysterious illness with thyroid medication. No one suspected a pregnant young woman of having HIV.

A visiting doctor from San Francisco treated Janice in the emergency room in San Jose. He said, "I've seen these symptoms before. This woman has AIDS." Only then was she given an HIV test. When the test came back positive, they moved her to the part of the hospital which was being used to quarantine people with AIDS. They stopped treating her like a regular person. The orderlies wouldn't bring food to her; they left her meals at the door of the room, too afraid to come in. A lot of people with AIDS were treated that way. If the patient was too sick to get out of bed to retrieve the food, they'd go hungry. No one came to visit her, to feed her. This was in 1990. By then, the level of fear was enormous, and ignorance was still massive, especially in counties that didn't have big numbers of HIV-positive gay men. Maybe the medical profession was better educated by the time Janice was in the hospital, but most people she met were just plain terrified of anybody who had HIV/AIDS. Today, people still blame others for being HIV-positive, but they aren't afraid to be around them.

Janice had the baby she was told she would never have—Derek, who she named after the father. Derek was born crying and never stopped.

He was sick with AIDS. The county ruled that Janice was too unwell to look after her baby. AIDS babies were unwanted in the foster care system as well. It wasn't long before Janice became too sick to visit him. Once the county had custody, they showed no interest in facilitating visits to reunite the mother with the child. Janice never got to spend much time with her son during both of their short lives.

The doctors gave Janice twenty pills a day to treat her AIDS in 1990. The meds didn't work. She had no income and no health insurance. She was living with the family of her best friend from elementary school, Virgie, but they didn't want her there anymore, now that she had this terrifying disease. Virgie's mother got my phone number from a postcard I had sent Janice from New York City. She called me: "Your sister has AIDS and she's pregnant." She told me Janice couldn't live with them anymore because she was going to make everyone sick. They let her sleep in the van on the driveway. When Janice went to give birth at the hospital, they quickly changed addresses without telling her. She returned from the hospital on the bus to the place she thought was home, only to find it empty. The police found her passed out on a bench with a crying baby next to her in St. James Park, at the end of the 66 bus route.

I was a college student thousands of miles away. I couldn't find any resources to help my sister—they didn't seem to exist. There were no relevant resources for homeless women with AIDS, let alone any resources for Native American women in that situation. There was no internet back then. I couldn't do a Google search. I was powerless.

Janice had nowhere to go. San Jose didn't have the services for people with AIDS that were available in cities with big gay communities like San Francisco. When people spoke about AIDS, they never thought about women with AIDS. She was fighting different and intersecting forms of discrimination. Not just AIDS stigma, but the exclusion of women from a health care system geared around treating HIV-positive men, and the invisibility of Native American people from basically every conversation about AIDS in the country.

The last time I saw her was Christmas 1990. I made it out to

California from New York. She was living with some new people by then, people I didn't know. I was relieved that she had a place to stay, but when I got to the house, it was terrible. She was sleeping on a mattress in the garage because they were too afraid to have her in the house. I was enraged. This family was getting money from the government to care for her, and they were keeping her in the garage like a caged animal. But Janice told me she wanted to stay there. She felt safe, she had a TV, and they'd bring her food. She was basically living in a storage shed in the yard. I tried to think of other places she could go, but she wanted to be with people she knew.

Janice told me she thought she was going to die soon. She was afraid and in pain. She worried about Derek. We knew that the baby was dying too. Janice and I would talk long-distance from California to New York. I paid a huge long-distance phone bill due to all the crying and all the long pauses. There I was on the other end of the line, powerless, with no idea what to say, no idea how to help my sister. I didn't have any resources. I didn't have anyone in the family I could turn to, because I was just as alone as she was. I was a college kid who'd also survived the foster care system, living on the other side of the country. I was too ashamed to tell anyone what I was going through.

Janice's death took the dilemma out of my hands. One day, I got back from an exam in my statistics class and saw the light flashing on the answering machine. That's how I learned of her passing. I just locked the hurt away in a time capsule in my mind.

At least I managed to have a small funeral for her. Six people in a run-down storefront church, just me and some people I didn't know. I was the only family member who attended. I have a blurry memory of someone offering me her ashes in a box. I refused the ashes. I wanted her back. None of the funeral homes in the county would accept her body because her death certificate said AIDS. We hadn't wanted a cremation, but by that point, cremation was just one more indignity on top of all the rest.

It's hard to talk about Janice. There's a sense of shame hanging over me because I was so powerless; I couldn't do what needed to be done, I couldn't help her. I wish I'd been there when she died. I wish I'd been able to bring her to live with me. I wouldn't have put her in the garage. I would have made sure she was comfortable. Similar tragedies were happening all over the country. New York City has Hart Island, an island filled with the unclaimed bodies of people who died from AIDS. Janice came close to being unclaimed.

Janice's death galvanized me to get involved in AIDS activism in Native American communities. I'd seen firsthand that Native Americans faced a difficult situation with HIV. Here's this invisible disease, and we were an invisible demographic. Most Americans know next to nothing about Native Americans. That's not by accident; it's part of the design. It's how the United States has handled its history: to eliminate the truth of how the country was founded. We can't tell a romantic story about democracy and freedom if we have to add, "Oh, by the way, we practiced genocide against the people who were already here. Our inheritance is trauma and we live with the side effects of past government policy and revisionist history."

In the mid-1980s, the government started to give out funding for HIV/AIDS, but Native American communities were pretty much always left out. AIDS was considered a "gay disease" so most of the first federal resources went to support white men. There were increasingly high rates of HIV in the Black community, in the Latine community, so money started to go in those directions too. Federal funding gets allocated by the spread of a population. The resources begin with the white community, then the Black community and the Latine community. But Native people often get categorized as "Other." When you're an "Other," you're not going to get the resources you need to thrive. You're invisible and there are still no HIV data available from the government that shows the actual rate of HIV in Native American populations. This lack of data makes it easier for government officials to not act, because there is no proof of the need without the data to evidence it. Even today, the tribes could still speak up and organize to bring more resources to fight

HIV and STIs in their communities but they remain silent. Stigma has the power to silence nations.

Before the AIDS crisis, Native Americans were already an invisible population. Then HIV came along. We had to make people realize it was killing us too. *Hey! It's us! The people you've ignored, the people you've pretended are already extinct. We still exist and we need resources to fight this plague, just like any other group.* I became an activist to fight this invisibility, to improve the lives of Native Americans living with HIV, and to help Native American people protect themselves from HIV and other STIs. The memory of the suffering of my sister and my nephew is the arthritic ache in my bones that forces me to exercise and give voice to their silent disappearance from a life they had a right to have.

Today, I work with a lot of recently diagnosed HIV+ people from very traumatic backgrounds. Like Janice, their lives have been shaped by abuse and neglect; they're hurting, and the hurt leads them to seek some way of escape from that aching feeling, those memories. Combine their pain with their need to earn money; it's a risky combination which makes HIV transmission more likely.

*Hurt.* That's the word I hear from many adults living with HIV or struggling with addictions. A pain that engulfs your existence and won't go away. When I think of Janice, I hurt. I hurt because of her absence. The opposite of hurt is hope. Hope that one day we will view the virus as the culprit and not the people it steals from us. One day I found a faded Polaroid picture of Janice as a baby and recognized my mother's messy handwriting. On the back of the picture, she'd written one word: *Hope.*

## SOURCE MATERIAL

## Letter to Roger

by Deryl K. Deese

*Deryl K. Deese was born in Texas in 1961. This letter first appeared in* Brother to Brother: New Writings by Black Gay Men *in 1991.*

Dear Roger,

It's been three weeks since you passed away, and it still hurts as much as it did when I saw you take your last breath. I promised you two and a half years ago that I would be there with you through the end. I'm glad I could keep my promise to you. Even though I had a long time to prepare for your passing, it didn't make it any easier for me. I remember telling you as you lay there in the hospice the last two days to let go and cross over and that I'd be okay. Well, I lied. I knew that I wouldn't be fine, but it tore me apart to see you like that. I was glad when you finally let go, only because you weren't in any more pain. You no longer had to deal with having needles stuck in you or a bedside full of medicines to take every four hours. No more hospital beds, no more crying. I have to admit, even though I was glad, I was also a little angry because I couldn't go with you, because I felt as though you left me, and also because no matter what I did or how many times I told you I loved you there was nothing I could do to keep the pain away or keep you here.

Over the course of your illness I felt so helpless, particularly this last year. Even though I rubbed your feet and hands, they continued to hurt. Each day I watched you get a bit more weak. As your appetite grew smaller, and you struggled to eat what little you did, I got angry and yelled at you, but it was only because I was frustrated. All I could do was watch you waste away. It killed me inside to watch you get weaker. There were days when I wanted to cry, but I had to be strong for you and your son, little Roger.

Remember when you asked me a few months ago if I would end your life for you if you began to suffer? I remember how angry you were when I said that I couldn't do it. But baby, as you lay there during your last two days I thought about taking the pillow and putting it over your face many times. I just couldn't bring myself to do that. I couldn't play God.

I miss you so much, honey. My life isn't the same without you anymore. Sometimes I get so lonely and hurt so much that all I do is curl up and hold myself until it passes. What should be home doesn't feel like home, not without you. It's only a place for me to lay my head at night. I avoid going "home" because if I do, I have to face the fact that you won't be there. I'm not motivated to do anything but get out of bed and go to the gym. It's funny, though, sometimes I can hear your voice pushing me like when we trained together. I miss the way we used to hold and kiss each other. I miss the love we made and the way we made each other feel so very special. Every time you looked at me I could see the love in your eyes; I could feel it every time we touched. I miss walking hand in hand with you, or kissing you in public. Roger, you were everything and more than I ever wanted in a mate. I'll never forget the day we stood in front of our family and friends and were married by Reverend Carl Bean. That was the happiest day of my life, being a gay man and marrying the man I loved.

I can't help but feel cheated that all we had was three years together, but then I look at other people and realize they never find the kind of love we shared. God truly blessed us by allowing us to find each other and to have the kind of love we had, even through AIDS.

I feel so empty without you. When you left, you took so much of me with you. I wish I could have gone with you, but unfortunately it isn't my time yet. I'm sure that with time I'll be able to go on, but right now it's very hard for me. All the memories, both good and bad, still hurt. Sometimes I cry and don't even realize that I'm crying. The love we shared was so powerful, baby.

Thank you for your love and courage to stand with me as my spouse and friend. Thank you for working out all of our problems with me and making our love stronger in the process. Thank you for fighting the virus the way you did, because each time I looked in your eyes, I found the strength to hang in there. You are the best thing that ever happened in my life. There is no one who could ever take your place and move me like you did. Because of you my life is so much better, but at the same time, the emptiness and loneliness I feel hurt so much.

I know that you are happy now with the Lord and I am happy for you. When you hear me crying at night, please come to me and hold me like you used to. You will always be a part of me and I guess now nothing can separate us. When it's my time to cross over, you'll be there to help me across. Until that time, my life goes on and I'll live it and love you as I always did. I love you, Roger.

Your baby,

Deryl

# Ricky Tucker

*Ricky Tucker is a writer and educator based in New York City. His nonfiction book* And the Category Is . . . : Inside New York's Vogue, House, and Ballroom Community *was a* Los Angeles Times *bestseller.*

They say the brightest stars burn out quickly. It's hard to imagine what my aunt Ronnie would be like if she were still here. She was a firecracker. She was a stereotypical Taurus—totally stubborn. But the flip side of her stubbornness was that she was incredibly loyal. She'd lived in New York. She'd lived in London. She'd visit us down in North Carolina and arrive at the house bearing gifts—trendy films, trendy music, stuff that hadn't made it to North Carolina yet. When I was a kid, she introduced me to musical artists like Neneh Cherry, Sade, Monie Love. She was just so hip.

My mom and Ronnie grew up in Brooklyn, and in the 1980s, they got caught up in the crack epidemic which was taking over the city. Addiction happened. Mom and Ronnie were dating two brothers who were both drug dealers. Ronnie's boyfriend was the oldest one, and he could be abusive towards her. One time, they were out partying. He attacked her. They had an altercation. She grabbed a gun, she shot him, he died. She was sentenced to prison for manslaughter.

Ronnie's prison was in Raleigh, the capital of North Carolina. We were two hours away in Winston-Salem. My family had been split between North Carolina and New York City for generations. Most Black people in America have a North and a South, because of Reconstruction after the Civil War. During Reconstruction, there was a huge migration of Black folks up north after they were freed from slavery. My great-grandmother's house in North Carolina was my anchor for me when Mom and Ronnie were addicted to crack, because I couldn't live with my mom while she was using drugs. But my great-grandmother was *strict*. My great-grandmother gave me consistency when my own mother was unable to, but never much nurturing. When Ronnie came to stay, it was always easier. Ronnie gave me a safety net. She stood up for me. She wouldn't stand it when my great-grandmother came down too hard on me.

Ronnie served two years for manslaughter. It was through being incarcerated that she found out she was HIV+. Ronnie's diagnosis was a wake-up call. My mom got sober, and this time, she managed to *stay* sober. Once my mom had a steady apartment, no more hopping around or relapsing, I was able to spend real time with her. She became an active member of Narcotics Anonymous, a twelve-step program for folks who are trying to stay sober. Eventually, she came down to live with me and my great-grandmother in North Carolina.

When I turned 13, I got my own room. But then six months later, Ronnie moved in with us and shared my room with me. I wasn't mad about it: I loved being around her, especially now that she was sober. She was an amazing roommate. Her health was up and down. She had AIDS. But she made the most of the good times. She'd stay up late with me, talking and watching TV shows. She'd go out to sober nightclubs and dance all night, then get Chinese food with me the next day.

I remember one time there was a birthday party for my cousin. One of his friends called me a faggot because I just didn't fit in with the other boys.

I was destroyed by it. But Ronnie came to me, and asked, "What's wrong?" So I told her what happened. She said, "Honey, I don't care if you're gay. I love you just the way you are. Don't listen to them."

Now that my mom was clean and Ronnie was HIV+, we all started to speak about AIDS at home. I got to know people who were living with AIDS, because the crisis was closely linked to drug use in underserved communities like ours. AIDS was really present in my mother's new community of people recovering from drug and alcohol addiction. It seemed like AIDS was always coming for one of my mom's recovery friends just as they were starting to get their life back together. By the time I turned fourteen, I had lost four people in my life to the epidemic.

Including Ronnie.

When someone has a terminal illness, there's a period when it feels like everything's okay. You're just waiting for the other side. When Ronnie got sick, she was hospitalized for a while and then she moved back to the house. This time, her bedroom was in the living room. I remember the exact moment she died. We were exhausted. I'd been off school for two weeks to help look after her and be around her. Then one day my sister and I were in my room in the basement, on my bed, and Ronnie's daughter comes down the stairs and says to us, "She's gone."

Time went by. I came out the closet. I grew up. When I was 20, I ran away from North Carolina to live in Boston with my art-school boyfriend. We watched tons of movies. One time, we rented a copy of a documentary called *Paris Is Burning* from Video Underground. It's about the ballroom scene in New York: a world of drag queens and voguing and Black queer community. As the opening titles came up on the screen back in our apartment, a bolt of lightning went through me. I knew I'd seen it before. And then I realized: It was with Aunt Ronnie. A VHS tape of *Paris Is Burning* was one of the cool things she'd brought back from the city to share with me when I was a kid. And here I was, in Boston, watching it with my boyfriend.

I was kind of punk rock back then. I lived in a Food Not Bombs community for a while. We were like the Hare Krishnas, providing food a couple times a week for folks in need in public parks. My experience growing up around AIDS played a part in why I felt at home in social justice movements. It seemed like the only people who understood AIDS were recovering addicts and older activists.

I think a lot about the death I saw earlier in my life. For the longest time, I just couldn't stop thinking about AIDS. I was so angry about it. I'm still angry. And then I got involved with the ballroom community when I moved to New York. I said to myself: *I'm not going to be sad anymore. I want to find my joy.* I loved ballroom immediately. How smart it was, how radical it was. Ballroom gave me freedom. And ballroom will always help me stay connected to my aunt Ronnie, when I remember how she showed me *Paris Is Burning* all those years ago.

## SOURCE MATERIAL

## Thousands of Angels

by Anna Forbes

*Anna Forbes has written many articles and children's books about HIV/AIDS. This poem first appeared in Fingernails Across the Chalkboard.*

I said to my father once, "I'll try."
And he said, "That's all the angels can do."
Thinking of him, I sat down in the street
In front of the White House, in front of my world.

Facing the cameras, we started to name them
The lovers and friends who were torn from our lives
As the names of the dead rang out and embraced us
All my cold nervousness started to fade

I'm here for you, Bill. I'm bringing your anger
I'm here, Baby Luz, small and clear in my mind
Tell Mama Consuela I'm here with the fury
I felt on the day that I heard you'd both died

And, Robby, I smile as I wait for the handcuffs
I'm hearing your cracks about great-looking cops
Your fabulous wit is still here to delight me
I borrow the courage to live with your style

Thousands of angels surrounding the White House
The millions of us who have already died
Call out in our voices for housing, protection,
Medicine, food and no more genocide

Jamaal, keep me safe as my body's dragged from here
Brenda, stay with me and help me to shine
Kesha, come chant with us as, for the living,
We press the demands that will keep us alive.

# The Names

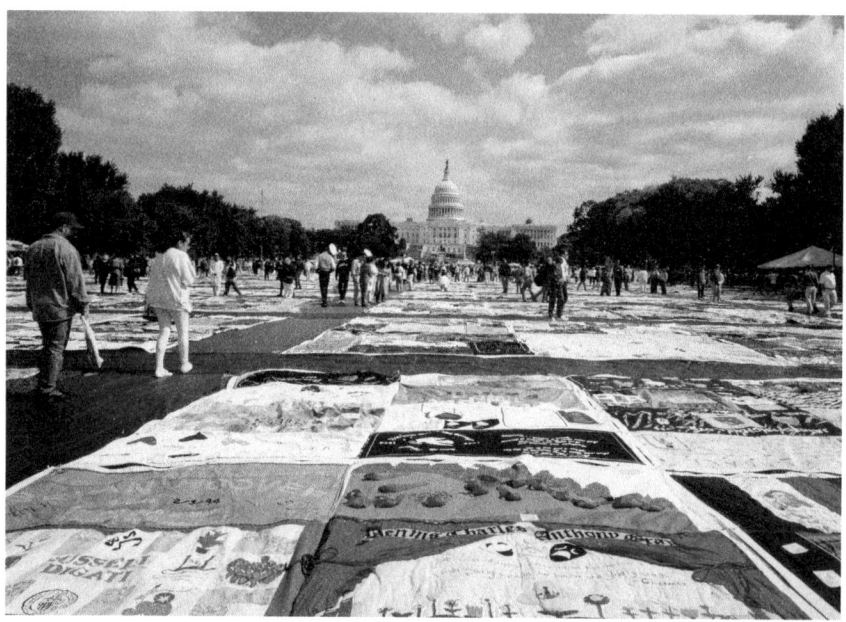

For a candlelight vigil in 1985, activist Cleve Jones asked those attending to bring small handwritten placards bearing the names of people who'd died because of AIDS. As the vigil passed the San Francisco Federal Building, marchers affixed these names to a wall. Seeing the squares of names assembled in this way, Jones was reminded of a quilt—all the separate pieces coming together in one powerful whole. It felt to him like a meaningful way to assemble the dead, to commemorate their lives and protest their deaths.

His idea became the NAMES Project. Jones and others put out a call for people who'd lost someone to AIDS to create a fabric panel, three feet by six feet, in some way marking that person's life. The NAMES Project set itself up in a storefront in San Francisco's Castro neighborhood, with the plan of joining the panels together into one large quilt.

The volunteers in that Castro storefront started with one sewing machine.

They would soon need many, many more.

Within weeks, panels were coming in from all over the country. Volunteers worked well into the night sewing them together, while at the same time reading the stories sent in with the panels about the people whose lives had been lost. The AIDS Memorial Quilt had, in a simple yet striking way, tapped into one of the greatest despairs that comes with grief—the despair that the dead will be forgotten, that your memories are the only things that will hold your loved one's name onto this earth. The Quilt was not only offering a place in history, it was offering company within that place—a memorial carved not out of impersonal, graveside stone, but drawn from all the fabrics that life could hold.

Anything that could be affixed onto a square was affixed onto a square. Mementos and symbols. Sequins and denim. Favorite T-shirts and childhood blankets. Vinyl records and gold necklaces. Costumes from stage productions and pockets holding ashes. Poems and flowers, in-jokes and nicknames. Pieces of opera house curtains and wartime flags. There for everyone to see: The names of the dead. The dates of their births. The dates of their deaths. The total years they had been given to live. From four months old to seventy years old. Worldwide celebrities and those who were buried in paupers' graves. All genders, all races. All having one devastating thing in common.

All across the country, they stitched. All around the world, they sewed.

A mother who'd watched one, then two of her sons die, putting them both on a single panel, because she knew that was what they would have wanted.

A twenty-one-year-old with AIDS creating a panel for his friend, knowing that one day soon, he would be getting a panel of his own. Then, after he died, another friend taking up the task and making that panel before he, too, died, to be stitched into the Quilt by someone else.

Family and friends coming together to commemorate someone they loved, each one taking a letter in his name, each using a fabric that reminded them of a time they'd shared with him—holidays they'd taken, shirts they'd worn together, love letters duplicated, their handwriting transformed into black thread.

A proud sister creating a panel in her younger brother's memory, only to have her parents insist that she cross out his last name so no one would have to know how their son died.

Other panels: anonymous. Out of fear. Out of desire to keep private things private. One daughter simply stitching *Love You, Dad*—because he had never wanted to talk about having AIDS and wouldn't have wanted his name to be there.

The entire display department of a department store coming together to sew panels for coworkers who've died. Later, the store will feature these panels in their windows as a show of support.

A man commemorating "the twelve men I expected to grow old with" by portraying them as twelve candles. Three remain lit. Nine have been snuffed out. (A year later, two more are gone.)

A teenage girl who reads in a newsmagazine about a man who died all alone, so she wants to create a panel for him, just in case no one else in his life would.

A woman who can't bear the thought of erasing a friend's name from her address book, so instead she cuts it out and sews it onto her piece of his Quilt.

Civil rights icon Rosa Parks creating a square for a friend, Deborah Haynes, who was one of the many people in her Black community who died because of AIDS.

Future Speaker of the House Nancy Pelosi reading out loud the name of her beloved niece as that niece's part of the Quilt is unveiled for the nation to see.

A grandmother sewing patch after patch after patch onto a panel for her thirty-seven-year-old grandson. "We were so close," she tells the NAMES Project. "I was there when he was born, and I was there when he passed away."

A man who made an annual Valentine's Day portrait of his lover asks in his dying days to be propped against the wall so his outline can be traced; after the lover's death, the man transfers the silhouette onto fabric, surrounding it with a multitude of small words telling their story.

On and on and on. Panels for children. Panels for parents. Panels for lovers, friends, coworkers. Panels for strangers. A panel for the near stranger who died in the hospital bed next to yours. A panel for the man next door, whose name you never knew. A panel for a musician whose piano playing brought you joy in low moments. Panels for drag queens using their drag names. Panels for drag queens using their offstage names. Panels for Republican politicians who never admitted what they were dying of. Panels for mentors, teachers, choir directors. Panels for men who lived on ranches. Panels for women who lived in ranch houses. Panels for those who died alone. Panels for those who died hearing voices that offered love, thanks, and release.

In 1987, in time for a giant queer march on Washington, DC, the Quilt is first shared on the National Mall, with 1,920 panels. It covers two city blocks' worth of space. It is a public catharsis and a political reckoning as the names are read aloud and the Quilt is revealed. People weep to see the names of those they've known, and they weep to see the expanse of names they never knew.

In 1988, the Quilt returns with 8,288 panels. In 1992, 12,000. In 1996, it is 40,000 panels strong, covering all eleven blocks from the Washington Monument to the US Capitol. An estimated 1.2 million people go to see it, including, for the first time, the president of the United States. In 2012, it is displayed in increments of 1,500 panels a day because the Quilt has become too large to show all at once.

It now has over 50,000 panels and continues to grow.

It covers 1.3 million square feet.

Parts of the Quilt still travel the country, and the entire Quilt can be seen at aidsmemorial.org/interactive-aids-quilt.

As was intended, the names live on.

*The following sequence is by award-winning illustrator Brian Selznick, created for this book.*

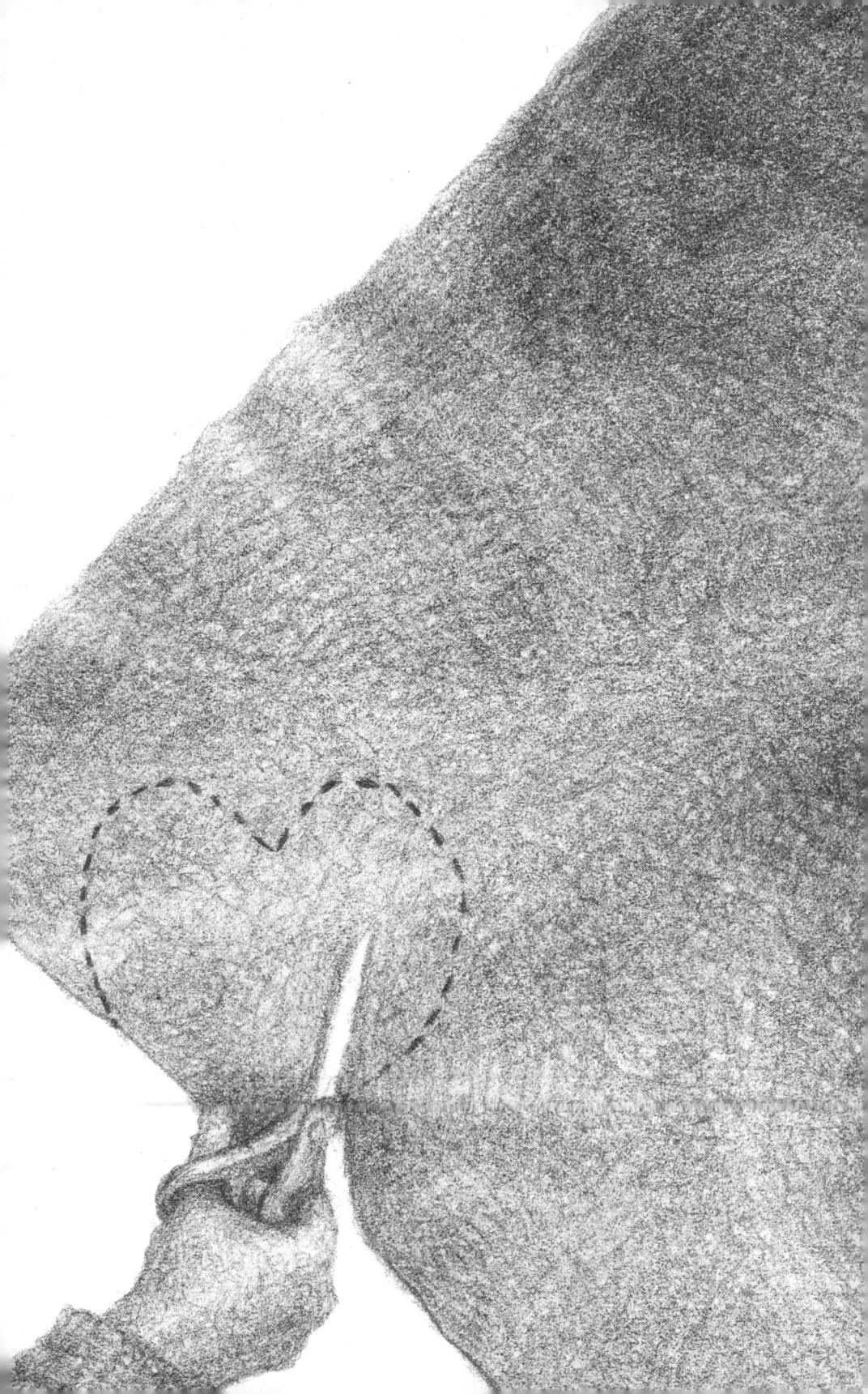

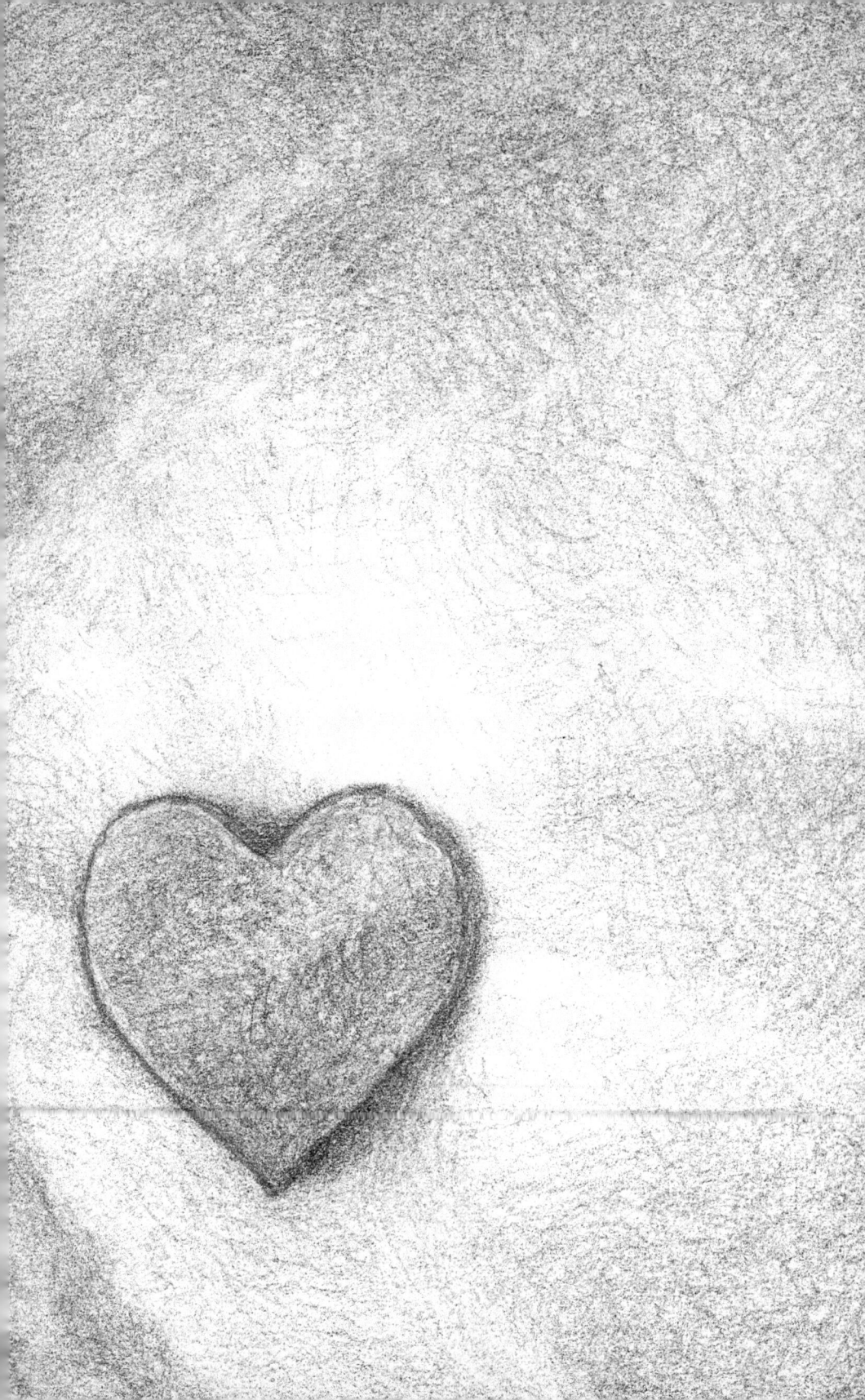

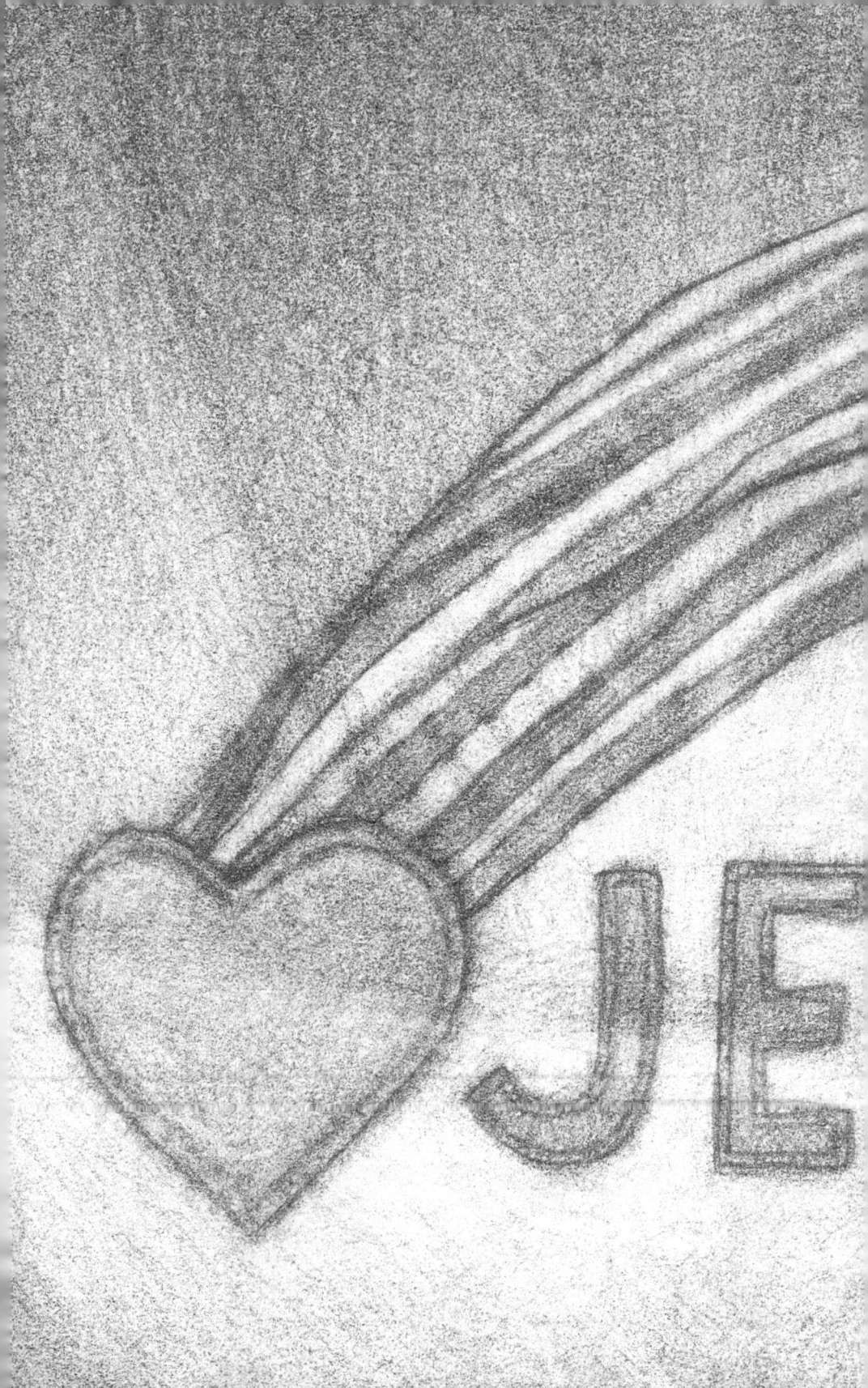

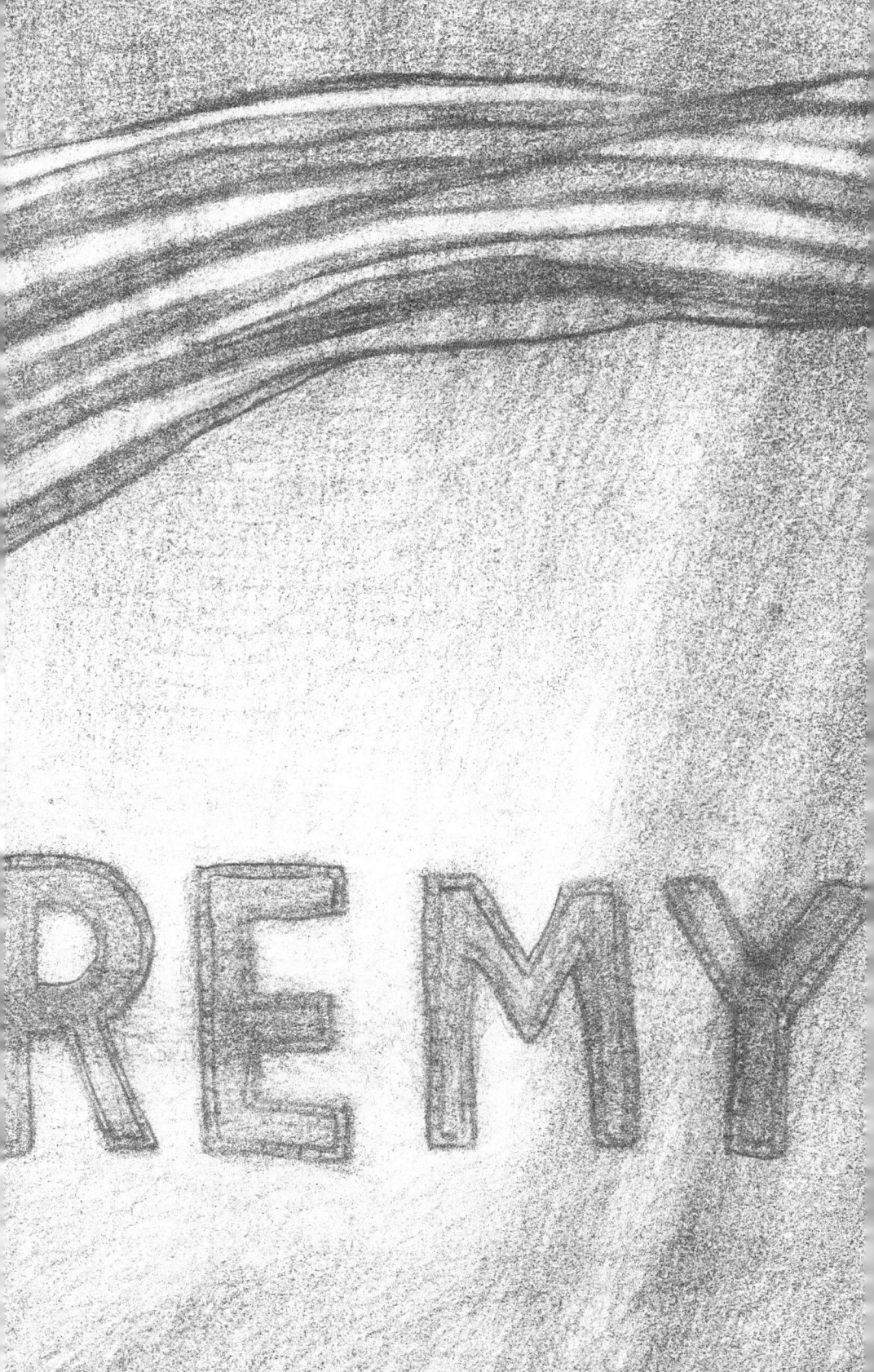

| | | |
|---|---|---|
| Ramiro Nunez | F. HOWARD COWELL | JOHN 8 12 42 ♥ 3 5 87 MIDDLEBROOK |
| LARRY RABBIT | Rod Carter | ROGER DBST 4 3 86 |
| Alini Kochs | MIKE PEARSON | HARVEY THOMPSON 1941-1996 |
| JIMMY CURRY | | Alan Paine SF CA |

| | | |
|---|---|---|
| BILL BUCHOLTZ | DANNY HARRIS | GREGG RICHARD |
| CHIP BALLINGER | | JAMIE |
| AARON HAYNES | | HENNING |
| | PAUL | |

| | | |
|---|---|---|
| | ROBERT MESSICK | MIKE TRUJILLO |
| | PABLO MAGALLANEZ | JERRY CURTIS |
| | JAVIER | JIMMY |

Tony Panico
JEREMY
ALPHONSE DE LAURA
BRAD SAWTELL
BRYCE HOLCOMBE
BRIAN HOVEY SEATTLE WA
RICHARD PARIS

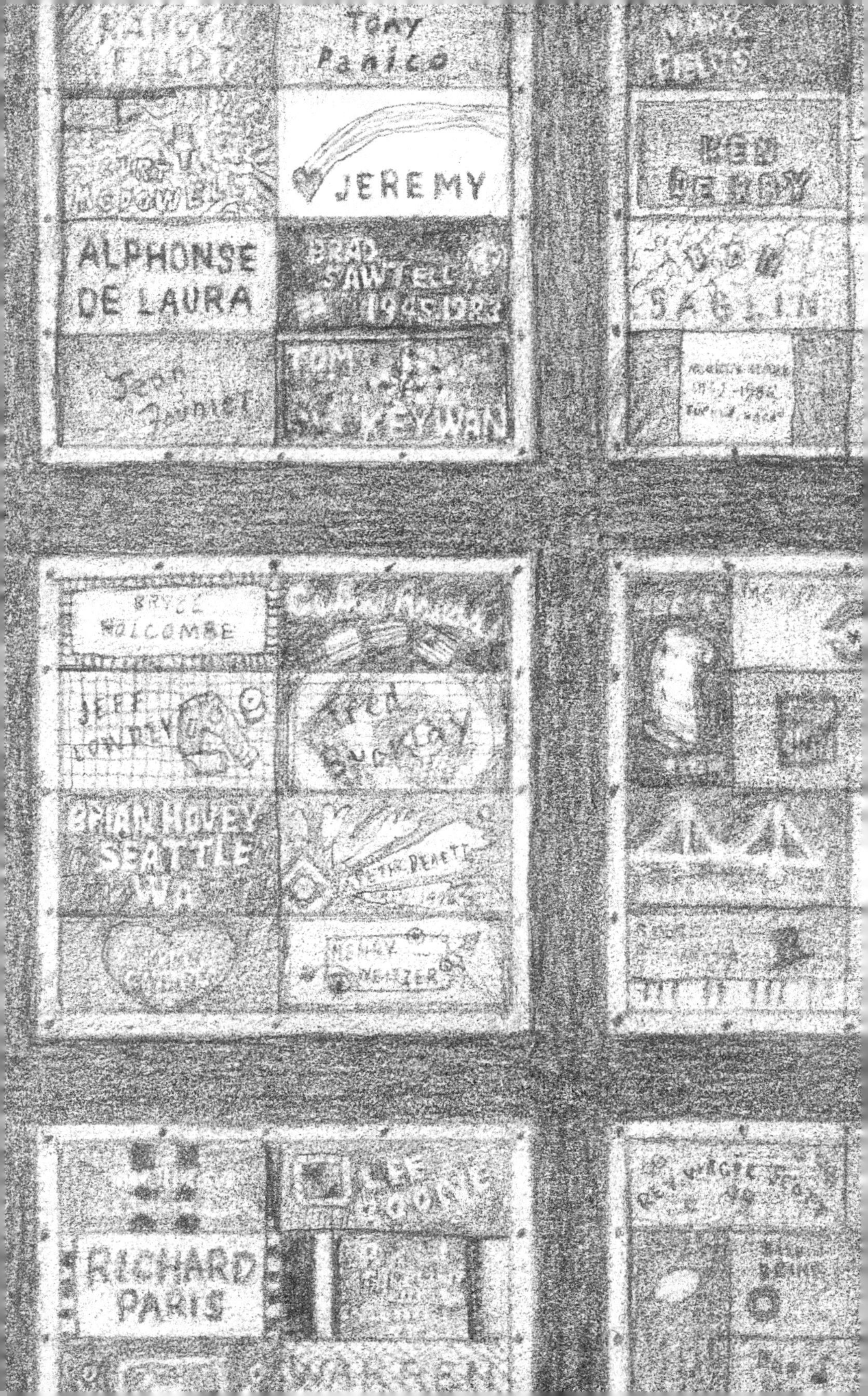

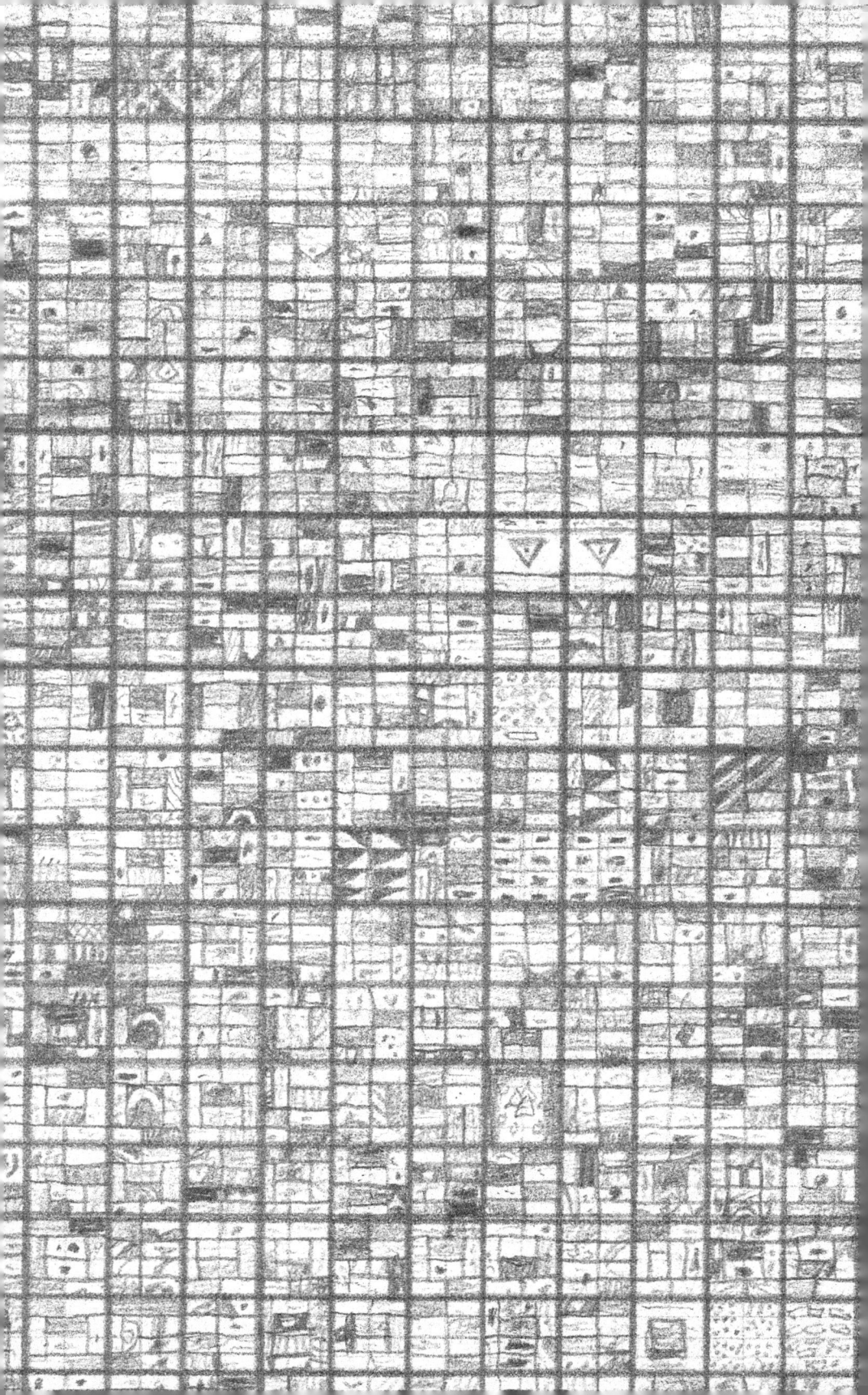

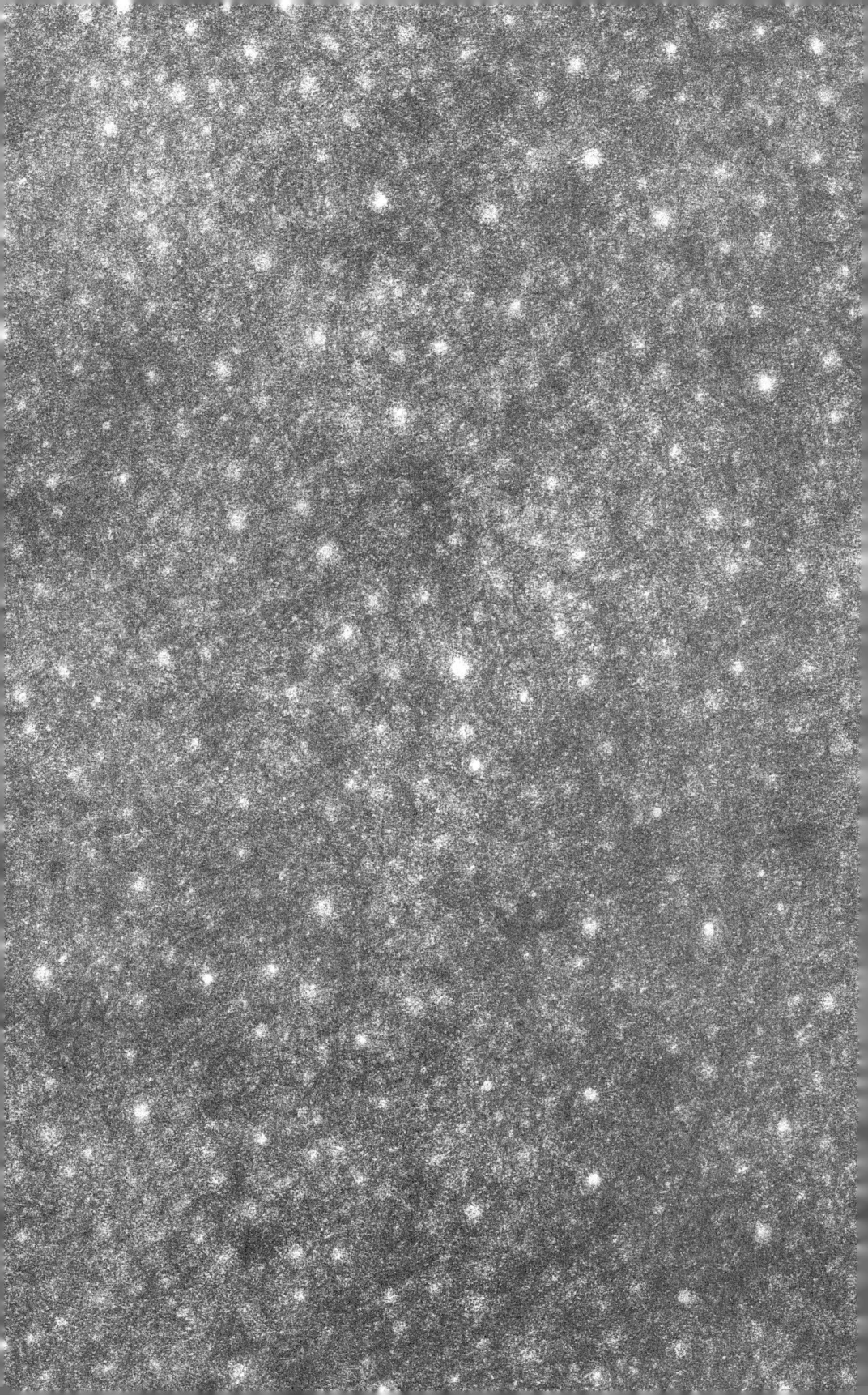

**SOURCE MATERIAL**

## Aunt Ida pieces a quilt

### by Melvin Dixon

*"As white gays deny multiculturalism among gays, so too do [B]lack communities deny multisexualism among their members. Against this double cremation, we must leave the legacy of our writing and our perspectives on gay and straight experiences." So said poet Melvin Dixon, addressing the Third National Lesbian and Gay Writers Conference in March 1992. He died of AIDS complications in October 1992, age forty-two.*

You are right, but your patch isn't big enough.

—Jesse Jackson

When a cure is found and the last panel is sewn into place, the Quilt will be displayed in a permanent home as a national monument to the individual, irreplaceable people lost to AIDS—and the people who knew and loved them most.

—Cleve Jones, founder, The NAMES Project

    They brought me some of his clothes. The hospital gown,
    those too-tight dungarees, his blue choir robe
    with the gold sash. How that boy could sing!
    His favorite color in a necktie. A Sunday shirt.
    What I'm gonna do with all this stuff?
    I can remember Junie without this business.

# Aunt Ida pieces a quilt

My niece Francine say they quilting all over the country.
So many good boys like her boy, gone.

At my age I ain't studying no needle and thread.
My eyes ain't so good now and my fingers lock in a fist,
they so eaten up with arthritis. This old back
don't take kindly to bending over a frame no more.
Francine say ain't I a mess carrying on like this.
I could make two quilts the time I spend running my mouth.

Just cut his name out the cloths, stitch something nice
about him. Something to bring him back. You can do it,
Francine say. Best sewing our family ever had.
Quilting ain't that easy, I say. Never was easy.
Y'all got to help me remember him good.

Most of my quilts was made down South. My mama
and my mama's mama taught me. Popped me on the tail
if I missed a stitch or threw the pattern out of line.
I did "Bright Star" and "Lonesome Square" and "Rally Round,"
what many folks don't bother with nowadays. Then Elmo and
me married and came North where the cold in Connecticut
cuts you like a knife. We was warm, though.
We had sackcloth and calico and cotton, 100% pure.
What they got now but polyester rayon. Factory made.

Let me tell you something. In all my quilts there's a secret
nobody knows. Every last one of them got my name Ida
stitched on the back side in red thread.
That's where Junie got his flair. Don't let nobody fool you.
When he got the Youth Choir standing up and singing
the whole church would rock. He'd throw up his hands
from them wide blue sleeves and the church would hush

right down to the funeral parlor fans whisking the air.
He'd toss his head back and holler and we'd all cry holy.

And nevermind his too-tight dungarees.
I caught him switching down the street one Saturday night,
And I seen him more than once. I said, Junie,
you ain't got to let the world know all your business.
Who cared where he went when he wanted to have fun.
He'd be singing his heart out come Sunday morning.

When Francine say she gonna hang this quilt in the church
I like to fall out. A quilt ain't no showpiece,
it's to keep you warm. Francine say it can do both.
Now I ain't so old-fashioned I can't change,
but I made Francine come over and bring her daughter
Belinda. We cut and tacked his name, *JUNIE*.
Just plain and simple. "*JUNIE*, our boy."
Cut the *J* in blue, the *U* in gold. *N* in dungarees
just as tight as you please. The *I* from the hospital gown
and the white shirt he wore First Sunday. Belinda
put the necktie *E* in the cross stitch I showed her.

Wouldn't you know we got to talking about Junie.
We could smell him in the cloth.
Underarm. Afro-Sheen pomade. Gravy stains.
I forgot all about my arthritis.
When Francine left me to finish up, I swear
I heard Junie giggling right along with me
as I stitched Ida on the back side in red thread.

Francine say she gonna send this quilt to Washington
like folks doing from all 'cross the country,
so many good people gone. Babies, mothers, fathers

and boys like our Junie. Francine say
they gonna piece this quilt to another one,
another name and another patch
all in a larger quilt getting larger and larger.

Maybe we all like that, patches waiting to be pieced.
Well, I don't know about Washington.
We need Junie here with us. And Maxine,
she cousin May's husband's sister's people,
she having a baby and here comes winter already.
The cold cutting like knives. Now where did I put that needle?

# Refuge in Their Final Days

At the height of the AIDS epidemic in the 1980s and 1990s, stigma and fear often eclipsed basic human compassion. While many people dying because of AIDS found support and care from their friends, families, and lovers, there were others whose families, friends, or lovers abandoned them in their time of need, or whose friends and lovers were too caught in their own struggles with the disease to provide the support and care needed. Except in cities like New York and San Francisco, hospitals were often unprepared for long-term AIDS care; besides hospitals, there were often few places for people with AIDS to go. Even after death, with many families refusing to bring bodies home for burial and many funeral homes refusing to handle AIDS-related deaths, people with AIDS needed a place to go.

When it opened in 1987, Bailey House was the largest residence in the US for homeless people with AIDS. Located at the corner of Christopher Street and West Street, it sat in the heart of gay Greenwich Village in New York City, on the site of (among other things) a former gay discotheque. The idea behind the forty-four-room residence was that lowering loneliness and housing uncertainty for people living with AIDS would give them more strength with which to face their medical challenges.

*The New York Times* featured a man named Angelo, who had been suicidal because of his status. He told the reporter, "I used to think, 'If I die, they won't find my body for three or four days.' It's tough to be by yourself. Loneliness is your worst enemy." Finding a "comfortable and warm" home at Bailey House changed his perspective. "We've got to treat each other as brothers and sisters," he said, "because we don't have anyone else."

Like those at a similar organization, Housing Works, that formed around the same time, the people running Bailey House knew that a sense of home was crucial to a sense of survival for its residents. Another organization, God's Love We Deliver, was formed to bring meals to people with AIDS who could not leave their homes because of illness; often, its volunteers found that it was the human interaction of the delivery that mattered as much as the food being delivered.

Sometimes more extreme measures had to be taken to give refuge, especially outside major cities. In 1986, Ruth Coker Burks was visiting a friend in a local hospital in Arkansas when she noticed a door with a big red plastic bag over it. She overheard a group of nurses reluctant to check on the man inside, dying because of AIDS and calling for his mother. Burks slipped into his room and sat with him for thirteen hours; when he thought she was his mother, arriving to be with him in his last hours, she didn't correct him. After he died, Burks discovered that his mother refused to take responsibility for burying him. So Burks found the only place that would cremate him (seventy miles away), paid for his cremation, put the ashes in a pottery jar, and buried him in her family plot.

She did not set out to build a refuge, but that was what happened. Rural hospitals from across the state sent patients her way. "They just started coming," she later told an interviewer. "Word got out that there was this kind of wacko woman in Hot Springs who wasn't afraid. . . . I was their hospice. Their gay friends were their hospice. Their companions were their hospice." Soon Burks's home was a way station for men with AIDS who had nowhere else to go. Along with her teenage daughter and any friends or partners they brought along, Burks ministered to them. And when they died, she gave them a place to be buried. (Accounts vary as to how many men were ministered to in this fashion; five have been named, and there are others who Burks says were buried there anonymously, as they'd requested.)

Paul Wineland, whose partner was cared for by Burks, told her on NPR, "You were the only person that we could call. There wasn't a doctor. There wasn't a nurse. There wasn't anyone. It was just you. . . .

You loved them more than their families could. You loved them more than their church could. Now it almost looks like looking back into another world."

In New Orleans it was, unexpectedly, two men from the Catholic Church who stepped in to give people with AIDS a caring home in their final days. In 1985, Father Paul Desrosiers, a Catholic priest, was overwhelmed by how HIV/AIDS was decimating his community. "It was tough," he said years later. "It was difficult because I was dealing with sick people, dying people, all the time, and it was a wide range of people, young people and older people. I had to deal with a lot of families who could not accept the reality."

Another local priest, Father Bob Pawell, was seeing the same thing in his parish, where many people on the margins of society were grappling with HIV/AIDS with nowhere to go. He and Desrosiers approached the archbishop to get permission to turn a former convent next to Desrosiers's church into a hospice. The archbishop granted their request, and ten beds were set up under the name Project Lazarus. For the first five years, there were no survivors, as the proper treatment had yet to be found. But better for these people to die being watched over by a staff who cared.

Father Desrosiers wanted to do more. He realized the rectory where he was living could be converted to expand the shelter—so he moved out, and twenty-four more beds were created for the ill.

Because of the stigma of HIV/AIDS, the location of Project Lazarus was kept secret. As Steve Rivera, a later director of Project Lazarus, said of Desrosiers, "Father Paul broached a very unpopular topic that was full of fear and he addressed it head-on. All he could see was beautiful people with beautiful souls."

In May 1987, Clara Hale, better known as Mother Hale, was eighty-two years old and legendary for starting Hale House, a Harlem home that over decades had raised hundreds of babies born addicted to drugs because of their parents' drug use. President Ronald Reagan called her "an American hero" in his 1985 State of the Union address, and no one would have faulted her for keeping to the same mission. But instead, she opened a home (said to be the first of its kind) to care for babies whose parents had died because of AIDS or could not help their children because of their disease. This was a significant problem in the 1980s; many hospitals had "boarder babies"—babies whose mothers had transmitted HIV to them while they were in the womb, and who survived when their parents did not. Many foster parents were nervous about bringing HIV+ babies into their homes, so sometimes nurses would take them under their own care, or hospitals would take care of the babies for as long as they could. Mother Hale felt it was her duty to care for these children, just as she did for those who were born addicted.

When asked the secret to her heroism, Hale said her way with the babies was simple. In truth, her instructions apply to the care given by anyone who gives refuge to people with AIDS, at any age. Whether they are coming into the world or leaving it, it is so essential to "hold them, rock them, love them and tell them how great they are."

## TIMELINE

# 1992-1996

### July and August 1992

As AIDS kills more and more people, it becomes impossible for politicians to ignore it. Both presidential candidates in 1992, Bill Clinton and the incumbent president, George H. W. Bush, want to show that they're compassionate to people with AIDS and committed to finding a treatment. As a result, both the Democratic and Republican National Conventions showcase speakers with AIDS.

At the Democratic convention, the first speaker to talk about AIDS (after an introduction by Representative Patricia Schroeder of Colorado) is Bob Hattoy, a gay man working on the Clinton campaign who has discovered only ten days earlier that he is HIV+. When he told Clinton about his test results, Clinton offered him a chance to talk to the world. And now here he is, in Madison Square Garden in New York City, talking to millions of viewers. After saying "AIDS does not discriminate, but George Bush's White House does" and "AIDS is a disease of the Reagan/Bush Years," he tells his audience:

> This is hard. I'm a Gay man with AIDS and if there's any honor in having this disease it's because it's an honor being part of the Gay and Lesbian community in America.
>
> We have watched our friends and lovers die, but we have not given up hope. Gay men and Lesbians created community health clinics, provided educational materials, opened food kitchens, and held the hands of the dying in hospices. The Gay and Lesbian community is an American family in the best sense of the word. . . .

President Bush, we are a million points of light; you are just too morally blind to see us. Mr. President, you don't see AIDS for what it is—it's a crisis in public health that demands medical experts, not moral judges—and it's time to move beyond your politics of denial, division and death. We need a President who isn't terrified of the word "condom."

Every single person with AIDS is someone worthy of caring for. After all, we are your sons and daughters, fathers and mothers. We are doctors and lawyers, folks in the military, ministers and priests and rabbis. We are Democrats, and yes, Mr. President, Republicans. We are part of the American family and, Mr. President, your family has AIDS and we're dying and you're doing nothing about it.

Listen. I don't want to die. I don't want to die. But I don't want to live in an America where the President sees me as the enemy. I can face dying because of a disease, but not because of politics.

Pediatric AIDS activist Elizabeth Glaser speaks next, defining the issue in her own human terms.

I'm Elizabeth Glaser. Eleven years ago, while giving birth to my first child, I hemorrhaged and was transfused with seven pints of blood. Four years later, I found out that I had been infected with the AIDS virus and had unknowingly passed it to my daughter, Ariel, through my breast milk, and my son, Jake, in utero.

Twenty years ago I wanted to be at the Democratic Convention because it was a way to participate in my country. Today, I am here because it's a matter of life and death. Exactly four years ago my daughter died of AIDS. She did not survive the Reagan Administration. I am here because my son and I may not survive four more years of leaders who say they care, but do nothing. I am in a race with the clock. This is not about being a Republican or an Independent or a Democrat. It's about the future—for each and every one of us.

I started out just a mom—fighting for the life of her child. But along the way I learned how unfair America can be today, not just for people who have HIV, but for many, many people—poor people, gay people, people of color, children. A strange spokesperson for such a group: a well-to-do white woman. But I have learned my lesson the hard way, and I know that America has lost her path and is at risk of losing her soul. America, wake up: We are all in a struggle between life and death.

I understand—I understand the sense of frustration and despair in our country, because I know firsthand about shouting for help and getting no answer. I went to Washington to tell Presidents Reagan and Bush that much, much more had to be done for AIDS research and care, and that children couldn't be forgotten. The first time, when nothing happened, I thought, "They just didn't hear me." The second time, when nothing happened, I thought, "Maybe I didn't shout loud enough." But now I realize they don't hear because they don't want to listen.

When you cry for help and no one listens, you start to lose your hope. I began to lose faith in America. I felt my country was letting me down—and it was. This is not the America I was raised to be proud of. I was raised to believe that others' problems were my problems as well. But when I tell most people about HIV, in hopes that they will help and care, I see the look in their eyes: "It's not my problem," they're thinking. Well, it's everyone's problem and we need a leader who will tell us that.

We need a visionary to guide us—to say it wasn't all right for Ryan White to be banned from school because he had AIDS, to say it wasn't all right for a man or a woman to be denied a job because they're infected with this virus. We need a leader who is truly committed to educating us.

I believe in America, but not with a leadership of selfishness and greed—where the wealthy get health care and insurance and the poor don't. Do you know how much my AIDS care costs? Over

> $40,000 a year. Someone without insurance can't afford this. Even the drugs that I hope will keep me alive are out of reach for others. Is their life any less valuable? Of course not. This is not the America I was raised to be proud of—where rich people get care and drugs that poor people can't. We need health care for all. We need a leader who will say this and do something about it.
>
> I believe in America, but not a leadership that talks about problems but is incapable of solving them—two HIV commission reports with recommendations about what to do to solve this crisis sitting on shelves, gathering dust. We need a leader who will not only listen to these recommendations, but implement them.
>
> I believe in America, but not with a leadership that doesn't hold government accountable. I go to Washington to the National Institutes of Health and say, "Show me what you're doing on HIV." They hate it when I come because I try to tell them how to do it better. But that's why I love being a taxpayer, because it's my money and they must feel accountable. . . .
>
> Once every generation, history brings us to an important crossroads. Sometimes in life there is that moment when it's possible to make a change for the better. This is one of those moments.
>
> For me, this is not politics. This is a crisis of caring.

Glaser concludes by saying, "I challenge you to make it happen, because all our lives, not just mine, depend on it."

A month later, at the Republican convention, it is Mary Fisher who addresses the crowd. She is an artist who contracted HIV from her husband and became an activist fighting the disease and the stigma around it. This is her speech in full:

> Less than three months ago at platform hearings in Salt Lake City, I asked the Republican Party to lift the shroud of silence which has been draped over the issue of HIV and AIDS. I have come tonight to

bring our silence to an end. I bear a message of challenge, not self-congratulation. I want your attention, not your applause.

I would never have asked to be HIV-positive, but I believe that in all things there is a purpose; and I stand before you and before the nation gladly. The reality of AIDS is brutally clear. Two hundred thousand Americans are dead or dying. A million more are infected. Worldwide, forty million, sixty million, or a hundred million infections will be counted in the coming few years. But despite science and research, White House meetings, and congressional hearings, despite good intentions and bold initiatives, campaign slogans, and hopeful promises, it is—despite it all—the epidemic which is winning tonight.

In the context of an election year, I ask you, here in this great hall, or listening in the quiet of your home, to recognize that AIDS virus is not a political creature. It does not care whether you are Democrat or Republican; it does not ask whether you are black or white, male or female, gay or straight, young or old.

Tonight, I represent an AIDS community whose members have been reluctantly drafted from every segment of American society. Though I am white and a mother, I am one with a black infant struggling with tubes in a Philadelphia hospital. Though I am female and contracted this disease in marriage and enjoy the warm support of my family, I am one with the lonely gay man sheltering a flickering candle from the cold wind of his family's rejection.

This is not a distant threat. It is a present danger. The rate of infection is increasing fastest among women and children. Largely unknown a decade ago, AIDS is the third leading killer of young adult Americans today. But it won't be third for long, because unlike other diseases, this one travels. Adolescents don't give each other cancer or heart disease because they believe they are in love, but HIV is different; and we have helped it along. We have killed each other with our ignorance, our prejudice, and our silence.

We may take refuge in our stereotypes, but we cannot hide there long, because HIV asks only one thing of those it attacks: Are you human? And this is the right question. Are you human? Because people with HIV have not entered some alien state of being. They are human. They have not earned cruelty, and they do not deserve meanness. They don't benefit from being isolated or treated as outcasts. Each of them is exactly what God made: a person; not evil, deserving of our judgment; not victims, longing for our pity—people, ready for support and worthy of compassion.

My call to you, my Party, is to take a public stand, no less compassionate than that of the President and Mrs. Bush. They have embraced me and my family in memorable ways. In the place of judgment, they have shown affection. In difficult moments, they have raised our spirits. In the darkest hours, I have seen them reaching not only to me, but also to my parents, armed with that stunning grief and special grace that comes only to parents who have themselves leaned too long over the bedside of a dying child.

With the President's leadership, much good has been done. Much of the good has gone unheralded, and as the President has insisted, much remains to be done. But we do the President's cause no good if we praise the American family but ignore a virus that destroys it.

We must be consistent if we are to be believed. We cannot love justice and ignore prejudice, love our children and fear to teach them. Whatever our role as parent or policymaker, we must act as eloquently as we speak—else we have no integrity. My call to the nation is a plea for awareness. If you believe you are safe, you are in danger. Because I was not hemophiliac, I was not at risk. Because I was not gay, I was not at risk. Because I did not inject drugs, I was not at risk.

My father has devoted much of his lifetime guarding against another holocaust. He is part of the generation who heard Pastor Niemöller come out of the Nazi death camps to say,

*They came after the Jews, and I was not a Jew, so, I did not protest. They came after the trade unionists, and I was not a trade unionist, so, I did not protest. Then they came after the Roman Catholics, and I was not a Roman Catholic, so, I did not protest. Then they came after me, and there was no one left to protest.*

The lesson history teaches is this: If you believe you are safe, you are at risk. If you do not see this killer stalking your children, look again. There is no family or community, no race or religion, no place left in America that is safe. Until we genuinely embrace this message, we are a nation at risk.

Tonight, HIV marches resolutely toward AIDS in more than a million American homes, littering its pathway with the bodies of the young—young men, young women, young parents, and young children. One of the families is mine. If it is true that HIV inevitably turns to AIDS, then my children will inevitably turn to orphans. My family has been a rock of support.

My 84-year-old father, who has pursued the healing of the nations, will not accept the premise that he cannot heal his daughter. My mother refuses to be broken. She still calls at midnight to tell wonderful jokes that make me laugh. Sisters and friends, and my brother Phillip, whose birthday is today, all have helped carry me over the hardest places. I am blessed, richly and deeply blessed, to have such a family.

But not all of you have been so blessed. You are HIV-positive, but dare not say it. You have lost loved ones, but you dare not whisper the word AIDS. You weep silently. You grieve alone. I have a message for you. It is not you who should feel shame. It is we—we who tolerate ignorance and practice prejudice, we who have taught you to fear. We must lift our shroud of silence, making it safe for you to reach out for compassion. It is our task to seek safety for our children, not in quiet denial, but in effective action.

Someday our children will be grown. My son Max, now four, will take the measure of his mother. My son Zachary, now two, will sort through his memories. I may not be here to hear their judgments, but I know already what I hope they are. I want my children to know that their mother was not a victim. She was a messenger. I do not want them to think, as I once did, that courage is the absence of fear. I want them to know that courage is the strength to act wisely when most we are afraid. I want them to have the courage to step forward when called by their nation or their Party and give leadership, no matter what the personal cost.

I ask no more of you than I ask of myself or of my children. To the millions of you who are grieving, who are frightened, who have suffered the ravages of AIDS firsthand: Have courage, and you will find support. To the millions who are strong, I issue the plea: Set aside prejudice and politics to make room for compassion and sound policy.

To my children, I make this pledge: I will not give in, Zachary, because I draw my courage from you. Your silly giggle gives me hope; your gentle prayers give me strength; and you, my child, give me the reason to say to America, "You are at risk." And I will not rest, Max, until I have done all I can to make your world safe. I will seek a place where intimacy is not the prelude to suffering. I will not hurry to leave you, my children, but when I go, I pray that you will not suffer shame on my account.

To all within the sound of my voice, I appeal: Learn with me the lessons of history and of grace, so my children will not be afraid to say the word "AIDS" when I am gone. Then, their children and yours may not need to whisper it at all.

God bless the children, and God bless us all.

Glaser remained involved in the Elizabeth Glaser Pediatric AIDS Foundation until her death from AIDS complications in 1994. After Bill Clinton's election, Hattoy served in his administration until 1999; he died in 2007, also from AIDS complications. Fisher founded the Mary Fisher Clinical AIDS Research and Education (CARE) Fund to support

HIV/AIDS research and education and in 2006 became a global emissary for the Joint United Nations Programme on HIV/AIDS.

## January 1993

Definitions are important. They're not neutral. They shape the world we live in. One of the ludicrous aspects of the AIDS crisis in the 1980s was that AIDS was defined by symptoms that affected people with penises, not people with vaginas. The root of this mistake was that most of the first people in whom AIDS was identified in the United States were in the first category, but HIV doesn't care about biological sex. By the late 1980s, it was abundantly clear that anyone, regardless of gender or sex, could contract HIV and develop AIDS-related illnesses. But the medical definition of AIDS was based on research into the way it manifested in men's bodies, not women's. (The fact that gender did not have to be defined by the presence of a penis or a vagina was not something that medical professionals were much engaged with at the time.)

A medical definition is a legal definition. By the late 1980s, there were some established protections and services for people with AIDS, especially in cities that had been hard-hit by the crisis, like New York and San Francisco. These services were always playing catch-up, because the latent period between HIV infection and AIDS meant that new cases were always appearing, increasingly. That meant it was a challenge for people with AIDS to access relevant services, either because of the county or state they lived in or because the services were overwhelmed by the growth in AIDS cases.

The narrow definition of AIDS made it even harder. Women experiencing AIDS could be told their symptoms didn't match the definition of AIDS, and that meant they weren't eligible for certain care or protections, like disability payments or sheltered accommodation. It meant that many women were kept in the dark about their condition, because the science of AIDS didn't incorporate the symptoms of people with bodies like theirs.

Activism played a huge role in pushing the CDC to update its definition. As the ACT UP protest slogan sarcastically observed: *Women don't get AIDS, they just die of it.*

At the start of January 1993, an updated definition of AIDS finally comes into effect, announced the previous month. Besides distinguishing HIV from AIDS by diagnosing AIDS when a person's HIV infection is marked by a CD4 cell count of below 200, the CDC adds pulmonary tuberculosis, recurrent pneumonia, and invasive cervical cancer to the list of AIDS-defining illnesses in HIV+ people. As a result, there is a 111 percent increase in the number of US AIDS cases, many of them among women. In particular, incorporating cervical cancer into the definition of AIDS means that HIV+ women can be tested and treated for this cancer before it becomes untreatable. It also means that people experiencing cervical cancer can be tested for HIV, in case the virus is causing the cancer.

An ugly truth of the AIDS crisis is that women have been, and continue to be, underdiagnosed with HIV until they're already experiencing AIDS. Changing the definition of AIDS to include symptoms associated with women helped to combat this issue.

## May 1993

> This disease will be the end of many of us, but not nearly all, and the dead will be commemorated and will struggle on with the living, and we are not going away. We won't die secret deaths anymore. The world only spins forward. We will be citizens. The time has come.
> Bye now.
> You are fabulous creatures, each and every one.
> And I bless you: More Life.
> The Great Work Begins.
> —Prior's final words from Tony Kushner's *Angels in America: A Gay Fantasia on National Themes*, the first part of which premieres on Broadway on May 4, 1993

## June 1993

In a stunning rebuke to the Clinton administration and America's treatment of immigrants with AIDS, US District Judge Sterling Johnson Jr. orders the closure of what he calls "nothing more than an H.I.V. prison camp" at the US naval base in Guantanamo, Cuba.

It has taken the imprisoned refugees over two years to get this decision.

In 1991, when Haitian President Jean-Bertrand Aristide's government was overthrown by the military, an estimated 40,000 Haitians fled the country. Of these, 10,500 were granted admission into the United States as political refugees. Over 25,000 were returned to Haiti. And approximately 200 were captured at sea and subject to a legal limbo: Their claims of political refugee status were deemed credible, but tests revealed that they were HIV+. US immigration law forbade the granting of permanent resident status to HIV+ people, and even though there was a loophole for immigrants seeking political asylum on American soil, Guantanamo was not considered American soil.

Judge Johnson does not hold back in the wording of his decision. He writes: "Although the defendants euphemistically refer to its Guantanamo operation as a 'humanitarian camp,' the facts disclose that it is nothing more than an H.I.V. prison camp presenting potential public health risks to the Haitians held there. The Haitians' plight is a tragedy of immense proportion, and their continued detainment is totally unacceptable to this court."

He describes the conditions at Guantanamo in this way:

"They live in camps surrounded by razor barbed wire. They tie plastic garbage bags to the sides of the building to keep the rain out. They sleep on cots and hang sheets to create some semblance of privacy. They are guarded by the military and are not permitted to leave the camp, except under military escort. The Haitian detainees have been subjected to pre-dawn military sweeps as they sleep by as many as 400 soldiers dressed in full riot gear. They are confined like prisoners and are subject to detention in the brig without hearing for camp rule infractions."

In an earlier decision, Judge Johnson allowed refugees with AIDS who needed medical treatment to come to the United States for treatment they could not get at the naval base. Now he frees the remaining 158 refugees—people with AIDS, HIV+ people, or the children or family members of HIV+ people who have been kept in Guantanamo as well.

The pressing question becomes: Where will these refugees go?

This is where the New York City government comes in. Prodded by ACT UP New York activists, who have been protesting the treatment of the Haitian prisoners for the past year, the city takes the refugees in, finds them housing, and provides for their medical care. It is not a happy ending—the refugees will still struggle to support themselves while dealing with their health issues—but it shows a positive, welcoming side of what governmental officials are capable of doing, in stark contrast to the horrendous treatment given in Guantanamo (which will soon be the site of even more notorious brutality during the Iraq War).

Once Judge Johnson issues his ruling, the refugees' lawyers call them in Cuba.

"They were screaming with joy," one lawyer tells the *Los Angeles Times*. "They were dancing in the camp they were so thrilled."

## February 1995

In an interview with celebrity journalist Barbara Walters, four-time Olympic gold medalist Greg Louganis tells the world he has AIDS. Louganis, who came out the year before at the Gay Games, becomes the first major openly gay sporting figure to disclose his HIV status.

Louganis reveals that he was diagnosed with HIV six months before the 1988 Summer Olympics in Seoul, South Korea, at age twenty-eight. He did not think he would live to the age of thirty. Still, he went on a taxing AZT regimen that had him taking medication every four hours—disrupting his sleep schedule as he trained for his events.

After Louganis reveals he has AIDS, much discussion centers on one of his dives in the 1988 Olympics, when he hit his head on the diving board and needed four stitches before reentering the competition. Many contend that he put the other divers in danger because his blood might have gone into the pool, though experts say the chance of transmission that way is virtually nonexistent. Even the doctor who treated his wound without gloves says it was highly unlikely he would have become infected in that moment. (The next year, the Olympics make it mandatory for doctors to wear gloves when dealing with blood.)

*Breaking the Surface*, Louganis's book about his experiences as a half-Samoan, half-white, dyslexic former outcast who became an Olympic star, is released shortly after the Barbara Walters interview. Louganis becomes one of the best-known people with AIDS in the world, and eventually combination therapy makes his viral load undetectable. In a later interview, the man who was sure he would die by thirty says that the achievement he is most proud of isn't his Olympic glory but his book tour, because on the book tour "people would come up and say that they were in an abusive relationship and that the book gave them the courage to leave, it gave them the courage to fight ahead dealing with HIV, . . . to come out to their parents about their sexuality." It is his glory that gets him the attention . . . but it is his story that leaves the mark.

## June 1995

*Sweet one, it's all okay. The birthday parties you won't be at, the shoes by the door. You helped your friends when it was their turn. It's your turn now, and everyone's here to help you, because people are mostly good. The bed next to you is empty again; the orderlies are getting it ready for the next patient. It's like Penn Station in here, this flow of arrivals and departures, hellos and goodbyes. It'll be your turn soon, your midnight train. Just you and the driver. Some days, you're at peace with that. You marvel at yourself: You've acquired a mystical power. You know how to walk toward the end with serenity. You've seen it firsthand—it's happening—the thread of sand falling through the hourglass. Accept it. Some people get hit by a car so fast they don't even know it's happening before the credits are rolling. Death doesn't have to be such a big deal; our lives are just video games we can't replay.*

*You are so beautiful. In and out of sleep in the darkness. Golden wings sprout from under your shoulder blades in the moonlight.*

*Then the sun begins to rise.*

The testimonies in this book are proof that the AIDS crisis didn't neatly end the moment protease inhibitors started to be used to fight AIDS in the mid-1990s. AIDS didn't vanish. HIV didn't vanish either. Combination therapy wasn't a magic wand that fixed everything. We still don't know how to bring back the dead. But it did help the living. The sun began to rise.

It's June 1995. The FDA approves the first protease inhibitor for use treating AIDS. It changes everything. It begins the transformation of HIV from an extreme and fatal illness to a long-term health condition. In the United States, the mid-1990s represented the darkest hour before dawn, which is a phrase people use to acknowledge that sometimes the solution seems to arrive only when the situation is dire. The worst and best parts of our lives are right next to each other.

*You will smile again. You will be lifted from the darkness and taken back into the light. Those little wings go back into your shoulder blades. You are going to live the life that you had made peace with losing.*

The first protease inhibitor is called saquinavir. In December 1995, this drug is approved for use in combination with other medications. When used alone, these medications can't consistently tackle the progression of AIDS. But scientists realize that if a combination of drugs are used together, the effects of AIDS dramatically recede. The teamwork of these drugs stops HIV from replicating itself in the body. If HIV can't replicate itself, then the immune system stops being as compromised, and the person living with HIV stops experiencing the symptoms and illnesses that define AIDS.

It's not a miracle cure. The treatment is complicated and expensive:

It feels like you spend every day managing an absurd timetable of pills. At first, there's a huge amount of anxiety that the virus will develop widespread resistance to this unprecedented treatment, sending us back to square one. But that doesn't happen. All the illness and death that seemed for so long inevitable are proven to be avoidable. For many, it's too late. Combination therapy won't be accessible in other parts of the world for more than five years, as scientists and governments wrestle with manufacturing rights and the problem of distributing expensive medications to vulnerable people. While that process drags on, millions of people around the world will continue to die.

*It's not a miracle until it's a miracle for everyone.*
*But you're leaving the hospital today. You feel good.*
*Let's dance.*

## December 1996

*Time* magazine's Person of the Year is usually a politician, a war leader, or an agent of great social change. In 1996, the magazine surprises many by naming Dr. David Ho its Man of the Year.

"Some ages are defined by their epidemics," the article, written by Philip Elmer-DeWitt, begins, noting that with nearly 30 million people infected worldwide by HIV at that point, "today we live in the shadow of AIDS."

Ho is bringing some light to dispel those shadows.

In July 1996, at an AIDS conference in Vancouver, Ho announced that his experiments showed that the cocktail of protease inhibitors and antiviral drugs was effective in containing HIV. And, for the first time, not only did the treatment stop the virus from replicating . . . it also began to weaken the virus, causing a rebound in patients' immune defenses.

Writes *Time*: "We have learned this year what may be the most important fact about AIDS: it is not invincible."

Ho is a virologist who understood early on that there was no real "dormant" stage when it came to HIV; as soon as it took hold in the body, it began to fight the body, aggressively growing wherever it could. Therefore, Ho determined, the best chance of treatment was getting in early and preventing the virus's spread. Although there are other doctors who were working on "combination therapy" (using multiple drugs in a cocktail), his team pinpoints its use in the earliest stages as the best remedy. And they get results. His patients are among the first to have their viral load declared undetectable, when the level of HIV within their blood is no longer measurable.

The success of the cocktail ushers in a new era of AIDS treatment. There is still a very high cost to the drugs (about $20,000 a year) at first, and accessibility is an issue. But this is the breakthrough that has been needed in order to bring hope back to the fight.

**TESTIMONY**

# Robert Levithan

**(1998)**

I want to be thoroughly used up.

Sometimes I wonder how Michael cannot somewhere be in a body. It is so simple to be alive—perhaps the illusion of death is simply a long-distance move. Michael is settled with framed spectacles on the border between Mongolia and China.

I can't follow this fantasy. It is like my refusal to go to LA since Michael died two and a half years ago—it is my not wanting to feel—to believe deep down that <u>he is dead</u>.

Michael died on Sept 18, 1996 at the age of 31. I am still here. These are the facts.

When he went, he seemed to not have used all his talents. When I die, I want to be thoroughly used up. Sometimes I think I'm trying to live for Michael and Carol and Peter and Mathew—that somehow I am obligated to live fully in order to make up for what they missed.

This is all clearly hubris. I am living as fast and as fully as I can for selfish reasons. I love the sensations, the taste, the caresses of living. The little murmurs and the great arias. I live to walk on a windy day at the beach with my dog and I live to sit talking about how we people work and I live to look another man in the eye and know that all these words are not necessary, that I am already wherever it is I am going.

## (2006)

I've outlived myself by a decade. Twelve years ago, when I entered the hospital with AIDS-related pneumonia, the result of a collapsed immune system, the prognosis was a couple of years of struggle and decline.

My official HIV diagnosis was already ten years old. I had been part of an early study of people with AIDS and others who didn't have the illness, but were from "risk" groups. I had been enrolled as an "other." Unbeknownst to me, I would be one of the first to be tested for HIV antibodies—more than a year before a test was available to the public. I don't know how long I was positive when that test was done—I have a memory of an unexplained flu-like illness in the Summer of 1975. . . . Who knows?

In April of 1994, a few days after my 43rd birthday and six months after my mother's death from ovarian cancer, I discovered that I had a T-cell count of 53. A few days later I arrived in NYC for my friend Cy's 60th birthday. I decided to take advantage of being on home turf, and called a family meeting.

Attending were my father, recently widowed, but staggeringly vital at 83; my two brothers, Allen & Jack (four and five years my senior); their wives, Beth, who I had known for thirty years and saw as a sister surrogate, and Carol, Jack's first wife—their 25-year marriage was on the brink of collapse, I later discovered.

There was neither a precedent nor a procedure for a meeting like this. They were already aware of my HIV status, but we had all lived in healthy denial regarding my condition. We had dealt with my mother's two bouts with cancer as a cohesive unit. My father was a rare man for his generation—nurturing and domestically capable. He had been my mother's main caretaker, but we had all participated, a team.

I knew what to expect. Did they?

"I have asked you here today to let you know that my immune system is seriously compromised, and if I am to survive, I will need support—emotionally and financially. I intend to seek out experimental, and if necessary, illegal, treatments. This could be expensive."

Not much more needed to be said. Their resources were pledged. From that moment until today, I have never chosen treatment options based on cost. There have been some high-ticket items: Gamma G at $1000 a monthly dose. $700 veal liver extract, cutting edge serums, and enough eastern medicine (Chinese and Tibetan), acupuncture and supplements to bankrupt me alone. But I was not alone.

Did these treatments work? I will never know for sure, but they were invaluable. My ability to be proactive helped me to maintain a sense of possibility and hope which carried me until I walked into my NY doctor's office in August of 1995 and saw an application for a lottery for early access to Crixivan, one of the first workable protease inhibitors. I had heard about it from my doctor, who had seen one of his patients return from the brink of death to reasonable health during a trial. Although I had said no to earlier trials, my inner voice said: *THIS IS IT.* I filled out the form and mailed it in. I won. I don't know what the odds were, but out of nearly a hundred patients in my doctor's office who applied, three of us got it.

On October 11 (a date I noted as the birthday of my dead ex, Peter Hujar) I began the regimen. Crixivan required an empty stomach—no food for two hours before and one hour after each dose, eight hours apart. My life became my schedule—meals, outings, sleep—everything timed for the best results. In a month, my T-cell count had doubled from 22 to 44. On December 7, Dr. Bellman and I were on *Charlie Rose* discussing the approval that day by the FDA of the first protease inhibitors. In January my T-cell count hit 212, so I threw a party—I had jokingly said if my T-cells ever went above 200 again, I would give a party. I wasn't going to tempt the fates. I hosted my dad and ten friends for a celebratory evening at Bar Pitti. An idle boast had become a reality. There have been peaks and dips along the way, but the climb has been consistent: My last count (2/06) was 879.

That fall of 1995, we didn't know what we were part of. We were creating the data for a new AIDS paradigm. Previously, it had not been known that when HIV is suppressed, the immune system can rebuild. At first it was hard to trust the results. A year into the cocktail, Dr. Bellman hesitated to take me off prophylaxis for opportunistic infections even though my T-cell count was over 300. "We don't know yet if these new T-cells are fully functional," he said.

Later that year, we took a leap of faith, and I have been HIV+ and healthy ever since.

A decade.

## (1999)

How many T-cells do you need to have a life?

I had 20. I stayed at the Hotel du Cap and sailed to Corsica, golden hair to my shoulders and the love of my life (so far) by my side. I was gallant, I was brave, I was in denial.

Then the miracle arrived. I won the lottery, which I knew I would, and took the pills, and worked and had sex with friends and pretty boys from the gym.

And then I had 140 and I got depressed! Now I had something to lose. But that didn't last. 212 and I gave a dinner party. 300 and I broke out the Veuve Clicquot. 400 was lost in mourning for Michael, who died at age 31, choosing the Shaman's drum over the cocktail. 501 was another celebration. And on It goes.

How many T-cells do you need to fall in love? Is 600 enough to withstand the struggle to remain myself?

Just today I said: I'm dating. Dating as opposed to chasing after or running away from. Maybe there are enough T-cells for me to slow down and believe that I have time, enough time to fall in love, to write a book, to sail the southern coast of Turkey nine months hence.

How many T-cells do you need to not be afraid?

It's all up to you.

## (1999)

My job is to walk Knick and sleep eight and a half hours a night and dress in one color and to smile at the lithe brown man in bed with me in the morning.

My job is to let myself be held and to let him walk the dog while I take a shower and let my hair dry.

My job is to sit in a well-lit room with eight other men, seven of whom have AIDS and one of whom has cancer in remission and a seeing-eye dog.

My job is to not put up with the acting-out client who calls fifteen minutes before a session for the second week in a row with a lame excuse for why he needs to cancel—and not feel the least bit of remorse.

My job is to write about what I am feeling. I am feeling warm in my heart and it's about all of my life—Dale, the man in bed, and Matthew, Sally, and Morgan sitting in black leather chairs, also writing, and Knick, a lump on his flank that will be prodded by a vet tomorrow at 12:15.

My job is to eat cholesterol-free oatmeal and drink Turkish tea and write and smile while other pens scratch and that dog lets out a sigh.

My job is to check the time on the watch I bought in St. Tropez in 1995. The saleslady said it had a two-year guarantee, and she didn't get it when I said, "I wish *I* had a two-year guarantee!"

## (2000)

Let me tell you about love.

You have to practice love like you practice God. It's a series of exercises, attempts, and repetitions. It's overcoming the inevitable lapses and breaches and messing up and continuing. It's an act of will matched by faith and selective reasoning, because eventually the mind must be outstripped by the inexorable, bloody, pure, and pitiless, unshakable, and wet heart.

**SOURCE MATERIAL**

## Non, Je Ne Regrette Rien

### by David Warren Frechette

*David Warren Frechette, born in 1948, was a native New Yorker whose writing appeared in magazines including* Essence, The Advocate, *and* Black Film Review. *He died in 1991.*

For Keith Barrow and Larry McKeithan

> *I had big fun if I don't get well no more.*
> —"Going Down Slow" as sung by
> Bobby "Blue" Bland

Sister Chitlin', Brother Neck Bone and
Several of their oxymoron minions
Circle round my sick room,
Swathed in paper surgical gowns.

Brandishing crosses, clutching bibles,
(God, *please* don't let them sing hymns!)
Pestering me to recant the
Wicked ways that brought me here.

"Renounce your sins and return to Jesus!"
Shouts one of the zealous flock.
"The truth is I never left Him,"

I reply with a fingersnap.
"Don't you wish you'd chosen a *normal* lifestyle?"
"Sister, for *me*, I'm *sure* I did."

Let the congregation work overtime
For my eleventh-hour conversion.
Their futile efforts fortify
My unrepentant resolve.

Though my body be racked by
Capricious pains and fevers,
I'm not even *about* to yield to
Fashionable gay Black temptation.

Mother Piaf's second greatest hit title
Is taped to the inside of my brain
And silently repeated like a mantra:
"Non, Je Ne Regrette Rien."

I don't regret the hot Latino boxer
I made love to on Riverside Drive
Prior to a Washington march.
I don't regret wild Jersey nights
Spent in the arms of conflicted satyrs;
I don't regret late night and early a.m.
Encounters with world-class insatiables.

My only regrets are being ill,
Bed-ridden and having no boyfriend
To pray over me.
And that now I'll never see Europe
Or my African homeland except
In photos in a book or magazine.

Engrave on my tombstone:
"Here sleeps a *happy* Black faggot
Who lived to love and died
With no guilt."

No, I regret nothing
Of the gay life I've led and
There's no way in Heaven or Hell
I'll let anyone make me.

**SOURCE MATERIAL**

## Litany

### by Christopher Gorman

> *Christopher Gorman's bio in* From a Burning House, *where this first appeared, concludes: "When Christopher left CBS in April 1995, he was Director, Motion Pictures for Television and Mini-Series. He turned forty in November 1995. The rest is unknown."*
> *He died May 20, 2001.*

**1995**   I live beyond the cure. I will die of AIDS, I say to myself. I know this like I know my phone number when asked—or the way I can pick out my car in a crowded parking lot. I have lived through all the medical breakthroughs in the war against AIDS. Still, not long ago, I threw a shovelful of Connecticut onto the casket of a friend who once wrote a Broadway play. The week he died, his doctors informed him he was cured of lymphoma—but the fevers got him anyway. Old joke: Dentist says, "The teeth look great, but the gums gotta go."

**1987**   Fortified with nine hundred T cells, I receive the breaking news about AZT with buoyant optimism. My sister calls to ask excitedly if I've seen the *New York Times*. I joke that now I might be alive for the publication of the sequel to *Gone with the Wind*.

**1988**   Infused with the spirit of my ancestors who had survived the potato famine, I drive through a rainstorm to Tijuana with six hundred dollars stuffed into my Calvin's. The latest AIDS treatment is available in

Mexico without prescription. Searching frantically for the Regis Pharmacia, I am pursued by small children who implore me to buy small packages of Chiclets. Fearful and determined, I speed on, past mothers rummaging in trash cans for discarded french fries and hot apple pies from McDonald's. One hour later, I drive through border customs with a three-month supply of ribavirin and Isoprinosene. "Anything to declare?" snarls a uniformed official who reminds me of Mandy Patinkin as Che Guevara. "No," I answer (flatly), having rehearsed several versions: "No" (detached); "No!" (emphatic); "No" (nonplussed); "No" (quizzical). He writes down my license plate number and glares at me through the dirty windshield of my Suzuki. I stare past him into the gray sky over San Diego. He waves me through—not knowing I am smuggling the AIDS cure into the United States wrapped in a brightly colored, hand-embroidered tablecloth.

**1989** I meet a friend of a friend at a restaurant on Beverly Boulevard. He knows an airline steward who is sneaking dextran sulfate into his luggage on return trips from Tokyo. I slip $400 across the table to this stranger. One month later, he completes the transaction, turning the drug over to me in the lobby of the Sports Connection.

**1990** My physician studies my most recent lab work and looks at me through a pair of glasses I recently admired at Oliver Peoples. "You have failed AZT," he says sternly, signing a form that would enroll me in a community-based trial of DDI. "This is a turning point in the treatment of this disease," he says, handing the form to me across a desk littered with phone messages. "A turning point," he repeats for emphasis. On the way home, I stop at Video West and rent the movie starring Shirley MacLaine and Anne Bancroft.

**1992** The Federal Drug Administration approves DDI. I have relocated to New York and am enrolled in a study of DDC—in combination with protease inhibitors and the aforementioned AZT. Every third

Tuesday I join the masses at Bellevue Hospital. Among the crack addicts and schizophrenics, I feel comparatively healthy and comfortably superior. One Tuesday, after spending an hour in the waiting room seated next to someone with penicillin-resistant tuberculosis, I treat myself to lunch at Arcadia, washing down the protease inhibitor, AZT, and DDC with a California cabernet.

**1993** "You failed dapsone," the emergency-room physician admonishes as I lie on a gurney in a basement hallway at New York University Hospital.

"Don't say I failed dapsone," I croak. "You sound like my high school guidance counselor. Dapsone failed me."

"Be that as it may, you have a mild case of Pneumocystis—or possibly, a severe case of asthma. We'll begin treatment with pentamidine immediately. I'll see you again Monday morning."

Delaying his exit, I whimper, "But . . . this is Friday."

Looking at me directly for the first time, he sheepishly explains, "I have a share on Fire Island. This is my weekend," and he's off, practically skipping down the hallway past linen carts and infectious-waste containers. I am left alone on the gurney to contemplate his diagnosis. Behind Door #1 is a ten-day $15,000 hospital stay. Behind Door #2 is a year's supply of Primatene Mist. Behind Door #3 is a full share in a house at the Fire Island Pines.

**1994** Back in Los Angeles. "I have the results of your viral sensitivity test," says the doctor with the thinning hair and the bulging biceps.

"Oh?" I respond tremulously—sounding like Mary Richards being interviewed for a job by Lou Grant.

"Yes," says the doctor with the thinning personality and the bulging bank account, "and the results are less than dazzling. Your particular strain of the virus has mutated to the extent that it is resistant to AZT, DDI, and DDC. Also D4T."

"Wait! I've never taken D4T."

"Well, now you won't have to," he answers without a trace of comic intention.

Driving away from UCLA, I recite the litany of drugs I am no longer sensitive to: AZT, DDC, DDI, D4T. Can R2D2 be far behind?

**Today** Recently, the *New York Times* broke the news that interleukin-2 therapy represented a significant breakthrough in the management of HIV disease. The article specifically mentioned that researchers believed the drug would not be an effective option for people with less than two hundred T cells. My T-cell count is now compatible with the song "One Hundred Bottles of Beer on the Wall." I've lived so long with this virus that I'm no longer available for the latest cure. My future is behind Door #4.

Was it Greta Garbo who said, "I'm tired"? Or Madeline Kahn?

I'm tired.

There.

Now *I* said it.

## TIMELINE

## 1997–Present

### 1997

The HAART treatment (the "cocktail") proves to be effective for many people with AIDS, as the CDC reports that AIDS-related deaths in the United States have declined by 47 percent compared with 1996.

During a commencement address at Morgan State University in Baltimore, President Bill Clinton calls for an AIDS vaccine by the year 2007, comparing it to President Kennedy's pledge to go to the moon in the 1960s. Clinton says, "With the strides of recent years, it is no longer a question of whether we can develop an AIDS vaccine—it is simply a question of when."

It does not happen by 2007. Or 2017. Or by the time of this book's publication.

Do we need a vaccine or a cure if science has already given us a selection of treatment options that keep the viral load in HIV+ people undetectable and untransmittable, meaning they are healthy? Do we need a cure if PrEP and PEP mean that HIV− people can essentially eliminate their chances of contracting HIV? Do we need more tools than the ones we have already?

The answer to these questions is simple. *Yes.* A cure would change lives in America and around the world—especially for those for whom ongoing medical care is arduous and hard to afford. For now, in the absence of that elusive cure, we need to ensure that everybody has access to the medications that make HIV both a manageable and a preventable health condition.

It's the usual culprits that stand in the way: shame, stigma, inequality.

## 1998

Even as the death rate declines, the racial inequity of those who have died increases. The CDC reports that African Americans account for 49 percent of US AIDS-related deaths while only making up just under 13 percent of the general population. AIDS-related mortality for African Americans is almost ten times that of whites and three times that of those classified as Hispanics.

In March, Black leaders develop a "Call to Action," insisting that the president and surgeon general declare HIV/AIDS a "State of Emergency" in the African American community. Following the leadership of the Congressional Black Caucus, Congress funds the Minority AIDS Initiative, giving $156 million to groups across the nation to prevent and treat HIV/AIDS in BIPOC communities.

Separately, in November, Congress enacts the Ricky Ray Hemophilia Relief Fund Act, authorizing payments to individuals with hemophilia and other blood-clotting disorders who were infected with HIV by unscreened blood-clotting agents between 1982 and 1987. But the payments are tangled up in budget battles and don't start to be made until late 2000, which is too late for Ricky Ray's brother, Robert, who dies in October 2000 of AIDS-related causes at the age of twenty-two. Ellis Sulser, a man who has lived with AIDS for over fifteen years and has spent over $6 million in insurance money on his illness, tells CBS News, "They help people that are victims of floods, they help people that are victims of earthquakes and other natural disasters. This is a disaster that was enacted by the government. We are still here waiting for help, and we haven't been given any."

## 1999

By the end of 1998, UNAIDS (the Joint United Nations Programme on HIV/AIDS) estimated that one-third of people living with HIV/AIDS around the world were between the ages of fifteen and twenty-four. And across the world, around half of new HIV diagnoses were happening in this age group. Teenagers and young adults, those at the age when most people are beginning to explore their sexuality, were contracting HIV at much higher rates than older demographics.

Even though scientists had invented drugs that worked, and these drugs symbolized a way to end the crisis, the task was only getting more immense. How do you scale up production and distribution as an epidemic gets worse, not better?

And how do you make a teenager understand the risk of contracting pretty much any illness, let alone something life-changing like HIV?

## 2002

Times have changed greatly since the early days, when HIV testing required agonizing waits of weeks (if not months) for results. In November, the FDA approves the first rapid HIV diagnostic test kit for use in the United States; it provides results with 99.6 percent accuracy in as little as twenty minutes. Even better, the test can be stored at room temperature, requires no specialized equipment, and may be used outside of traditional laboratory or clinical settings, which makes testing much more accessible to the general population. According to the CDC, half of American adults ages fifteen to forty-four report that they've been tested, with 15.1 percent tested in the last twelve months.

## 2003

During his State of the Union address, President George W. Bush announces his President's Emergency Plan for AIDS Relief (PEPFAR), a five-year, $15 billion initiative to fight HIV/AIDS, primarily in Africa and the Caribbean. The president tells Congress:

> Today, on the continent of Africa, nearly 30 million people have the AIDS virus—including 3 million children under the age 15. There are

whole countries in Africa where more than one-third of the adult population carries the infection. More than 4 million require immediate drug treatment. Yet across that continent, only 50,000 AIDS victims—only 50,000—are receiving the medicine they need.

Because the AIDS diagnosis is considered a death sentence, many do not seek treatment. Almost all who do are turned away. A doctor in rural South Africa describes his frustration. He says, "We have no medicines. Many hospitals tell people, you've got AIDS, we can't help you. Go home and die." In an age of miraculous medicines, no person should have to hear those words.

AIDS can be prevented. Anti-retroviral drugs can extend life for many years. And the cost of those drugs has dropped from $12,000 a year to under $300 a year—which places a tremendous possibility within our grasp. Ladies and gentlemen, seldom has history offered a greater opportunity to do so much for so many.

The president goes on to say that this plan "will prevent 7 million new AIDS infections, treat at least 2 million people with life-extending drugs, and provide humane care for millions of people suffering from AIDS, and for children orphaned by AIDS." This ends up being a massive understatement, as PEPFAR becomes the largest global health initiative in American history, with over $100 billion being spent. On the legislation's twentieth anniversary, it is estimated that the initiative has saved over 25 million lives, having provided antiretroviral treatment to over 20 million people and the treatment that allowed 5.5 million babies to be born to mothers with HIV without having the virus themselves.

"There needed to be something major, something big, something unprecedented, to be able to tackle this level of despair, this level of hopelessness," Dr. Wafaa El-Sadr, director of the International Center for AIDS Care and Treatment Programs (ICAP) at Columbia University and professor of epidemiology and medicine at Columbia Mailman School of Public Health, told NPR. "It was kind of a remarkable moment. I was thinking, 'Oh, my. This might be it.'"

## 2005

Staying on top of any treatment for any condition means changing your routine to make sure you don't forget about it. Wake up, take a pill. Time for bed, take a pill. When people describe the first treatment for HIV/AIDS as a "regimen," it's because you had to attempt military-level precision to keep up with your doses. Some of the early drugs had to be kept in the refrigerator. One you had to take on an empty stomach, another you took with food. Some you took twice a day; others, three times. One drug even had to be taken in the middle of the night, to ensure it was always ticking away, doing its thing in your system. There were no smartphones, just the drone of electronic alarms to remind you: a ritual of beep-beep-beeps, nagging you to take your pills, confronting you with their necessity.

This reality could make it hard to stay healthy, because it's hard to schedule life around a convoluted, unforgiving treatment plan—sometimes with an added sense of secrecy because you might not want friends or colleagues to guess you have HIV. You're scared you'll lose your job if a coworker sees you take your pills on your lunch break.

Drug providers knew they needed to make HIV treatment simpler. In 2005, a new version of an HIV/AIDS drug, Kaletra, becomes available. This drug combines two drugs to reduce the need for multiple doses. People who are newly diagnosed and have never taken antiretroviral drugs before ("treatment-naïve") have to take only one dose a day; the dose suppresses HIV without needing a cocktail of other drugs. You don't have to refrigerate it. It doesn't matter if you have it with or without food. You don't have to wake up at three a.m. for a late-night dose. The introduction of Kaletra is a game-changing moment. Kaletra heralds the arrival of a more efficient, tolerable category of anti-HIV drugs. The easier it is to treat HIV, the easier it is for people to take their medication without anxiety or confusion. Simpler forms of treatment make it easier for people with HIV to keep the virus suppressed, and simpler forms of treatment allow HIV+ people to have the same quality of life as anybody else.

## 2007

Timothy Ray Brown was diagnosed with HIV in 1995. His life, like those of most HIV+ people, went pretty much back to normal after he was able to start combination therapy. He was HIV+, and that had its challenges, but life was okay with medication.

Eleven years later, his doctor told him he had acute leukemia, a cancer of the blood that starts in the bone marrow. In February 2007, Brown undergoes his first of two stem cell transplants to treat the cancer: a dangerous procedure, reserved for life-threatening illnesses. Stem cells are baby blood cells—they start in the bone marrow and grow up to be white blood cells, which fight viruses and other pathogens; red blood cells, which carry oxygen; or platelets, which stop bleeding. Leukemia starts in a single bone marrow stem cell; much like HIV, this one rogue cell multiplies and replaces normal bone marrow and blood cells with cancer. The aim of a stem cell transplant is to repopulate the patient's bone marrow and immune system with stem cells donated by someone who doesn't have cancer, through an invasive and complex operation.

Brown's transplants are successful. In fact, they are so successful that Brown stops testing positive for HIV. The stem cell donor carries a rare genetic mutation that prevents the person from contracting HIV. When the media begins reporting the fact that someone has been cured of HIV, Brown's name is withheld, and he is known only as the "Berlin Patient." Three years later, Brown waives his right to anonymity because he wants people to understand: "I did not want to be the only person in the world cured of HIV; I wanted other HIV-positive patients to join my club. I want to dedicate my life to supporting research to search for a cure or cures for HIV!"

It's huge to think that somebody has been cured of HIV after all these years, even if this cure is so specific to one extremely rare scenario. Millions of people wait to see if Brown's cure can be replicated for other individuals, but it's not readily transferrable. Brown nearly dies as a consequence of the stem cell transplants. It isn't sustainable or affordable to locate individuals who carry a rare genetic mutation and persuade them to donate bone marrow. But still, the trail is there for researchers to follow: For the first time on record, HIV has been erased from a person's body.

## 2008

Dr. Pietro Vernazza was working at the Division of Infectious Diseases at the Cantonal Hospital in Switzerland when he started to develop a theory that would change the way people talked about HIV. He was working on the Swiss HIV Cohort Study—a large-scale study of HIV+ people in the country. The study had 8,000 participants, who were all receiving antiretroviral therapy, or ART for short (otherwise known as combination therapy). Vernazza knew from his research that a minority of the participants weren't using condoms with their partners. But it didn't seem to be causing an uptick in new HIV cases.

A few years went by. There still hadn't been a single instance of somebody contracting HIV after having sexual contact with one of the participants. Vernazza worked with heterosexual participants, some of whom were desperate to conceive a child with their partners. His clinic began a trial to work with, and closely monitor, serodiscordant couples (couples where one person was HIV+ and one was HIV–) who wanted to conceive naturally. It was a success. Not a single parent or child related to the trial contracted HIV.

By 2008, Vernazza's team had swapped notes with scientists in Uganda and Brazil who had reached the same hypothesis in their clinics. On January 30, the Swiss Federal Commission for HIV/AIDS releases a statement in the *Bulletin of Swiss Medicine* to alert the world to their findings. It becomes known as the Swiss Statement:

> An HIV-infected person with potent ART is not <u>sexually</u> infectious, i.e. does not transmit the virus via sexual contacts as long as
> - the therapy is practiced consistently and monitored regularly by the treating physician;

- the viral load on ART has been below the limit of detection for at least 6 months;
- no infections with other STI are present.

Under these circumstances, potent ART therefore definitely prevents HIV transmission as safely as condoms.

The statement sends shock waves through the international health community. Health agencies like WHO and UNAIDS reject Vernazza's claims as irresponsible and reckless. Anthony Fauci speaks out against them. Some people argue that, even if the findings are right, this information shouldn't be made public because it will encourage unsafe sex. But further scientific study proves Vernazza correct. Today it's widely understood that the vast majority of HIV+ people are able to have an undetectable viral load thanks to combination therapy. And if your HIV load is undetectable, you can't transmit the virus to anybody.

## 2009

Twenty years after it was first passed, and long after data has disproven fears that needle exchange greatly increases substance abuse, Congress lifts its ban on federal funding for syringe-exchange programs. According to House Speaker Nancy Pelosi, "Sound science is an essential component of good public health policy, and science must come first in our public health policy decisions. The language lifting the ban on the use of federal funds for syringe exchange appropriately allows local public health and law enforcement officials to determine where exchanges should operate in their communities."

Unfortunately, "sound science" does not win the day for long, because a Republican Congress reinstates the ban in 2011. It is not until 2016, as the opioid epidemic hits the home states of congressmen like Senate Majority Leader Mitch McConnell, that the ban is lifted again. And even then, there's a hitch: Funding can go to local needle-exchange organizations, and can be spent on anything . . . except needles and syringes.

The local programs figure out ways to work around this.

## 2010

Saying that he "look[s] forward to working with Congress, State, tribal, and local governments, and other stakeholders to support the implementation of a Strategy that is innovative, grounded in the best science, focuses on the areas of greatest need, and that provides a clear direction for moving forward together," President Obama unveils the first-ever National HIV/AIDS Strategy, setting goals for reducing the number of HIV cases and increasing access to care in an equitable way.

## 2012

*The Washington Post* and the Kaiser Family Foundation release a survey of attitudes toward HIV across the American population. There is good news. The data shows that most Americans believe access to treatment should be equitable; drugs to treat HIV shouldn't be determined by someone's ability to pay for them. The survey shows signs of less fear and less intolerance—but less awareness, too. A quarter of surveyed Americans think you can contract HIV from sharing a drinking glass. That's pretty much the same percentage of the population that had that mistaken belief in 1987.

There's a clear message here: Understanding how you can and cannot contract HIV is just as important today as it was in the 1980s.

Also this year, Truvada becomes the first drug that the FDA approves for pre-exposure prophylaxis (PrEP). A Truvada pill is actually the combination of two drugs, tenofovir disoproxil fumarate and emtricitabine. It has already been used as part of the cocktail to treat people who have HIV, but now it is being approved as a preventive measure. (For more on how PrEP works, see page 30.)

Some activists are concerned that the availability of Truvada will cause a false feeling of security (since it is not, at the time, 100 percent effective), and others say the need to stick to the regimen may be hard for many people to do. Also, the cost for a year's worth of the medication is $13,900—which is very hard to afford if insurance does not cover it.

Still, the introduction of Truvada is met with a great deal of hope. "Truvada for (prevention) won't end AIDS by itself, but we certainly can't end the HIV epidemic without it," James Loduca, spokesman for the San Francisco AIDS Foundation, tells *SFGate*.

## 2015

The Strategic Timing of Antiretroviral Treatment (START) trial releases its results. After ten years of research across thirty-five countries, it's proven that starting antiretroviral medication early will help save and improve lives. Previously, treatment wasn't recommended for healthy people living with HIV. It was thought better to wait until their T-cell counts fell to an AIDS-defining number. Another reason the START trial is so important is that it adds further proof that people who are receiving treatment have a suppressed viral load, and that having a suppressed viral load means you can't pass on HIV.

"We now have clear-cut proof that it is of significantly greater health benefit to an HIV-infected person to start antiretroviral therapy sooner rather than later," says Anthony Fauci, director of the US National Institute of Allergy and Infectious Diseases (NIAID). He points out that early therapy gives a "double benefit" because it not only helps the health of infected individuals but also lowers their viral count, making transmission rarer. Fauci concludes, "These findings have global implications for the treatment of HIV."

## 2017

The concepts of "undetectable" and "untransmittable" are legitimized in an announcement by the CDC stating that people who are HIV+ and on treatment that makes their viral load undetectable have "effectively no risk" of passing the virus along to sexual partners.

Still, the CDC notes, "Among gay and bisexual men living with diagnosed HIV, 61% have achieved viral suppression, more than in previous years, but well short of where we want to be."

## 2019

We're all connected. Technology connects us, but so do viruses. When people start to get sick and die in China at the end of 2019, the world at first thinks the sickness can be contained. But by the time the virus, COVID-19, is being reported in China, it has already spread around the world, traveling with us on planes and trains. Soon the world is under its sway.

The COVID-19 pandemic is strikingly different from the AIDS crisis, because COVID-19 explodes dramatically across the globe in the months after it first appears. It isn't a sneaky virus like HIV; it doesn't sit inside your body waiting to show its effects. It's much easier to contract COVID-19 than HIV, and infinitely easier for your body to deal with it on its own. With COVID-19, you get sick a few days after you pick up the virus; most people make a full recovery, and drug companies roll out the first vaccines within a year or so of the outbreak.

When COVID-19 starts, much of the world responds: Cities shut down, schools close, airports sit empty. People are scared to be near each other, scared that showing physical intimacy might make them sick. Global efforts to solve the problem remind survivors and activists how little action was taken to deal with AIDS in the early 1980s—back when marginalized communities of people affected by AIDS were fighting for their lives, fighting for their governments to do something.

This time, governments listen, because the virus is too widespread. The US government turns to Anthony Fauci to be its point person in combatting COVID-19, and all of his lessons from the war on AIDS come in handy. The death toll is still horrifyingly large—but the norms set down by AIDS activism help keep it from being even larger.

## 2022

For many queer people, the alarm is an eerily familiar one: A disease is spreading through sexual contact, primarily in the gay community. No one knows why it started—but they know it can cause harm.

This time, the disease is mpox (earlier known as "monkey pox"), and although it is rarely deadly, it is still painful . . . and threatens to grow worse.

This time, we don't need Bobbi Campbell to put up photos of his lesions in the front window of a store in the Castro. Word spreads over the internet—on news sites, dating apps, DMs to friends. Luckily, a vaccine is already available from a governmental store of vaccine to guard against smallpox. Inoculation centers are set up in major cities and some (but not enough) rural areas. People at risk come out in droves, with vaccination sites becoming de facto queer centers.

We've learned our lesson. There will be no silence this time. And the government delivers the care we need, when we need it.

## 2023

According to the government's most recent report, there are approximately 1.2 million people in the US who are HIV+, and 13 percent of them do not know they have it. In the CDC's HIV Surveillance Report for 2023, the last year covered before the deadline for this book, over 39,000 people were newly diagnosed with HIV in the U.S. and six territories and freely associated states. Over 80 percent were men, with 66 percent attributed to male-to-male sexual contact. Hispanic and Black individuals each accounted for more than a third. Ages 25 to 44 accounted for 60 percent of diagnoses, and the South region represented 51 percent. As the CDC noted in its 2022 report: "Racism, HIV stigma, discrimination, homophobia, poverty, and other barriers to health care continue to drive disparities in HIV diagnoses."

## 2025

There is currently uncertainty as to when we will next see full governmental figures on HIV/AIDS, including data on PrEP. In September 2025, a note on the CDC website reads: "In 2024, CDC paused PrEP coverage reporting for one year to update overall PrEP coverage estimates using newly available data sets and determine the best way to present PrEP coverage. However, CDC is unable to resume PrEP coverage reporting at this time, due to a reduction in force affecting the Division of HIV Prevention (DHP). As part of this staffing reduction, the DHP branches that produced HIV incidence estimates and provided the statistical expertise needed to assess PrEP coverage were eliminated. CDC is currently evaluating plans and capacity to resume this work."

You wake up one morning in 2025 and before you make coffee you grab your iPhone and switch it off airplane mode and news notifications bounce up on the screen like a video game.

*Radical changes in US policy threaten two decades' progress in HIV.*

*Trump's PEPFAR cuts upend the lives of Kenyan families battling HIV. Withdrawal of HIV funding hits hard in the South. Risk of 2,000 new HIV infections a day after US aid freeze.*

*UN says, "A bloodbath": HIV field is reeling after billions in US funding are axed.*

*US shutdown of HIV/AIDS funding "could lead to 500,000 deaths in South Africa."*

*"It's back to drug rationing": the end of HIV was in sight. Then came the cuts.*

The story of AIDS in America is a story of life and death, ignorance and truth, neglect and community, steps forward and, now, steps back.

Welcome to the next chapter of the fight.

A couple of weeks into the second Trump presidency, the newly formed Department of Government Efficiency (DOGE) announces mass firings and funding freezes across numerous federal agencies. One of the targets is the US Agency for International Development (USAID). For more than two decades, USAID has helped to provide health care for people affected by HIV/AIDS all around the world. Federal funding for international aid is compassionate, but it's also pragmatic; the healthier the rest of the world is, the healthier Americans are. PEPFAR, the proudest achievement of a previous Republican administration, is completely gutted.

Under these unprecedented cuts, the global HIV/AIDS community is thrown into chaos, as international agencies struggle to ensure access to lifesaving treatments and testing for millions and millions of people. Money stops flowing. Clinics stop working. People start dying. Within the United States, DOGE's cuts to federal budgets create fear and confusion among HIV/AIDS providers, with the half a million HIV+ Americans accessing treatment through the Ryan White CARE Act every year wondering if their care will still have governmental support.

There are immediate legal challenges to most of the Trump administration's actions and many members of Congress try to save PEPFAR. As we write this in August 2025, there are no conclusions—only chaos.

In the middle of the chaos there is good news—although the good news is compromised by politics. In June 2025 the FDA approves Lenacapavir, made by Gilead Sciences and to be marketed as Yeztugo. This is a twice-yearly injection that provides a nearly complete shield against HIV infection in clinical trials. It's not a cure, but it is a treatment that would be more accessible than any treatment that's come before. The hitch, as always, is how to get it to the people who need it the most around the world—and this is where the good news turns bad, because cuts to Medicaid (for people in the US) and the shutting down of PEPFAR and USAID (for people in countries outside the US) will make it exponentially harder to get the treatment to the people who need it. Mitchell Warren, the executive director of the international HIV prevention organization AVAC, tells *The New York Times,* "We're on the precipice of now being able to deliver the greatest prevention option we've had in 44 years of this epidemic. And it's as if that opportunity is being snatched out of our hands by the politics of the last five months."

On February 26, 2025, dozens of activists and USAID employees stage a die-in at the Cannon House Office Building, the oldest federal building in Washington, DC. They lie down on the ground, blocking the rotunda, chanting "Congress has blood on its hands, unfreeze aid now" to protest the extraordinary cuts being made to HIV/AIDS services. Their actions and voices echo those of earlier generations of activists, particularly the members of ACT UP who lay on the ground outside the FDA in October 1988.

How quickly can we build something? How fast can it be destroyed? The February 2025 die-in resurrects a long history of AIDS activism. The past and the present are always tumbling against each other, a dance you only learn by doing. You can hear the voices of history joining in with the chant. The ones who died. The ones who lived. Those who were born after.

It's 1987. It's 1993. It's 2025.

ACT UP, FIGHT BACK, FIGHT AIDS!

Our work continues.

While today there is no cure for HIV/AIDS, there is a treatment ... for those who are aware of it, and those who can afford it, particularly in America. This does not mean the virus has gone away. This does not mean that no one dies from AIDS complications anymore. They do. And even though, for many, living with HIV has become easier, that doesn't mean it's easy.

Because even if there is a treatment for HIV, homophobia endures. Racism endures. Medical inequity endures. Ignorance—particularly the willful ignorance of a certain breed of politician—endures. American society's inability to treat all those who are sick with care and dignity endures. The complications of homelessness and mental health endure, and the opioid epidemic and the COVID-19 pandemic add new complications into the mix.

Vigilance and activism are still required.

*I didn't understand HIV, and I didn't want to understand it. HIV didn't tie into my lived experience; it didn't fit into how I saw myself and my future. But HIV happened to me anyway....*

# Mallery Jenna Robinson

*When Mallery Jenna Robinson learned she was living with HIV in 2011, she began a journey to become a trailblazing advocate for HIV+ Black trans women. In addition to her work as a transgender and HIV health care advocate, Mallery hosts a podcast,* A Hateful Homicide, *that examines the epidemic of violence faced by trans women.*

I found out I was HIV+ in 2011. I was twenty-one years old in Alabama, working my way through college waiting tables at a barbecue restaurant. One day, I was over by the soda fountain, making a drink for a customer. A wave of exhaustion came over me. The next thing I know, I'm waking up in the hospital. I'd fainted and been rushed to the ER in an ambulance. The doctors did some hematology work; my blood came back positive for HIV.

I was shocked, confused, upset. Before my diagnosis, I didn't understand HIV, and I didn't *want* to understand it. HIV didn't tie into my lived experience; it didn't fit into how I saw myself and my future. But HIV happened to me anyway. I went straight into treatment and met the most amazing care providers at the clinic in Alabama. My viral load became undetectable. I came to see my daily medication as nothing more than a multivitamin which helps me stay healthy and strong.

But the emotions were hard. I'd already had to learn to love myself as a trans woman. Now I had to learn to love myself all over again as a person living with HIV. I came out as trans to my parents back when I was sixteen years old. One night I overheard my mom and dad talking about me. "Who's going to love our child? Who's going to fall in love with a transgender woman?" I carried their doubt with me for a long time. After my HIV diagnosis, all those thoughts got worse. I'd think to myself: *Who's going to love me as a trans woman living with HIV?*

My family had supported me in my gender journey. I have four brothers, so gaining a daughter was like winning the lotto for my mom. But I kept silent about having HIV. Was my family going to be okay with it? Would they finally tell me it was too much for them to cope with? But everyone was supportive. I told my mom after six months. I'd been nurtured by the treatment center in Alabama; my viral load was undetectable. I even got to a place where I could tell my grandparents. I wanted to be able to have as much information as possible; to be able to say to them, "It isn't the 1980s anymore. The treatment is easy and it works. I've been living with HIV successfully. You don't have to worry about me. I'm healthy, I'm undetectable, I'm happy."

I finished college. I fell in love. I got married. I trained to be a teacher. I moved to Florida and taught in a school; it was empowering to be an openly trans teacher in the classroom. I learned that life will surprise you. It's easy to expect the people around you to show the worst of themselves when they hear those three letters, H-I-V, or when they learn that you're transgender. But a lot of people are kind.

Five years ago, I left Florida and moved to Los Angeles. I got a job working as an advocate for trans people who are living with HIV or at risk of contracting HIV. There's a high proportion of Black and Brown trans women who are living with HIV. Especially in the younger age group; the numbers are skyrocketing. As an advocate, it became my job to go out to nightclubs which attract a trans crowd and talk to the girls. My aim was to encourage these women to come in and get tested for HIV. Trans people in Los Angeles are disproportionately impacted by HIV but less likely to access testing and treatment. I might be a Black trans woman, but my life has been different from most of these women.

One of the girls said to me, "Mallery, I love you. I love your bubbly spirit. But I'm so tired of people coming out to the club to persuade the Black and Brown trans folks to get tested. You give us an incentive to get tested, a twenty-five-dollar gift card, but what happens if the test comes back positive? What help do we get then?" These women were sick of being treated like they were just data for the government. They were sick of providers not recognizing the challenges they faced accessing and staying connected to treatment.

I sat down with her. "What is it that you need? What can I do to help you feel recognized?" And then the conversations started.

Storytelling is an important part of my culture. My maternal grandfather is Haitian. When I was a child, he told me about coming over from Haiti with his parents. He passed on the stories he was told by his parents and by their parents. My family can keep telling those stories to the next generations. This storytelling is called griot, and it's rooted in a West African tradition that predates the slave trade. Griot is the art of preserving the lived experiences of members of the Black community. Let's be real: For Black people in America, our histories have been whitewashed. We hold onto our histories by telling the stories we pass down from generation to generation about people whose lives could otherwise be forgotten. Griot gives you a connection to the community you never got the chance to meet. Griot is about making sure the next generation knows the truth. You keep telling the story. You tell the story the way you were told it. You don't change it.

Working with these trans women in Los Angeles reminded me of my grandfather's stories. It reminded me to show my respect to the experiences these women were sharing with me about their lives and their relationship to HIV. I sat with these girls at the club. I thought to myself, *What if we saw some of the most marginalized people in our society as griots who can teach us about the truth of their lives and what they need to thrive?*

We need to enshrine Black trans women's experiences as part of our ancestral narrative of telling stories, passing the truth down from generation to generation. So many of our community members have either succumbed to HIV or been murdered. Once they're gone, they can no longer tell their stories. Sometimes I don't know if the client is still going to be here tomorrow. I don't know if they're going to move. I don't know if they're going to be missing or murdered. If the worst-case scenario is murder, I definitely want to make sure that I have a living record of their story, something that I can take with me.

I knew a beautiful Black trans woman. She was twenty-three years old and she was a sex worker. She stopped working the streets and got a job at a queer health care organization. But she was outspoken. Anytime she felt that discrimination was happening, she would advocate. People are happy to say Marsha P. Johnson's name and Sylvia Rivera's name. It's easy to support trans women in theory, right? But a lot of people have a problem when they see a trans woman advocate for herself. This woman became a problem for her boss and she was fired. Around the time COVID-19 was starting, she went back out onto the streets. And then the worst thing happened. She was murdered.

This woman's best friend was another trans woman, a young woman who engaged in survival sex work and who was living with HIV. This friend was so devastated by her sister's murder that she went into depression. We tried everything. She wouldn't eat. She wouldn't take her medicine. If we're battling depression, no one can get us out of it except ourselves. Some of us can manage to do that. We take antidepressants. We go to therapy. We start journaling. We do yoga. But it isn't always that easy. This woman was so haunted by her sister's death that she just gave up. The official cause of her death was AIDS but it felt like she really just died of a broken heart.

Those two women existed. They were young, they were full of life, and their lives were cut short. I wish the woman who was murdered was still here, telling us how she managed to survive her abuser. I wish her friend was still here, telling us she's living proudly with HIV and taking her medication. I want a light at the end of the tunnel for both of them. But there wasn't one. That's the ugly side of what many Black and Brown trans women have to go through. HIV/AIDS is just one part of the picture.

Just presenting as trans in public makes it hard to get a regular job. If you manage to get a job, you're likely to encounter harassment and discrimination. Unless you're already set up for success, trans women can get trapped in sex work for survival. You agree to have sex for some cash; the guy pays more not to use a condom. Money talks. That cash is going to stop you being hungry and cold; you get something off the dollar menu at McDonald's, you get a cheap motel room for a few nights. But survival sex work increases your risk of contracting HIV. And if you're relying on sex work to survive, you're unlikely to be in a position where you can consistently access PrEP to protect yourself from contracting HIV in the process. It's a vicious circle. Sex work to survive. You contract HIV. You get diagnosed. You start treatment. You fall out of treatment, for reasons beyond your control. And it's not like you're sick—yet. This narrative doesn't just apply to trans women. We're seeing an increase in HIV in young trans men too. Some trans guys sleep with cis gay men for money. Survival sex work puts you in situations where your chance of contracting HIV is just higher.

Housing. Transportation. Food. Water. These essential services are available for some, but not for others, especially the most marginalized. Sometimes people have to stop their HIV treatment because they have to move at short notice to protect themselves from danger. Or the money you'd spend getting all the way to the clinic has to go to food or debt. Immediate threats to your life are more pressing than staying on a lifelong course of antiretroviral medication. Maybe you were living with your family but they told you to leave because they found out you're trans. They put you on the streets. You're moving from shelter to shelter. You're on Skid Row. Without a secure address, you don't have a safe space to maintain treatment. In a city like Los Angeles, it's a challenge to get to the clinic when it's miles away and you don't have a dollar. You can't walk it.

In my job as an advocate, I'm always telling clients who do sex work that they should be taking PrEP to minimize the risk of contracting HIV and getting PEP if not. PrEP is kind of like birth control. You take PrEP to ensure you can't contract HIV, or it's useful if you're having a romantic relationship with someone who has HIV. PEP is like the morning-after pill, right? If you've slept with someone who you think has HIV, and you didn't use a condom and you're not on PrEP, you take PEP to protect yourself.

But it's too simple to assume that everyone can get PrEP or PEP. If you don't have a steady home, if you don't have steady transportation, you're facing barriers. Most sex work is initiated online, but there are still plenty of sex workers who work the streets in the red-light district. Some of my clients leave suddenly because they're fleeing domestic partners. Often the "boyfriend" is really the pimp.

What I'm trying to say is that it's not unusual for people in my community to be literally fleeing for their lives. Can we judge them for struggling to maintain a long-term treatment program when there are so many immediate dangers? Can we listen to their stories and help them find solutions which work for them instead?

The recent wave of anti-trans laws which we're seeing in some states doesn't help any of these problems. Anti-trans laws make it harder to be trans in public life. When politicians try to ban drag queen story time or ban drag shows, they reduce the opportunities for trans people to make money. When you take away their livelihoods, some trans folks are left with that age-old narrative: engaging in sex work simply to survive. Anti-trans laws make it that much harder for trans people to avoid contracting HIV, and that much harder for HIV+ trans women to stay in treatment.

Sometimes I think the ultimate goal for anti-trans politicians is for our communities to become extinct. They want us to take our own lives when we're left with no opportunities for employment. Trans kids need to know that their lives matter. I've been out and proud as a trans woman since I was sixteen years old. Yes, this life has come with its fair share of challenges, but it also comes with its fair share of changes. I've seen states turn around and become pro-trans, I've seen anti-trans politicians go out of office and new ones come in who are ready to create the change they want to see.

Yes, it's hard, it's heavy, it's hurtful, it's harmful.

But please. Don't give up.

# Q

*Q is a drag performer and designer based in Kansas City, Missouri. She was a contestant on the sixteenth season of* RuPaul's Drag Race, *which aired in 2024.*

When you get the call for *Drag Race,* you only have three weeks to get ready before filming. Every episode has a different runway with a different weekly theme. One of the themes for our season was "The 1980s." When I saw the prompt, I knew immediately that I wanted my dress to be inspired by AIDS activism. So many queer people were lost to AIDS in the 1980s. I wanted my outfit to be a beautiful homage to that chapter of queer history. But it was also an homage to the fact I was HIV+ myself.

I wanted the dress to contain multiple elements that evoked the history of the HIV/AIDS activism movement. The dress was cut in a 1980s silhouette with a Keith Haring–inspired print. Keith Haring was a big activist for HIV/AIDS until his AIDS-related death in the early 1990s. I juxtaposed the Keith Haring print with a red ribbon as my neckline. The red ribbon is the symbol of AIDS awareness.

Halfway through the competition, it was time for the 1980s theme. I was so nervous when I woke up that morning, because I knew I'd be talking about being HIV+ on television. *RuPaul's Drag Race* is watched by so many people around the world. Some of those fans will be HIV+. Some might become HIV+ in the future. I figured being open about my HIV status on *Drag Race* might help one person feel less alone. It might educate some fans of the show who don't understand HIV.

As we were getting in drag to go out onto the runway, I spoke to the other contestants about being HIV+.

"I am doing something very sentimental for the runway today," I said. "It's inspired by the generation of gay people that we lost to the AIDS epidemic in the 1980s. It's really, really special to me."

The cameras were on me.

"I've been HIV-positive for two years now. When I first got my diagnosis I felt really lost and super alone." I spoke about the ignorance and dehumanization I've had to face as an HIV+ person. "But I'm here, I'm on *Drag Race*, I'm living my dreams."

When I stepped out onto the main stage, the lights and cameras ahead of me, RuPaul and Michelle Visage and the other judges, I felt myself opening up. All the anxiety melted away. It was suddenly so freeing to talk about it openly during the judges' critiques, even though I also felt like, "Oh my God, I'm talking about being HIV-positive on national television!"

Talking about HIV on *Drag Race* gave me an ultimatum I needed in my personal life. I'd been so supported by my drag family and queer friends after my diagnosis, but I still hadn't told my biological family. Now I had to tell them I was HIV+ before the episode aired. I'd already come out as gay in high school; now I needed to come out as HIV+. I'm from a small, rural town in Kansas; it's the kind of town where queer kids have to figure out everything on their own. No one talks about HIV. My family isn't familiar with the queer community, let alone knowledgeable about HIV. They didn't understand it, and until now, they'd had no reason to try. Telling my family I was living with HIV was powerful. Sharing my life and my truth with them has made them so much more informed about what it means to be LGBTQ+ and HIV-positive today.

Since the episode aired, it's been amazing meeting other people who are affected by HIV/AIDS. I've met people who lost friends and family during the worst years of the AIDS epidemic. Older gay people who've been living with HIV for a long time as well as younger folks too. I found out that some of my friends in my queer community are also HIV+. It's amazing to feel a sense of community with other people who've experienced HIV across the decades.

When I was diagnosed, it was terrifying. As a queer person, I was well-informed about HIV before my diagnosis. I knew I could live a normal life. I knew being HIV+ no longer meant developing AIDS. But it was still scary. Today, I feel proud to be someone who is openly HIV+. I feel proud to talk about it. I feel proud to connect with people about it. I feel proud to be representing a community of people who are still marginalized, mistreated, and misunderstood.

# Justin Smith

*Justin Smith is the director of the Campaign to End AIDS at Positive Impact Health Centers in the Atlanta region. From 2019 to 2023, he served on the Presidential Advisory Council on HIV/AIDS.*

You could say I started working in HIV because of my great-uncle. He was a remarkable man. I didn't get to know him super well—I was still a child when he died—but what I do know is that he was very educated. He did his master's at Columbia at a time when there weren't a lot of Black people going to Columbia. He became a high school principal in New Rochelle, just north of Manhattan. He had a partner, but unfortunately, I don't know much about him. I just know they were two very cultured Black men living together in New York.

My great-uncle had this grace about him. When I was a child, I didn't know that he was gay—we didn't speak about it—but I remember I was always so drawn to that quality of him—his elegance. He died because of AIDS in 1989. Everyone was so, so sad when he died. I was nine years old. I didn't understand what had happened to him. I just knew it must have been something devastating, but no one ever said anything about it.

It wasn't until I was older that I finally had a conversation with my grandmother. Then she told me he had been gay and he'd died of AIDS. It all made sense to me then.

This knowledge helped me to understand myself as a gay man. I wasn't the first one in my family. He made space for me to exist. And that's powerful.

The work I do today in HIV is kind of a love letter to him.

\* \* \*

As a teenager in Atlanta and New Jersey in the mid-1990s, it felt like HIV was everywhere around me. You'd turn on the radio and hear songs about AIDS like "Waterfalls" by TLC and "Let's Talk About Sex" by Salt-N-Pepa. AIDS was so present in the public imagination. The message I got as a sixteen-year-old gay boy was that if you were gay, you were going to "get AIDS." Be sure to use condoms for every possible thing. Make sure you're covered in latex from head to toe. Otherwise, you "get AIDS" and you die. I was hyperconscious of that risk; contracting HIV was one of the things I was most afraid of.

AIDS was something which was whispered about. Oh, so-and-so, she's *ill*—that's how people would say it. AIDS was always in the ether. I remember there was another Black gay man—one of my mother's friends—who died of AIDS around that time. His name was Otis. I'd met him a couple times, but I never got to know him well. After he died, she told me about it, and I recognized it: He's a Black gay man just like me, and he died. The threat of AIDS was just always a part of my consciousness.

In 1998, I started college at Brown. That first day, my dad had just left me, I was unpacking my stuff, and this guy called over to me and shoved a flyer in my face. It was a flyer for the local HIV service organization in Providence.

He was like, "I think you might need this."

Basically, he was clocking me. That was terrifying! I still wasn't 100 percent sure if I wanted to be openly gay in college. I'd chosen Brown because it had a queer students of color organization; I knew there'd be other queer people of color there. Initially I'd wanted to come to school and be totally out from day one. But when I arrived, my roommate was a straight Black man from New York, and he reminded me of homophobic guys from my high school, which made me nervous about being out because I didn't want him to find out that his roommate was gay. And now this random guy had literally clocked me on the first day of school! But thanks to him, I ended up going down to the meeting that was listed on the flyer later that week. And that's how I started working in HIV.

At the meeting, I met Jim West. He was this quintessential Black leather daddy, but he was also the prevention director for AIDS Project Rhode Island. He mentioned to me that he was starting this new program called the Messengers, which focused on getting the message about HIV out to other young gay men of color.

We'd go out and do outreach in the nightclubs. You know, go to the club, give out condoms, lube, all that kind of stuff. At that point, Jim was the first Black gay man I knew—other than my uncle—living with HIV. It meant a lot to me to meet a Black man who was living proudly and out as gay and HIV+. And hey, he was also the first Black leather daddy that I'd ever met, you know, so he represented a lot of firsts for me.

In my sophomore year, I met a woman who went to my church in Montclair, New Jersey. She was the daughter of one of my grandmother's church lady friends. This woman was a medical doctor and a professor at Brown specializing in HIV care. Knowing that I had an interest in this area of medicine, my grandmother was like, "You should talk to Dr. Stone." So I emailed her and I was like, "Hey, we go to the same church, blah, blah, blah," and through these conversations, she ended up asking, "Do you want to do an internship with me over the summer? You can come and work in my clinic."

Working in the clinic humanized HIV for me in a different way. It was the first time I'd met women living with HIV. I met people who used drugs who were living with HIV. I started to see firsthand that HIV doesn't just affect gay people, which had been my mentality before I started working there.

I'll always vividly remember a woman I met at the clinic that summer. She'd just immigrated from the Dominican Republic and found out she was HIV+. She was so young, maybe 22 years old, not much older than I was at the time. I remember her being so scared. She didn't speak English at all, but I was able to speak a little Spanish with her, and that helped her relax some. I recall absorbing just how scared she was. But over time, working with Dr. Stone, she went on medication, and she started to feel better. She became so much more vibrant. But I'll never forget the fear on her face that first day: She really thought she was going to die. She felt that she would never be able to tell her family, and she couldn't even speak English. There were so many things she was carrying in that moment.

By the late 1990s as a college student, I still wasn't really aware of the advances in treatment for people living with HIV/AIDS. After I started at the clinic, that was my first understanding of how the new medication worked. I'll never forget walking into the conference room in Dr. Stone's clinic for the first time. There was a poster which listed all of the HIV medications. As the years went on, the doctors would slowly add new pills to this poster. At one point, I could memorize them all. But today, that poster is probably three times as big as it was back in 2000, which is fantastic. It shows how many treatment options there are today to support people living with HIV.

When I was younger, the threat of AIDS had made me too afraid to have sex at all. I just didn't. Over time, that changed. Slowly, condoms became something which I was more comfortable with. I started to gain much more knowledge about the actual risk of contracting HIV from different types of sexual behavior, and that knowledge made me more comfortable about my sexuality. Knowledge gave me power and agency; it helped me to determine what I wanted to do, because then I was able to understand the risks which were or weren't involved. It taught me that I could make choices.

Around 2007, several of my friends started testing positive for HIV. I think that for a lot of my friends, taking the medications wasn't actually that hard for them. It was around the time Atripla came out: Just one pill a day and you're good. My conversations with them were less about treatment, and more about navigating HIV in their personal and professional lives, because there was still so much stigma about being positive.

How do I tell my friends?

How do I tell my boyfriend?

How do I tell my family?

What will professional life look like?

What will my romantic future look like?

There was an incredible amount of stigma for a man to be living with HIV. The stigma still persists today, for sure, but I think it was worse then. My friends had to wrestle with that. Navigating dating apps, do you disclose, or do you not? In the mid-2000s, this technology was still really new; people were just figuring it out as they went. So how do you figure that out at the same time as you deal with an HIV diagnosis?

PrEP is a very powerful HIV prevention tool that we now have which we didn't have in the 1980s, or the 1990s, or the 2000s. It came on the scene in 2012. You take one pill a day, and it essentially eliminates your risk of contracting HIV. The more people we have taking PrEP, the more chains of transmission are broken. I feel like when a new technology becomes a meme or a joke on the internet, that's when you know it's everywhere. Seeing people joking about PrEP on the internet makes me feel confident that it's part of our culture. But only for a specific subset, right? In the United States, PrEP has reached something crazy like 90 percent coverage among white gay men, but only 15 percent in other groups. That needs to change.

Being "undetectable" is much more part of the gay lexicon nowadays too. If you're living with HIV and taking treatment consistently, you're extremely likely to have an undetectable viral load, which means you can't pass on the virus to someone. The knowledge that being undetectable = being untransmittable still isn't universal, but there's undoubtedly been a huge increase over the last ten years in public knowledge of PrEP and U=U. That knowledge helps to lessen the fears that people have about HIV. That's life-changing. It's empowering for people who are living with HIV and for people who might yet contract the virus.

# Kay Poyer

*Kay Poyer is a content creator in Dallas, Texas. She learned she was living with HIV in 2019, when she was eighteen years old.*

I was a freshman at college when my mom committed suicide. Having somebody close to you die like that . . . it's creepy. Like living inside a scary movie. After her funeral, I finished the school year, then quit college and moved back to Texas to live with my dad. This was in 2019.

Grief can put you in weird positions. I was eighteen and just starting to experiment with dating apps. One night, I was talking to this random man and I agreed to go to his apartment to hook up. I didn't really know what I was doing and I never consented for him to go as far as he did. Something happened that I did not say yes to.

When I left his apartment, I had this feeling in my heart and in my body: *A violation just happened. That wasn't okay. I think he's given me HIV.*

It was two in the morning. I was frantically Googling stuff and reading about HIV on my phone. I learned about PEP, a drug you can take in an emergency if you think you've been exposed to HIV. If you take PEP immediately, there's a good chance it will protect you from contracting HIV. I thought, *Oh shit, this could save me.* I called every hospital and every emergency clinic in my area. I asked all of them if they could give me PEP, but they all said, "No, sorry, we don't have that." There was probably an LGBT health center that could have helped me, but at the time, I didn't know places like that existed.

I had to accept that I wasn't going to get PEP. I tried to just hope it would all be fine. But I still had this gut feeling that something bad had happened. It takes four weeks for HIV to show up in a test. So I waited, paralyzed by fear. I was eighteen years old and I got super depressed. I wasn't eating. I was still grieving my mom. I stayed at home, chain-smoked, watched three horror movies a day. I didn't diverge from my strict chain-smoking schedule except to worry about HIV and read about it online.

My friends were telling me it was all going to be okay. I tried really hard to believe them. But then I started to seroconvert. I'd been reading about what happens after you contract HIV, so when the symptoms began, I knew my intuition must have been right. The weird part is that I knew there was good treatment. I knew you could live a normal life with HIV. But I was still attached to the sense that my life would be over if I became HIV+. That feeling is powerful; it was very hard to let go of.

I had to wait another two weeks for the results, and then it was confirmed: I had HIV. Thankfully, my viral load hadn't gotten crazy. It was very easy to get under control once I entered treatment.

A lot of medical professionals cannot swing it about HIV; they look at you like you're crazy and treat you like shit and don't know how to have any decorum about it. There are medical professionals who still treat HIV like it's gross. They act like we don't have gay people in Texas or people who get HIV in Texas. When I was calling the clinics and asking for PEP, I felt like the people answering the phone thought what I was asking for was gross and nasty.

But I found a good doctor. She'd put gold stars on my blood results and her nurse would always tell me how her son was doing. I think if everything hadn't sailed super smoothly after being diagnosed, I would be more pissed about the fact I couldn't access PEP. I knew about PrEP, but only because I was a very online teenager. When I started having sex, I didn't want to talk to my dad about PrEP, especially with my mom gone. I wasn't exactly going to talk to my dad about my teenage sexcapades and ask if we could add PrEP to the family health insurance. Maybe I'd have gone on PrEP if been able to think ahead a little and had the opportunity to sit down and be honest. I kick myself more about not being on PrEP than anything else, because I could have probably found a way to make it happen. But let's be real. You cannot be doing foresight at eighteen. You haven't unlocked that skill yet.

Once I started treatment, I realized that I was fine and my body was going to be fine and my life was going to be fine. After that realization, all the fear I'd been carrying started to seem silly. HIV is a human thing that just happens to some people. I learned firsthand that HIV is not the big deal that it was for so many people who came before me. All the fear I'd felt began to be replaced by a better feeling. I started to feel blessed to have been born in a time when HIV could happen to me and I could keep on living.

The Texas health department was on my ass immediately. The second I got that diagnosis, they came to my house and stuck a pink slip on my door that very plainly said, "You've been diagnosed with HIV, you have to call us." I had this archaic phone conversation about how I got HIV, what position I was in, who gave it to me, what their home address was. I get that it's important to track transmission, but the way they went about it felt so hostile and judgmental. As time went on, it started to seem morbidly funny to me. I take this pill every day. And I'm . . . completely fine? I have no symptoms. I can't transmit HIV. I live a normal life. So why is there all this bullshit and stigma around me? It was like gaining infrared vision. I started to see through all the crap around this virus.

People expect Texas to be all dirt roads and the honky-tonk and the Piggly Wiggly. The South is renowned for being very racist towards Black people and immigrants—especially Mexican immigrants. Yet there are thriving Mexican communities, thriving Black communities, thriving queer and trans communities. A lot of the most iconic queens from *RuPaul's Drag Race* come out of Texas. There's a joke people say here about wanting to be a natural-born Texan. If a pregnant woman has to give birth out of state, she'll ask for someone to bring a pan of Texas soil so the baby can be born on Texan land. I feel comfortable in the South. I know my way around here. I know how to talk to people. I know how to get old people who might hate me for being trans to at least joke around with me. Texas raises tough queer people. Sure, I wish the adversity wasn't there. It would be wonderful if we weren't constantly being attacked by our government. But even without the hostility, just being Southern gives you a little bit of grittiness. We make it work and we make it fun.

But here's the thing about Texas: At school, you're going to get the 1980s version of the facts. We learned about HIV at school, but we didn't learn anything real. We didn't learn about how good the treatment is. We didn't learn about PEP or PrEP. We didn't learn about the disability rights movement. We didn't learn about all the activists who took part in die-ins and fought for the rights of people with HIV/AIDS.

I grew up being taught that abstinence was the best policy. Abstinence-first sex education is bullshit; they don't teach you anything important. People get kinks about stuff because it's taboo! I remember sitting through our sex education class and thinking, *Y'all are literally setting horny teenagers up to be stupid, because you're making sex seem like this crazy thing that you're not allowed to do.*

The teacher had one kid brush their teeth and offer the toothbrush to someone else. You're supposed to realize that this person has already used this toothbrush, so nobody else would want to use it; it's supposed to be a symbol for virginity. That part of the class was very specifically geared towards the girls in the class. "He's already put it in his mouth, so who else is going to want to put it in their mouth?" Great analogy, guys. But when it comes to the Great Toothbrush of People Having Sex with Each Other, it's actually not that big of a deal when people have sex. People are always going to have sex.

This so-called education doesn't help queer or trans kids either. When I was six years old, kids at school were asking me if I was a girl or telling me I was gay. I became hardened as a way to protect myself. I learned to be mean to people when they were mean to me. There's an active battle against trans kids and their parents in Texas. Some politicians would love for young queer kids to be thrown to the wolves and eaten by them. You come out of that experience pretty scratched up. The system is set up to funnel gay and trans kids into the worst possible lives for themselves so that they can be disposed of more easily. I truly believe that from what I saw and experienced as I was growing up.

So I had to learn everything online. But even then, so much of what gets said about HIV by queer people on the internet is still from folks who don't have HIV. The stories they share never seem to involve treatment. They never seem to involve HIV+ people and they seldom talk about post-diagnosis living. It's always about how to prevent yourself from getting HIV and then talking about how many people died.

An HIV diagnosis is a dunk in ice-cold water. If people only talk about prevention, then we don't get to learn about what happens if you get diagnosed, and that can unintentionally lead to a lot of fear. So many people have experiences with HIV. So many people have experiences with all kinds of illnesses, sexually transmitted or otherwise. But in our society, we don't often get to hear people with HIV, or herpes, or HPV, talking about what happened and explaining, "This part was hard, this part was hard, this part was hard, but overall, I'm very happy." I want people to know that we don't get put in a vault and cryogenically frozen when we get diagnosed. Our lives go on.

I told my dad I had HIV as soon as I got the results back in August 2019. I had no other option because I needed to use his insurance to get on medication. By the time the COVID-19 pandemic was beginning, it was clear I had to move out of my dad's house. We'd never been close, but since my mom died, our relationship was strained. He didn't want to deal with me having HIV. I knew I needed to transition. I knew I needed to go on hormones. But I knew my dad would get mad if he saw that on the health insurance.

Not long after I told him I was a trans woman, he cut me off the insurance plan.

I texted my friend's mom: "I have to move out. I don't have anywhere to go. Could I come and live with you for a while?" I had good people around me and they became a new kind of family to me. Queer people having chosen families feels like a cliché. It feels corny. But it's literally been true for me. You build a new family. I would not trade it for anything.

It was so much to handle. Getting diagnosed with HIV after I lost my mom to suicide. Leaving my dad's house at the start of COVID-19. Losing access to his insurance after my transition. Eventually it started to seem like everything I'd been afraid of losing was actually holding me back from being myself. I was afraid of being cut off from my dad. I was scared of not having parents. I was afraid of being rejected by people because I had HIV. I was so scared before I transitioned: *What if he cuts me off? What then?* After I moved out, I was really, really poor for a while. In the end, pizza delivery was what changed everything for me. I made a bit of money. I got a little more comfortable in my own skin. I realized that I could make it without my dad. The world felt less scary.

When I lost my insurance, Gilead provided me with a free year of HIV medication. I got enrolled at the LGBTQ health center in Dallas and now I get my treatment through the Ryan White CARE Act. There's this guy at the center whose whole job is to be your friend when you're at the clinic. He talked to me about a period in his life when he stopped taking his HIV medication because he got super depressed. I don't know that I would have learned so much about the importance of community if I hadn't gone through this experience. There are a lot of people I wouldn't have met and a lot of conclusions I wouldn't have reached as soon as I did if I hadn't had to deal with having HIV.

It might sound macabre, but becoming HIV+ gave me a greater sense of being connected to our past as queer people. It's forced me to look at that history. It's made me feel connected to parts of the community that I'm not a part of, like when I read about how many lesbians showed up for dying gay men during the crisis. My boss is an older gay guy. One day I mentioned I had HIV and he told me about his youth in the 1980s. He was kicked out of his home at the age of fifteen and he lost a lot of friends to AIDS. There are these two older trans women I know on TikTok—very much your classic fled-to-New-York-in-the-1980s beautiful dolls. They talked to me about being a trans woman in New York back then; all the shit they had to deal with to survive. I look at my life from a trans perspective and an HIV+ perspective. Even when I've been broke, no parents, dead mom, delivering pizzas in the fucking boonies in a car with no AC, I'm still just so lucky.

There's so much discourse online today amongst young LGBTQ+ people who just don't feel connected to the queer community. They don't have a conception of why we all decided to make an acronym and a rainbow flag and hang out in the same neighborhood despite our differences. It's strange, but HIV gives us an actual, material reason to value the connections we have with each other, because queer people have always been on the front line of the crisis. Having HIV does not feel like a blessing—it's not like I'm part of a special club or anything. But learning about the history of HIV as I adjusted to living with the virus made me feel more connected to my ancestors, whether as a trans woman or as an HIV+ person. It's the silver lining.

But before you can recognize that silver lining, you have to deal with the anger. You have to deal with the pain and the depression. The hard feelings. After that, you get to make a decision. *What happens now? What am I going to make out of this?* You have to take a shitty experience like getting HIV at the age of eighteen and create something out of it. I've had older trans people or gay men say to me, "You're so lucky to be HIV-positive now. It wasn't like this in my time." That's a heavy thing to hear. But it reminds me that I've been very lucky overall. There's a lot of hope for HIV+ people nowadays—if we're only given the guiding hand to see that when we're diagnosed.

# Antonio Boone

*Compassion goes a long way toward helping individuals accept a new HIV diagnosis. Antonio Boone learned this firsthand as a college student in 2011.*

When I found out I was HIV+, I was in my senior year at Temple University in Philadelphia. I remember the date it happened because it was around World AIDS Day: the fifth of December 2011. It was finals week. I was in my room getting ready for class when I got the call from Student Health Services.

"Your results are in. Can you come in, please?"

In Philly, I'd been exploring my sexuality. By senior year, I could count on one hand—okay, maybe two—my number of sexual partners. I knew condoms were important, but I struggled to use them. I couldn't stay hard when I was wearing one. Some people just can't use condoms perfectly—that's why PrEP is so important. But PrEP wasn't available in 2011. So I'd manage the risk as best as I could, balancing caution with desire, having conversations with any potential partner: "When were you last tested? When did you last have unprotected sex?"

I knew the phone call meant bad news. If the results had been negative, they'd have told me on the phone. I went over to the clinic and met with the provider who broke the news. My test had come back positive for syphilis, gonorrhea, and chlamydia. And HIV, too. Back then, I leaned on the traditional Baptist Christian faith values instilled in me by my family. I leaned my head back to the ceiling and spoke to God: "Whatever direction we're going with this, I'm running with it. I will follow your lead wherever this goes."

At the clinic, I got connected to treatment and support services. I was given antibiotics for chlamydia, gonorrhea, and syphilis—three easily treatable sexually transmitted infections. And I started medication for HIV pretty much immediately. The clinic rang an outreach worker, and she came over to meet me literally ten minutes later. The stars don't align like that for everyone in my situation, and people don't always act with the decent amount of compassion. Not everyone is as lucky as I was.

I knew I wasn't going to die. I knew HIV wasn't a "death sentence" anymore, but the stigma was still heavy on my shoulders at first. I was worried about what my new life would look like. I worried nobody would want me, like I should just be happy with whatever I could get.

Nowadays, I know better. Fuck that!

In Philly, if you contract HIV or an STI, you have to go to a city health center and report what you've acquired.

I showed up at the Philadelphia Public Health Department, and the person I spoke with was cold and unkind.

"Okay, so you have chlamydia, gonorrhea, syphilis . . ."

She read it like a grocery list, dryly and without empathy, like I was another item being checked off of her to-do list. Her tone lacked compassion. But I was a human being in the middle of a terrible start to his finals week. I was resilient enough to rise above it. I didn't let that experience stand in the way of accessing the support and treatment that I needed and was entitled to. But some people don't have that resilience. Some people lose their trust in the health system when they are treated like numbers and not human beings. They retreat into themselves. They choose not to engage in health care services and resources. Individuals and communities suffer when that happens. It's not enough for providers to understand the science: They need to be culturally competent and administer holistic care like human beings.

After my diagnosis, I went to see a good friend. We met on the corner of 21st Street and Spring Garden, and I told her what had happened. She didn't have to say anything: She just held me and I knew she was on my side. I kept busy. I successfully passed all of my finals. I found friends, allies, and built a strong support network. My diagnosis happened as I was trying to figure what I wanted to do with my life. After graduation, I joined the HIV workforce. I joined a global community of amazing people, working to end new HIV diagnoses and support people with lived experiences all over the world. It feels like the closest thing I can get to being a superhero.

That's the thing about living with HIV: Life goes on.

If you find out you have HIV, don't let internal or external stigma limit you from living your life and pursuing your dreams.

Because you deserve everything.

## Sarah Schulman

*Writer and activist Sarah Schulman has played a major role in documenting the history of ACT UP. With Jim Hubbard, Sarah led the ACT UP Oral History Project, interviewing the surviving members of ACT UP over eighteen years—many excerpts from which you will find across this book. Their project culminated in* United in Anger: A History of ACT UP, *a documentary released in 2012, and* Let the Record Show: A Political History of ACT UP New York, 1987–1993, *Sarah's book on ACT UP New York, which was published in 2021. Today, Sarah is one of a small number of surviving writers who have been covering AIDS from the surfacing of the epidemic in the 1980s to the present. We wanted to find out what Sarah thinks about the legacy of AIDS activism and the changes still needed to confront the reality of AIDS-related inequality.*

The real problem today is that we don't have a functional health care system for the entire world. We see this every time there's a new virus. Every time some new medication is invented, it doesn't solve the problem, because there's no equity in distribution. We have more refugees in the world than we've ever had in history, more homeless people, more people without access to basic services. So as long as there's this brutal reality, health care is compromised, and that affects HIV/AIDS.

But that's a more sophisticated way of conceptualizing the problem than I had access to when I was twenty-three, back when it all started.

I was born in 1958. AIDS was identified in 1981. It's not called AIDS yet, but they see the virus emerging. At that time in New York City, you didn't have to work a million hours a week to survive. My rent was two hundred and five dollars, so I only had to work ten hours a week as a waitress. I was living in a bohemian subculture. We had fun, all the time. When friends started to get sick, it took a while to understand what was happening. Partially because we were so young back then, but also because the mainstream press was completely ignoring it. And that meant that we were having a lived experience that was not being represented in the media.

To deal with it, first you have to understand what you're actually experiencing. You're not learning about what's happening to you and your friends by reading about it. You're only learning it by living it.

And then you have to produce the materials that other people read so that they can start to comprehend what's happening.

And *then* you have to force the mainstream media to represent it.

But to represent it *accurately*—that's even more difficult.

*In the early 1980s, access to information about AIDS was hindered—and precious time was squandered—because not enough people cared about a condition that only seemed to be affecting people who were already oppressed and excluded from the mainstream. Although the gay press played a crucial role in reporting the emerging outbreak of AIDS among gay men in the first part of the 1980s, it remained challenging to get people to understand what was happening to other groups of people, too. As a lesbian writer in downtown Manhattan, Sarah was on the front lines when AIDS hit the city's gay community. Once she understood what was going on, she knew she needed to make people understand that AIDS was impacting people beyond this demographic, and so she started covering the specific experiences of women with HIV, newborns, and homeless people.*

AIDS has been distorted from the very first day. It was a distortion when it was initially called GRID, because "Gay-Related Immune Deficiency" never existed. There was never any such thing as a gay-related immune deficiency. No one has ever shown a biological marker for queerness. It was stigma that made HIV associated with being gay, not any biological source or origin.

I was involved with AIDS for six years before ACT UP was founded. I wanted to make people understand what was happening through my writing and journalism. In New York City, at the early part of the earliest period of the epidemic before there were any treatments, there was a lot of pediatric AIDS: children living with AIDS. Back then, there wasn't even an HIV test. Certainly, when the HIV test was invented, low-income people didn't have access to it, and they didn't have health care, either. So babies were born HIV+ or with pediatric AIDS. Their mothers didn't even know they had it, because the mothers didn't know that they themselves had AIDS.

These newborns were often funneled into a double-blind study: Half the patients got whatever medicine was being tested; the other half got placebo. Scientists like these kinds of studies because they have clear data: The comparative is clean.

But from the point of view of people with AIDS, you don't want that. You don't want to be the person who gets that sugar pill. You want to get the medication. These newborns, of course, were people with AIDS, but as babies, they didn't have a voice of their own. They couldn't advocate for themselves. Often, their mothers felt so guilty that they had unwittingly infected them with HIV that they would consent to use their children in these studies—studies which many people felt were unethical, because they required that 50 percent of participants would receive no treatment at all.

I wrote a piece about this issue. I sent it to a leading journalist in the progressive press, *The Village Voice,* at the time, but he didn't want to broadcast this perspective, because he believed in double-blind studies. He might have been gay, but that didn't mean he was looking at it from the point of view of people with AIDS. He was looking at it from the point of view of science. So he objected to my perspective and wouldn't publish the piece.

Unlike him, I was imagining the patient's perspective. My politics had developed out of the reproductive rights movement of the 1970s—the feminist women's health movement—in which everything was looked at from the patient's perspective. After all, there were very few women doctors or high-level researchers and administrators. Women were the patients. The situation called for patient-centered politics: We needed to look at the issue from the view of people with AIDS. Later, in '87, that was a core belief of ACT UP: that people with AIDS are the experts.

Is it ethical to subject people with terminal illnesses to a double-blind study? Especially if they're newborns who cannot consent, and whose mothers are consenting under emotional pressure. What is "a mother's consent" when mothers were made to feel guilty for giving birth to infected children?

Eventually, through the effort of activists, double-blind studies were changed so that instead of placebo, people were given the standard of care. But early on, there was no standard of care. As they began to find treatments that they thought might help in some way, those became the placebo.

And then whatever new experimental drug they were testing was the comparative.

You know, all those early drugs—none of them worked anyway. That was part of the tragedy. People fought very hard for drugs that didn't work.

*As people fought for drugs that didn't work, the death count climbed and climbed. Hundreds of cases became thousands; thousands became tens of thousands. By the late 1980s, AIDS had become a leading cause of death within the American population. Sarah was one of hundreds of members of ACT UP New York who took part in direct action to demand greater attention to AIDS-related injustice, more drug research and access, more social services and housing. Being a member of ACT UP during this critical period was an opportunity to redirect your feelings of grief, fear, hopelessness, and frustration into collective outrage. It was about wanting to change the world because the status quo was killing people.*

After ACT UP had started, I was surrounded by other people who cared. It's one thing when you're twenty-three and you know three people who have AIDS, but when you're in ACT UP, you're suddenly surrounded by many young people who are dying. One of the things about AIDS is that you learn how to talk about it because you're surrounded by it. It becomes part of your casual daily conversation.

We're bonded for life, the surviving ACT UP people. Even if we don't particularly like each other. We see each other all the time, in all kinds of capacities.

We're bonded because we changed the world. Very few people have had that experience. You know, that's one of the reasons I'm an optimist politically—because I've been part of a movement that *actually made things better*. That's a special experience, because it gives you the knowledge that change is possible.

When Jim and I started the ACT UP Oral History Project in 2001, every single one of the 188 people we interviewed was very proud of what they did. Everybody. They understood what they achieved. Not many other movements can say that.

There are some aspects of AIDS that people now just can't comprehend. There are experiences that we can have empathy with, but unless you're in it, you can't really fully grasp. Because they're singular experiences—like being Palestinian right now. It's almost impossible to convey what it was like to someone who isn't there with you. Today, people who are very knowledgeable about HIV, people who are HIV+ themselves, they still cannot truly conceptualize that earlier period. When they try to talk about it, they misunderstand it, because that mass death experience, and the indifference we faced, is so impossible to imagine.

I think people in ACT UP thought they were going to end the AIDS crisis. And let's be clear: They didn't. We didn't. We expected a different kind of future. There's a famous speech by Vito Russo called "Why We Fight" where he's like, "First, we're going to kick the shit out of this virus, and then we're going to kick the shit out of the system!" But neither of those things has occurred, even though ACT UP did so much in widening access to treatment, diagnoses, education, and support.

*Despite the life-changing (and lifesaving) success of combination therapy in the mid-1990s, there was still no cure for HIV. Today, a cure remains elusive. Instead, people living with HIV and AIDS depend upon a lifetime supply of medications—a need that generates revenue for pharmaceutical companies. For that reason, access to combination therapy has always been uneven and inequitable, whether in different parts of the US or around the rest of the world. People with low incomes and living in precarious circumstances are more likely than others to come into contact with HIV and, simultaneously, less likely to have access to consistent health coverage. The worst of the crisis in the United States ended once combination therapy started, but huge inequalities and stigmas continue to shape the reality of AIDS in America and in the world.*

There was disappointment. We had to understand what our actual victories really were, how these victories had been compromised by capitalism, because capitalism turned out to be more powerful than HIV. None of us anticipated that. People thought that by getting treatments and securing services, they would end AIDS. They didn't understand that capitalism was going to inhibit that. Having the treatments was not enough when so many were not going to have health care, and when pharmaceutical companies were going to have unchecked greed as AIDS worsened around the world. These unexpected realities were going to obstruct people getting access to the treatment, but we didn't understand that back then. We thought our main problem was HIV, not the relentless greed of a number of global pharmaceutical corporations.

PrEP is a good example of this greed. Obviously, everyone should have access to PrEP to prevent new transmissions of HIV, and PrEP should be 100 percent covered by whatever form of insurance anybody can get access to. But why does it seem like PrEP is only marketed to gay men? What about women?

Most women don't even know what PrEP is. They don't know whether they can or should take it. And the big irony of the PrEP market is that it's dependent on people continuing to be infected with HIV. If everybody who was HIV+ received the standard of care, they'd be undetectable. Current medication renders HIV+ people virally suppressed, which means that they become biologically incapable of passing on the virus. So if everyone who's living with HIV today has good access to the current standard of care, there would be no more new HIV infections and no market for PrEP. From this perspective, you could say that the huge profits which pharmaceutical companies continue to reap from selling PrEP are only available because we don't have an equitable health care system in the first place.

That has to change.

## SOURCE MATERIAL

## Remembrance

### by Kenneth McCreary

*This piece first appeared in* Brother to Brother. *At the time, Kenneth McCreary taught English literature in Northern Virginia.*

> I am distressed for thee: . . . thy love to me was wonderful, passing the love of women.
> —I Samuel 1:26

He said he wanted his body burned and thrown where I would not go to that pile of nothing and weep. He also said he wanted all of his possessions given to the poor.

I have pictures of us on our vacation in the Keys. He was a strong 190 pounds; I have no pictures of him at 93 pounds. He had such a soothing and persuasive voice that it was difficult to disagree with him, but I will never forget the hoarseness and rattle of his voice when he had pneumonia. Even in the hospital, I cared for him because the nurses were afraid. AZT was only a false hope. What am I going to tell his parents?

Last Sunday, I rode a ferry to Mayport to release his ashes. Except for the helmsman and two fishermen, I was alone. Only the muffled rattle of the engine and the lapping of water against the sides of the boat intruded into my thoughts. It was a beautiful morning. The gentle breeze caused his ashes to float several seconds before landing in the water. My tears burned as they streamed down my face; I could not see through this liquid veil.

Several weeks later I was cleaning the garage and found one of his old shirts tossed in a corner. It still smelled like him—that light orange odor. I also found our old beach ball, but I could not let the air out—his breath was in it.

**SOURCE MATERIAL**

# Happy Anniversary

### by Robert Vazquez-Pacheco

*When this was published in* Sojourner, *Robert Vazquez-Pacheco had been living with HIV for about ten years. In his bio he described himself as "Puerto Rican, third generation mainland, and single." You can find more of his story in the ACT UP Oral History Project.*

I was brushing my teeth in my boyfriend's bathroom. As usual there was a little blood. I don't floss enough. It's hard to think of my blood as something potentially fatal. As I rinsed the brush, the sounds from the TV came into focus. Some morning show was discussing the tenth anniversary of the AIDS crisis. The footage was depressingly familiar: white gay men in San Francisco and in hospitals, Latinos and African-Americans shooting up, white teens, emaciated Africans, children of color in hospitals and white doctors, white journalists, and white government officials. They spent about five minutes on it and then followed with a cheery ten-minute piece about jugglers. Some things haven't changed.

Ten years of crisis. Ten years under siege. Ten years of my life. In 1981, my lover Jeff was diagnosed with Kaposi's sarcoma. A PWA on his thirtieth birthday. We had been together six months. He told me I could end our relationship if I wanted to. He would understand. I didn't. How could I leave my man?

Our doctor was surprised that Jeff was the one diagnosed. If Doc were a gambler, he would have bet on me. A sure thing? After all, I was the one who didn't take care of himself. I was the "bad guy." On some level, I felt a bizarre sense of smugness. So much for modern medicine and Dr. Thing's diagnostic ability. I have learned there are very few sure things in this epidemic.

A miracle of survival, I'm told. An inspiration to us all. I watched the inspiration climb five flights to our apartment with lesions on his hip and behind his knee. I tied the inspiration's shoes. I was relieved when he died. The suffering became too much for us both. The miracle of survival, like all miracles, only works in the realm of the fabulous. They don't play in real life.

I learned I was HIV-positive in 1987. I've probably been seropositive for longer than that. I've outlasted my lovers, my friends, some of my exes, my tricks, my relatives, even some of the queens I couldn't stand. I've outlasted our doctor. I've even outlasted the guilt of still being alive and healthy. It's funny. There is no satisfaction in that word: outlasted. There is no satisfaction in living longer than friends and loved ones. No catharsis crying at yet another memorial service. I don't go to them anymore. The miracle of survival. Survival is a spot between the rock of guilt and the hard place of memory.

I wander through the city and pass places so loaded with memory it's surprising there's no sinkhole there. The past is evermore and to quote Gladys Knight, those memories get in my way. A kind of Puerto Rican ancient mariner, dragging the albatross of memory through bars and clubs. I live the *Twilight Zone* episode where all disappear except for one. For me, New York is a ghost town. History is written by survivors.

I remain asymptomatic. A swollen lymph node is the most visible sign of my seropositivity. I like to think of it as my dueling scar. A reminder of my daily duel with my own fear and hopelessness. My fight with my growing alienation. A battle at dawn with myself. The prize: another day. The goal: not to shut down and shut everyone out. Every day I must convince myself that love is not loss, that friendship is not desertion, and that long-term relationships with other gay men are not exercises in futility. Every day I fight to remain optimistic as I hear I've outlasted someone else. Every day I am surprised to find that I still do things like hope and dream and even love. I'm in love now and it fills me with fear. I love with an intensity beyond the obsessions of my youth. I have to. There's nothing else.

**SOURCE MATERIAL**

# Little Prayer

## by Danez Smith

*Danez Smith is an acclaimed queer, nonbinary, HIV+ poet from St. Paul, Minnesota. Their books include the National Book Award finalist* Don't Call Us Dead, *from which this poem comes.*

let ruin end here

let him find honey
where there was once a slaughter

let him enter the lion's cage
& find a field of lilacs

let this be the healing
& if not   let it be

## SOURCE MATERIAL

## Excerpt from **Committing to Memory**

### by Paul Monette

*Paul Monette's many works about living with AIDS include* Borrowed Time: An AIDS Memoir *and* Love Alone: Eighteen Elegies for Rog, *which he wrote for his partner Roger Horwitz. Monette died in 1995, at age forty-nine.*

Sometimes like Vincent and his burning sky
I'm so far out of myself I'm
a cypress, clanging a thousand green
bells. Especially now with the solstice
coming on, druidical and perm-frosted,
we crave a chill in the air who have been
sunstruck too long. What you must remember
is the reason we are on fire like this
is to light our way to New Year's. Nobody
knows how many are lost, how many more
will follow. There is the narrowest zone
between the ices of winter and the deep
freeze of the black chamber. Nevertheless,
here is where we have to skate, waltzing
on a sheet of ice membrane-thin. Enough
of summer. Give me the smoke of your breath,
this longest night with the stars erupting,
kin to those priests of the waning sun
dancing in their stone circles. Didn't we
meet on the brink of winter? So, give us
bare branches and birds thronging south,

a great horned owl on our telephone pole.
We'll fuck in the snow and come in for tea,
safe in the winter harbor of the heart.
Druid brother, pagan mate, ours be the hard
flame, ours the silver fields of frost
and a pair of cypresses crowning the hill,
reaching to graze the sky. Men can love like that.

**SOURCE MATERIAL**

## Excerpt from **The Tomb of Sorrow**

### by Essex Hemphill

*for Mahomet*

When I die,
honey chil',
my angels
will be tall
Black drag queens.

I will eat their stockings
as they fling them
into the blue
shadows of dawn.
I will suck
their purple lips
to anoint my mouth
for the utterance of prayers.

My witnesses
will have to answer
to go-go music.
Dancing and sweat
will be required
at my funeral.

Someone will have to answer
the mail I leave,
the messages

on my phone service;
someone else
will have to tend
to the aching
that drove me
to seek soul.

Everything different
tests my faith.
I have stood in places
where the absence of light
allowed me to live longer,
while at the same time
it rendered me blind.

I struggle against
plagues, plots,
pressure, paranoia.
Everyone wants a price
for my living.

When I die,
my angels,
immaculate
Black diva
drag queens,
all of them
sequined
and seductive,
some of them
will come back
to haunt you,
I promise,
honey chil'.

# TESTIMONY

## Robert Levithan

**(2001)**

Twenty years ago I was thirty and people like me began to die. Oh, at first we looked for how they weren't like me. They went to the baths, they did poppers, they . . . they . . . they. But within a couple of years it was clear—it wasn't them, it was us. Us was at first friends of friends, people I'd had dinner with or spent a night at their house in Sag Harbor or, even worse, had sex with one afternoon after we'd met at a useless audition. There was a waiter who worked for me. And then there were terrifyingly skinny men on the streets everywhere. And then Bob and Peter and my first GMHC buddy and my second. By 1985 they were dying and sex had begun to equal death. Some of us didn't test—for political reasons, out of fear. I had been part of a study, but didn't know the results for years. When I found out, I found out that I had been positive for at least seven years, that my T-cell count had dropped from 1250 to 535 over these years. And there was still nothing to do except go on with my life. I changed careers, moved, and started and finished many relationships. I was dumped, I was left, I parted amicably, but the pesky specter of AIDS always lived in the house. It didn't go.

AIDS brought me friends and colleagues, satisfying work leading groups and workshops and eventually a degree as a therapist.

It brought me to my knees. Seven years ago my T-cell count was 56 and pneumonia took over my lungs and nearly ended my body.

Almost six years ago I won a lottery (literally) and began experimental drugs on a compassionate access program and my T-cells went from 20 to 40 to 110 to 212 (I gave a party) and then 301 and then on to today.

Aswan died and Carol and Felicity and Rob and Rick and Jeffrey Johnson and Louis and dear young Michael.

And then people weren't dying so much. We were making a living and salvaging not only immune systems but careers and relationships and dreams.

Risen from the dead, we remember. But others don't seem to know. They act like it's only a pesky condition that is easily treated. They overlook side effects and viral mutations and livers that can't process one more chemical. They play, and we hold our breaths, waiting for eyes to open and hearts to break.

It would be easier not to know but it's only a sorry game of waiting—after twenty years the good news and the bad news is that it's not over—there is more life but there will be more and more suffering and loss.

## (1998)

"This *is* normal!" I reply when a client talks about the fantasy of a normal life with AIDS. Why would I devalue the last seventeen years of my life? All of my thirties and now most of my forties have been lived on the journey: GRID, fear that it might be me, living as if it was me, then the certainty that it is me. Readjustments and the discovery of just how adaptable the human heart is. The unthinkable becomes day-to-day business and what others often consider heroic is as ordinary as flossing morning and evening. Some of my comrades don't agree, but I am fully alive in midst of being a man with AIDS. It is no more certain than my hair color, certainly less constant than the blue of my eyes when I'm in love. I no longer have a non-AIDS sense of my life. There is no longing to go back to the way it was before because then I was twentysomething and certain that if I lived past thirty, I would have already proved myself wrong.

I remember. It's 1977 and I'm at a psychic in Rockland County. Peter

Hujar and I are sitting with Jacki Apple, a downtown artist/slash/arts administrator. She is reading my palm. I remember one phrase: "In your forties there is a break in your lifeline. You will have a choice—to live or die. It is up to you." I don't like her saying this, but it stayed with me, buried with other unwanted sights. And then, this many years later, I remember that phrase. Long before AIDS my palm predicted the moment almost four years ago when I chose not to believe I would die, even though I was a dozen years into this AIDS thing in my body, my immune system was virtually gone and I was lying in a bed on the second floor of St. Vincent's Hospital in Santa Fe struggling to breathe.

Somehow I was always certain that I didn't have to die from this. How often I saw that slightly condescending smile, the shared glance that bespoke of my delusional state, but I knew, I was not yet dying—any more than anyone else, that is. So I have crossed the divide. I have found the certainty to travel beyond an easy out, outliving myself, reinventing normal, living this ordinary, extraordinary life with a slight case of AIDS.

## (2011)

"I jumped into the East River the day I found out I was HIV-positive." R.J.

"I went on a drug binge that lasted two weeks." P.

"I thought I'd feel relieved. I feel stupid." G.

"I can't get my mind out of 1985 thinking—even though it's 2011." S.

I have never counseled a newly HIV-positive man or woman who didn't wish that they had done things differently.

I am 60. I have lived half my life with HIV/AIDS. This is my normal. When I tested positive, no one would have expected me to be here—let alone to be thriving. Not many of the first wave are here.

In 2011 (in the developed world) we have left the era of AIDS. We are however still very much in the age of HIV. There is an entire generation that did not live through the dark days of AIDS. Some of them have little or no fear of HIV: "You just take a pill every day." Or, they might consider it a part of the landscape: "I'm going to get it eventually, so I might as well have fun while doing it."

This is tricky territory. One can have a wonderful life living with HIV. And, it is at least a major inconvenience and sometimes a danger to well-being that can usually be avoided. I want people with HIV to not feel stigmatized while I want those who are negative to remain so. Therefore, I speak out as an AIDS elder.

Long-term survival is a combination of luck, genetics, resiliency, attitude and the interplay amongst them all. As a psychotherapist and workshop facilitator, in private practice and at Friends in Deed, I get to observe firsthand the extraordinary capacity for adaptation and reinvention that manifests for many when faced with catastrophe. I have also lived it.

AIDS brought the true challenges. First there was terror: Will it be me? Then it was activism: I'll save myself by being at the front lines. Then it was me: Live for now. And then I outlived myself. I doubted, however, that I would ever have a partner again, that I would ever feel sexy again, that I would ever believe that a future was possible. And then it did get better: The life I am living today—gay, HIV-positive, and at the top of my game as I reach 60.

When AIDS was first identified, 30 years ago, I knew it was going to impact my life. I remember the first person I knew who died, a charming handsome young writer and editor. How am I different from him? Did he do something I didn't do—can I dodge this bullet? In my case, no. As my brother once said to me, it must be odd to find out in retrospect that you were playing Russian Roulette without even knowing it—today's youth, in contrast, should know it.

I figured the best way to know what was happening was to be on the front lines, so I began to volunteer, first at GMHC and then as an active member of the alternative support community. Hope and possibility were radical concepts in the dark days of AIDS.

I would love for the younger generation to learn their lessons from another teacher. Being HIV-positive is to be avoided.

I am fortunate. I have the privilege and honor to work with men and women facing their biggest challenges and that helps keep me awake to the importance of life now in the present. I still get caught up in petty problems and vanities, and my life is filled with constant reminders: Does this really matter? Will I even remember this in a year?

I am sure that if I had been HIV-negative, my life would have been interesting and challenging. That just wasn't my life to live.

## (2014)

When I am feeling true joy, I'm experiencing the sum total of every part of this beautifully complicated journey. I cannot selectively leave out the painful parts—not illness, not the decimation of my generation of gay men, nor the aftereffects of my familial history. My joy includes all of it.

I grew up as an outsider doing a very good imitation of an insider. Today I strive for an authenticity that celebrates a particular path: surviving a plague, facing mortality, losing so many and yet being granted so many privileges. I get to work with extraordinary men and women who have found exquisite power through their challenges.

I carry my history and the history of my fallen brothers. Surviving catastrophe is a teaching. And I remain simply a man who has had the good fortune to cultivate the necessary resilience to thrive into his sixties, eager to discover what might be the next opportunity to serve, the next challenge while striving to enjoy the pleasures of being here now—in the twenty-first century.

What was unknown territory for me is now assumed: We can come back from the brink and not only survive, but thrive. Life is full of surprises.

# Notes and Sources

**A Brief Overview of the AIDS Epidemic** (p. 9) A number of timelines were consulted in putting this together. The timeline at hiv.gov was the most definitive, but timelines at historyofhiv.org, nycaidsmemorial.org, and amfar.org were also valuable. Many different timelines cite different figures for the number of cases and deaths each year; our numbers in this section come from the CDC's HIV Surveillance Report, vol. 13, no. 2, 2001, p. 14. Statistics and trends for 2002 to 2025 come from hiv.gov at hiv.gov/hiv-basics/overview/data-and-trends/statistics.

**A Brief Overview of the AIDS Epidemic, Through the Story of My Uncle, Robert Levithan** (p. 15) *A note from David:* My uncle was a very active self-documentarian throughout his life, leaving behind many handwritten journals and authoring many essays and columns about his life. Some of these columns were written for *The Huffington Post* and some were collected in his book *The New 60: Outliving Yourself and Reinventing a Future*, which is still in print. For this book, I read all of Bobby's journals, read every applicable file on his laptops, and went through the folders he kept of his writing. The timelines here and in all his sections later in the book come from these writings. Bobby was not shy about sharing his experiences and his emotions with readers, and we feel his inclusion in this book is a fitting extension of all the work he did while he was with us. (p. 18) The lyric from *Rent* shared here is from the song "Will I?" written by Jonathan Larson. Larson's father, Al, was friends with my grandfather Lou, and the musical's history is deeply entwined with that of Friends in Deed. During the pandemic in 2021, the New York Theatre Workshop streamed *25 Years of Rent: Measured in Love*, and I was moved to see Bobby's face in the documentary footage. It is hard to understate the effect *Rent* had in terms of inviting its audience into the world of living with HIV.

**A Boy, Lost in History: Robert Rayford** (p. 23) Elvin-Lewis is quoted in "Boy's 1969 Death Suggests AIDS Invaded U.S. Several Times," *New York Times*, October 28, 1987. (p. 26) We are grateful to Ted Kerr for his research on Robert Rayford, particularly "AIDS 1969: HIV, History, and Race," *Drain*, vol. 13, no. 2, 2016. We also refer to "Systemic Chlamydial Infection Associated with Generalized Lymphedema and Lymphangiosarcoma," *Lymphology*, vol. 6, no. 3, 1973 by Elvin-Lewis et al.

**HIV and AIDS: The Basics** (p. 30) Information here about HIV and AIDS comes from many sources, including cdc.gov/hiv/about, hivcare.org/hiv-basics, healthysexuals.com/about-prep, hivinfo.nih.gov/understanding-hiv, kidshealth.org/en/teens/aids, and hopkinsmedicine.org.

**Timeline 1978–1982: 1978** (p. 31) Landesman's comments come from his interview in the Physicians and AIDS Oral History Collection at the Columbia Center for Oral History. (p. 32) We are indebted to the ACT UP Oral History Project, founded by Sarah Schulman and Jim Hubbard, which gave us permission to freely quote from its firsthand accounts. We urge you to check out the full collection at actuporalhistory.org. When we cite the ACT UP Oral History Project, we will give you both the name of the interviewee and the number of the interview. In this case, the quote from Betty Williams comes from interview 099. **June 1981** (p. 33) We are also grateful to the *Bay Area Reporter* for permission to quote from its articles throughout the book. This passage comes from the July 2, 1982, issue, page 34. **August 1981** (pp. 33–34) Humm's quote is from "40 Years Ago: Meeting at Larry Kramer's House as a Pandemic Began," *Philadelphia Gay News*, October 6, 2021. (p. 34) Mass is quoted from "GMHC Founders Day: Dr. Larry Mass Reflects on Early Days of AIDS Crisis," gmhc.org, August 7, 2024. **December 1981** (p. 35) Bobbi Campbell is quoted in "I WILL SURVIVE," *San Francisco Sentinel*, vol. 9, no. 2, December 10, 1981, p. 1. **January 1982** (p. 36) Waxman's opening statement is from the House Subcommittee on Health and the Environment's hearing on Kaposi's Sarcoma and Opportunistic Infections, April 13, 1982. **May 1982** (p. 38) The "GRID" quote is from Laurence K. Altman's now legendary "New Homosexual Disorder Worries Health Officials," *New York Times*, May 11, 1982, sec. C, p. 1. Vazquez-Pacheco is quoted from the ACT UP Oral History Project, interview 002. **October 1982** (p. 41) Our transcription of the press conference is based on the audio presented here: youtube.com/watch?v=yAzDn7tE1lU.

**The Accidental, Deliberate Poster Boy: Ryan White** (p. 45) Markel's words are from "Remembering Ryan White, the teen who fought against the stigma of AIDS," *PBS Newshour*, April 8, 2016. (p. 46) Smith and White quotes are from "Officials Fear Hemophiliac Will Spread Disease: School in Indiana Bars Boy with AIDS," *Los Angeles Times*, July 31, 1985. The "Ryan White joke" is recounted in the memoir that White completed before he died, *Ryan White: My Own Story*, which was cowritten with Ann Marie Cunningham and published by Dial, a division of Penguin Random House, in 1991. It remains the fullest account of Ryan's life, largely in his own words. All quotes from the book included in this chapter are used by permission from Penguin Random House and the GMA Agency. (p. 47) The *People* quote is from an August 3, 1987, interview. The *Indianapolis Star* quote is from Tim Evans's "Retro Indy. Ryan White (1971–1990)," April 8, 2010. The "Why were they so scared?" quote is from "Ryan White, Who Died of AIDS at 18, Would Have Turned 50 Today: 'He Made the World Better,'" *People*, December 6, 2021. (pp. 48–49) All the *People* covers are as cited; the "24 Hours in the Crisis That Is Breaking America's Heart" cover story is from August 3, 1987. (p. 50) Decades later, in 2017, an adult Milano told *NBC News*, "There is nothing about my activism that isn't directly motivated by my love for Ryan White . . . He taught me that I had a power as a celebrity to change things and to stand up for what's right, and he gave me the courage to do that. My activism today is a direct reflection of that little boy." ("Before #MeToo, Before Doug Jones, Alyssa Milano's Activism Started with a Kiss on TV" by Elizabeth Chuck, *NBC News*, December 16, 2017). (pp. 50–52) White's testimony is reprinted in Ryan White and Ann Marie Cunningham's *Ryan White: My Own Story* and also part of the congressional record. (p. 53) Irene Emerson's quote is from Geoff Boucher's "Untimely End to a Turbulent Life: Memorial: Death of Channon Phipps, Who as an HIV-Positive Hemophiliac Fought to Attend Public School, Is Mourned," *Los Angeles Times*, September 14, 1995. (p. 54) The transcript of Reagan's news conference is from the archives at reaganlibrary.gov. (p. 55) Ryan White's quote is from *Ryan White: My Own Story*, cited above. *People* quote from its April 23, 1990, issue; Kramer's quote is from an interview he gave to *Playboy*, September 9, 1993. (pp. 55–56) Reagan's eulogy was titled "We Owe It to Ryan" and can be found in the April 10, 1990, edition of *The Washington Post*. (p. 56) David Robinson's response, titled "He Should Have Spoken Sooner," *Washington Post*, April 13, 1990, reprinted with permission from the author. (p. 57) Excerpts from Alan Daniels, Daniel Warner, and Frances J. Mac Guire all in "Ryan White's Battle Against Ignorance, AIDS," *Los Angeles Times*, April 14, 1990; Jeanne White's quote is shared in "Ryan's Mom to Promote Book," *Deseret News*, April 1, 1991.

**Complications** (p. 61) Tichane is quoted from Benjamin Heim Shepard's *White Nights and Ascending Shadows: An Oral History of the San Francisco AIDS Epidemic* (Cassell, 1997), p. 191. (p. 63) Poem from Thom Gunn's *The Man with Night Sweats: Poems* (Farrar, Straus & Giroux, 1992), reprinted by permission of Farrar, Straus & Giroux. (p. 67) "The valley of death" is from *Poets for Life: Seventy-Six Poets Respond to AIDS*, edited by Michael Klein (Persea Books, 1992), reprinted by permission of HLP. (p. 70) Top Photo: *Bill with His Partner, Jimmy* by Bromberger Hoover Photography. Caption: "Portrait of Bailey-Boushay AIDS inpatient Bill Blackmar (left) embraced by his partner, Jimmy, Seattle, Washington, 1993. Blackmar had twelve 'Burial Bears' (one seen on his lap here), teddy bears [that] will eventually contain his ashes and be given to his family and friends. He said, 'When I'm gone they're still going to have me.' Learning he had full blown AIDS in 1989, he arrived at the Bailey-Boushay House, America's first AIDS hospice, weighing 138 pounds; here he weighed 108 pounds. Speaking about his partner Jimmy, he said, 'I'd never make it through the night without him . . . if it hadn't been for Jimmy I might have died a long time ago. We've been together for five years and I've been sick for three of those years. He takes good care of me.' He died, in Jimmy's arms, in May 1993. Nurse Margot Rosen later recalled it was 'a very gentle death.'" Reprinted by permission of Bromberger Hoover Photography / Getty Images. Middle Photo: *AIDS Patient with Hickman Catheter* by Thomas McGovern. Caption: "AIDS patient lying in bed with Hickman catheter on his chest in 1991 in New York City." Reprinted by permission of Thomas McGovern / Getty Images. Bottom Photo: *Mark's Family During His Last Days* by Bromberger Hoover Photography. Caption: "Bailey-Boushay House AIDS inpatient Mark Gittings (left) is embraced by his mother, June, and brother during the last days of his life, Seattle, Washington, 1993. The thirty-year-old Gittings, fourth of five siblings, had lived with AIDS for seven years. His mother said, 'He is my baby.'" Reprinted by permission of Bromberger Hoover Photography / Getty Images.

**Health Care** (p. 71) This essay first appeared in *Still Here: A Post-Cocktail AIDS Anthology*, edited by Allan Peterkin and Julie Hann (Life Rattle Press, 2008). Reprinted by permission of Dr. Allan Peterkin.

**June 25** (p. 73) This excerpt is drawn from an essay that first appeared in *Life Sentences: Writers, Artists, and AIDS*, edited by Thomas Avena (Mercury House, 1994). Reprinted by permission of the Frances Goldin Literary Agency.

**Timeline 1983–1986: March 1983** (p. 103) Kramer's essay can be found in his book *Reports from the Holocaust: The Making of an AIDS Activist* (St. Martin's Press, 1989), p. 50. You can also see the cover of this issue of the *New York Native* at historyofhiv.org/1983. **May 1983** (p. 104) Wilson is quoted in "Candlelight Memorial" by Carol Ness, *SFGate*, May 13, 1998. **August 1983** (p. 105) Photograph courtesy of AP, reprinted with permission. (pp. 105–7) Transcripts of Callen's, Lyon's, and Ferrara's congressional testimony can be found at historymatters.gmu.edu/d/6894. **September 1983** (p. 107) Quotes from "First-of-a-Kind AIDS Forum for Black Gays Held at Clubhouse" by Lisa M. Keen, *Washington Blade*, September 30, 1983. **September 1984** (pp. 108–9) We are indebted to the article "Enola Gay and the Witchy Origin of the First AIDS Protest" by Marke B. at *48hills*, September 19, 2019, for the quotes and the information about this undersung protest. **October 1984** (p. 111) Breaux's quote (and much more information about this topic) can be found in "The Bathhouse Battle of 1984" by Hank Trout, posted on the San Francisco AIDS Foundation's website December 22, 2021. **March 1985** (p. 111) The article cited here is "This Is How the HIV Test Was Invented" by Merrill Fabry, *Time*, June 27, 2016. **June 1985** (p. 113) Photograph by Jack Davis, reprinted with his permission. Davis was one of the activists at the Enola Gay protest mentioned on pp. 109–10, and we are grateful to him for documenting so much HIV/AIDS history with his camera. **November 1985** (p. 114) White's quote is from "A Shattering AIDS TV Movie Mirrors a Family's Pain" by Jane Hall, *People*, November 18, 1985. (p. 115) Cowan's and Lipman's quotes are from the *People* magazine article cited above. **November 1985** (p. 115) The quote from the doctor appears in "Rev. Stephen Pieters, Interviewed by Tammy Faye Bakker About AIDS, Dies" by Brian Bromberger, *Bay Area Reporter*, July 26, 2023. (pp. 115–16) Quotes from the interview are from the video embedded at nbcnews.com/nbc-out/out-pop-culture/televangelist-tammy-faye-bakker-became-unlikely-ally-aids-crisis-rcna2059. (p. 116) Pieters's final quote is from the *Bay Area Reporter* obituary cited above. **December 1985** (p. 117) Boan's quote is from "Minority Gays Find Strength in Unity" by Ginger Thompson, *Los Angeles Times*, April 30, 1989. **March 1986** (p. 117) Buckley's op-ed piece is "Crucial Steps in Combating the AIDS Epidemic; Identify All the Carriers," *New York Times*, March 18, 1986. Buchanan's quote is from "Patrick Buchanan: In His Own Words, the Presidential Hopeful's Writings and Comments Shed Light on His Claims That Mainstream Media Have Distorted His Views," *Baltimore Sun*, October 3, 1999. Falwell's quote is cited in "The Legacy of Falwell's Bully Pulpit" by Hans Johnson and William Eskridge, *Washington Post*, May 19, 2007. Robertson's quote is in "Pat Robertson Defends His Warning of Gay AIDS Handshake Ring" by

Abby Ohlheiser, *Atlantic*, August 27, 2013. (p. 118) Helms is quoted in "AIDS Booklet Stirs Senate to Halt Funds," *Los Angeles Times*, October 14, 1987. Photo *ACT UP Protest at FDA* by Catherine McGann. Caption: "ROCKVILLE – OCTOBER 11: Members of AIDS activist group ACT UP (AIDS Coalition to Unleash Power) hold up signs of George [H.W.] Bush, Ronald Reagan, Nancy Reagan, Jesse Helms and others with the word 'Guilty' stamped on their foreheads, along with a banner stating 'Silence Equals Death' at a protest at the headquarters of the Food and Drug Administration (FDA) on October 11, 1988 in Rockville, Maryland. The action, called SEIZE CONTROL OF THE FDA by the group, shut down the FDA for the day." Reprinted by permission of Catherine McGann / Getty Images. **October 1986** (pp. 118–19) All figures are from cdc.gov. (p. 119) Harris's actions are described in "The Invisible Man: Distribution of Blame for the Spread of HIV in African American Communities" by Debby Cheng, *Tortoise*, Spring 2020. **October 1986** (p. 120) The "dogmatic Christian" quote is from "Putting Public Health First," *Boston Globe*, March 1, 2013. The "if there ever were" quote is from Koop's article "The Early Days of AIDS, As I Remember Them" in the March 29, 2011, issue of *Annals of the Forum for Collaborative HIV Research*. (p. 121) Levi's quote is from "Doctor, Not Chaplain: How a Deeply Religious Surgeon General Taught a Nation About HIV" by John-Manuel Andriote, *Atlantic*, March 4, 2013. A full version of Koop's "Understanding AIDS" report can be seen at https://digital.library.unt.edu/ark:/67531/metadc1584361. Schlafly's criticism and Koop's response to it can be found in "Koop's Crusade: The Surgeon General Made Public Health a Divine Commandment" by Anthony Petro, *Slate*, February 27, 2013. Koop's conversation with Maureen Dowd can be found in her column "Washington Talk: The Surgeon General; Dr. Koop Defends His Crusade on AIDS," *New York Times*, April 6, 1987. Figures for the pamphlet's distribution come from "As AIDS Epidemic Raged, a Rogue Reagan Official Taught America the Truth" by Alexandra M. Lord, *Washington Post*, June 8, 2023. (p. 122) Information on follow-up surveys is also from Lord's article. Koop's "my whole career" quote is from the *Annals* piece cited above. The colleague quoted at the end is Peter I. Hartsock from his letter to the editor, "C. Everett Koop, a public servant above politics," *Washington Post*, February 27, 2013.

**Young People Schoolin' Other Young People** (p. 124) Image of ephemera created by the AIDS and Adolescents Network of New York, Education Task Force, 1991–1993. From the AIDS and Adolescents Network of New York Records, 1987–1999, at the New York Public Library, Manuscripts and Archives Division, Box 11, folder 9. Reprinted with permission. (p. 126) Spreads from *YELL* Zine #1, used with permission from ACT UP. (p. 127) Spread from *YELL* Zine #2, used with permission from ACT UP. The second issue of *YELL* led with the tagline "Students Are Dying for Sex Ed" and even contained information to help readers arrange their own demonstrations in their schools. (p. 128) Cover of *New Youth Connections*, December 1987 issue, from the AIDS and Adolescents Network of New York Records, 1987–1999, at the New York Public Library, Manuscripts and Archives Division, Box 54, folder 8–9. Reprinted with permission. (p. 129) "The Twelve Days of Christmas" ephemera created by Youth Agenda. From the AIDS and Adolescents Network of New York Records, 1987–1999, at the New York Public Library, Manuscripts and Archives

Division, Box 33, folder 3–5. (p. 130) Sweeney is quoted in "Rap Star Eazy-E Says He Has AIDS" by Lisa Respers, *Los Angeles Times*, March 17, 1995. (p. 131) Teen rap from San Francisco AIDS Foundation Records, MSS 94–60, box 19, folder 53. (p. 132) Howard Cruse, *Safe Sex* first generation copies with screen, 1983. Howard Cruse Papers, 1941–2019. Columbia University Libraries. Box 27, folder 6. Reprinted with permission of International Literary Properties LLC. (pp. 133–34) Pages from *YELL's The Foster Kid's Guide to HIV Testing!* zine reprinted courtesy of ACT UP. (p. 135) Willmore quote from "TikTok Creator Zack Willmore Is Vlogging His Life Living with HIV" by Uwa Ede-Osifo, *NBC News*, March 13, 2023.

**How to Have Sex in an Epidemic and the Denver Principles** (pp. 136–37) Quotes from *How to Have Sex in an Epidemic: One Approach* by Richard Berkowitz and Michael Callen, News from the Front Publications, 1983, Tower Press, pp. 3–4, p. 40. (p. 138) We are grateful to Richard Berkowitz for sending us this personal photo from Denver and giving us permission to use it. The Denver Principles statement is from "The Denver Principles: 40 years on," *UNAIDS*, June 26, 2023. (p. 140) Image from the Library of Congress, Prints & Photographs Division, *U.S. News and World Report* Magazine Collection, by John T. Bledsoe. Caption: "Marchers, some holding banners reading 'Fighting for our lives' and 'NY AIDS Network' during a gay rights march dedicated to the victims of AIDS, New York City, June 26, 1983." Used with permission of the Library of Congress.

**How to ACT UP When SILENCE=DEATH** (p. 142) Cylar quote is taken from his obituary in *Gay City News*, "Keith Cylar Is Dead at 45" by Paul Schindler, April 14, 2004. (p. 143) Larry Kramer quotes are taken from his essay "The Beginning of ACTing UP," which is reprinted in *Reports from the Holocaust* cited above. (pp. 143–44) Avram Finkelstein is quoted from his contribution to the ACT UP Oral History Project, 108. Repeated thanks to the OHP for allowing us to quote freely from their incredible work. (p. 144) Kramer's "At the rate" quote is cited in Masha Gessen's "Larry Kramer Had the Courage to Act on His Fear," *New Yorker*, May 28, 2020. (p. 145) Kramer's "Do we want to start" is quoted in "ACT UP" by Craig Rimmerman, *The Body*, January 1, 1998. (p. 146) AZT protest quotes are from "AIDS Drug's Prices to be Cut 20%" by Michael Specter, *Washington Post*, December 14, 1987. (p. 147) Kramer is again quoted here from "The Beginning of ACTing UP," cited above. AZT protest quotes taken from *Washington Post*, cited above. (pp. 149–50) Robinson quotes are taken from the essay "Allan Robinson, AIDS Activist" by B. Michael Hunter in *Sojourner: Black Gay Voices in the Age of AIDS*, Other Countries Press, 1993. Reprinted with permission. (p. 151) Emily Nahmanson's testimony is interview 023 in the ACT UP Oral History Project. (p. 152) Footage of ACT UP protests can be found here: actuporalhistory.org/actions. The "NO MORE BUSINESS AS USUAL!" ACT UP flyer is found here: actupny.org/documents/1stFlyer.html. Reprinted with permission from ACT UP. (p. 154) Top Photo: *ACT UP Protest at FDA* by Catherine McGann. Caption: "ROCKVILLE – OCTOBER 11: AIDS activist group ACT UP protest at the headquarters of the Food and Drug Administration on October 11, 1988 in Rockville, Maryland. The action, called SEIZE CONTROL OF THE FDA by the group, shut down the FDA for the day." Used with permission from Catherine

McGann / Getty Images. Bottom Photo: *AIDS Protestor Being Arrested* by Thomas McGovern. Caption: "AIDS protestor wearing an ACT UP T-shirt being arrested by police in 1989 at the New York City Department of Social Services in New York City." Used with permission from Thomas McGovern / Getty Images. (p. 155) Top Photo: *AIDS Activists Stage Die-In* by Thomas McGovern. Caption: "AIDS activists stage a die-in at Grand Central Station in 1991 in New York." Used with permission from Thomas McGovern / Getty Images. Bottom Photo: *ACT UP Demonstrators Protest and Take Over the FDA Headquarters* by Peter Ansin. Caption: "ROCKVILLE, MD – OCTOBER, 1988: ACT UP protesters close the Federal Drug Administration building to demand the release of experimental medication for those living with HIV/AIDS. Their slogans read: 'Never Had a Chance'; 'Dead from Lack of Aerosol Pentamadine'; 'I Got the Placebo'; 'I Died for the Sins of the FDA.' The demonstration was held outside the FDA headquarters in Rockville, Maryland on October 11, 1988." Used with permission of Peter Ansin / Getty Images.

**Peggy Sue** (p. 165) Photo by Rick Gerharter from the June 21, 1990, issue of the *Bay Area Reporter*. Reprinted with blanket permission from the *Bay Area Reporter* through their partnership with the GLBT Archive.

**"STOP THE CHURCH"** (p. 171) Protest chants and speeches are transcribed from the ACT UP Oral History Project archive of video documentation, available here: actuporalhistory.org/actions. (p. 172) "STOP THE CHURCH" from the ACT UP Oral History Project, reprinted with permission. (p. 173) The first two O'Connor quotes are from *After the Wrath of God: AIDS, Sexuality, & American Religion* by Anthony M. Petro, Oxford University Press, 2015, pp. 123 and 91; the third is from "Here Is the Church: Scenes from the Documentary PBS Yanked" by Kim Masters, *Washington Post*, August 13, 1991; the fourth is from "What Are We Doing to the Young?" by Cardinal O'Connor, *Celebrate Life*, March–April 1994. (pp. 174–75) Navarro's quotes are from the ACT UP Oral History Project footage at actuporalhistory.org/actions/stop-the-church. (p. 176) The first Nahmanson quote ("After all . . .") is taken from *Let the Record Show: A Political History of ACT UP New York, 1987–1993* by Sarah Schulman; Farrar, Straus & Giroux, 2021, p. 149. (pp. 176–80) Testimonies here are taken from the ACT UP Oral History Project: Emily Nahmanson's testimony is interview 023, Michael Petrelis's is 020, Tom Keane's is 176, Ann Northrop's is 027. (p. 181) Ann Northrop is quoted here from "Here's the Story Behind the St. Patrick's Cathedral Action Depicted in 'Pose'" by Mathew Rodriguez, *Body*, June 12, 2019. Additional quotes from inside St. Patrick's Cathedral are taken from Petro's *After the Wrath of God* cited above, p. 150. (p. 182) The final quote of the chapter is from "Rude, Rash, Effective, Act-Up Shifts AIDS Policy" by Jason Deparle, *New York Times*, January 3, 1990.

**Fighting Words: Larry Kramer vs. Anthony Fauci** (p. 189) Kramer quote ("I discovered") from "Remembering Larry Kramer Through His Most Powerful Words" by Belle Hutton, *AnOther Magazine*, May 28, 2020. Used with permission. Fauci is quoted ("My entire existence") from "Exclusive: Anthony Fauci on the Aids Crisis, Monkeypox, Trans Rights and His Retirement" by Io Dodds, *Independent*, June 16, 2022.

(pp. 189–90) Kramer's "An Open Letter to Fauci" (*The Village Voice*, May 31, 1988) can be found here: villagevoice.com/an-open-letter-to-dr-anthony-fauci. (p. 193) Fauci quote ("I was a little bit shocked") from "Dr. Anthony Fauci on His 'Dear, Deep Friendship' with Larry Kramer," interview by Brett Lang, *Variety*, May 28, 2020. Peter Staley quote from his opinion piece in *The New York Times*, "Anthony Fauci Quietly Shocked Us All," December 31, 2022. Fauci quote ("I was pushing") from "Three Decades Before Coronavirus, Anthony Fauci Took Heat from AIDS Protesters" by Diane Bernard, *Washington Post*, May 20, 2020. (p. 194) Staley's story about Fauci asking him if he's all right is from his *New York Times* piece cited above; the *Washington Post* coverage is from "1,000 Rally for More Vigorous AIDS Effort: 82 Arrested at NIH in Demonstration to Support Additional Research, Expanded Testing" by Veronica T. Jennings and Malcolm Gladwell, May 21, 1990. Fauci's quote about protesters is from an interview with the American Association for the Advancement of Science: "Anthony Fauci: A View from the Maelstrom of HIV/AIDS Research Policy," by Bob Roehr, May 16, 2011. (p. 195) Kramer is quoted from a PBS interview; the full interview can be found here: pbs.org/wgbh/pages/frontline/aids/interviews/kramer.html. Fauci's "like two generals" quote is from "Looking Back at Dr. Fauci's Enduring Bond with AIDS Activist Larry Kramer—and Their Final Phone Call" by Adam Carlson, *People*, June 2, 2020. (p. 196) Kramer's "Actually it was his idea" quote is from the PBS interview cited above. Fauci's recollections of Kramer (including the two quotes on this page) can be found in "'We Loved Each Other': Fauci Recalls Larry Kramer, Friend and Nemesis" by Donald G. McNeil Jr., *New York Times*, May 27, 2020. Kramer's response ("I concede") and Fauci's "He wants to kill me more than I want to kill him" are documented in Jacob Bernstein's "Larry Kramer Revives 'A Normal Heart,'" *Daily Beast*, April 27, 2011. (p. 197) The "blood on his hands" quote is cited in "AIDS Epidemic Veterans Recall 'Long and Complex History' of Dr. Tony Fauci" by Rob Phelps, *Boston Spirit*, April 4, 2020. Kramer's "Tony, more than anyone in the world" quote comes from Adam Carlson's *People* article, cited above. Fauci's recollection ("All of a sudden") is from "He Was a 'Force of Nature': Anthony Fauci, Tom Frieden, and Others Remember Larry Kramer" by Patrick Skerrett, *STAT News*, May 28, 2020, reprinted with permission from *STAT News*. Kramer's quote about Fauci as the "consummate manipulative bureaucrat" and Fauci's response are from Carlson's *People* article cited above. (p. 198) Fauci's full appreciation of Kramer, "Anthony Fauci on Larry Kramer and Loving Difficult People," *New York Times*, July 4, 2023, can be found here: nytimes.com/2023/07/04/opinion/anthony-fauci-larry-kramer.html. (pp. 198–99) His "It's hard to fine-tunedly" is quoted from the Io Dodds interview in the *Independent*, cited above. (p. 199) The Peter Staley quote is from his *New York Times* piece cited above. The Michael Specter quote is from his article "Larry Kramer, Public Nuisance," *New Yorker*, May 5, 2002, quoted with permission of the author. Kramer's "being gay" quote is from the *AnOther Magazine* interview cited above. (p. 200) Fauci's "brothers in arms" quote is from his *New York Times* article cited above.

**Addressing the Need: Needle Exchange and HIV/AIDS** (p. 203) CDC and other figures are from naco.org, "The Benefits and Challenges of Needle Exchange Programs," February 20, 2019. "Research over the past" quote from "Syringe Services Programs'

Role in Ending the HIV Epidemic in the U.S.: Why We Cannot Do It Without Them" by Dita Broz et al., *American Journal of Preventive Medicine*, November 2021. (p. 204) "The Johnny Appleseed of needles" is from Bruce Lambert's *New York Times* article "AIDS Battler Gives Needles Illicitly to Addicts," November 20, 1989. The *Chicago Tribune* quote is from "AIDS Guerrilla," May 7, 1989. Parker and Judge Kelly are quoted in Lambert's *New York Times* article. (p. 205) Statistics on Prevention Point are from sfaf.org/resource-library/needle-exchange-in-san-francisco. "The worst drug-fueled outbreak ever to hit rural America" is from "5 Years After Indiana's Historic HIV Outbreak, Many Rural Places Remain at Risk" by Laura Unger, NPR, February 16, 2020, which also features Pence's quote. (p. 206) The March 2021 NPR piece quoted is "Indiana Needle Exchange That Helped Contain a Historic HIV Outbreak to Be Shut Down" from *Morning Edition* by Mitch Legan. Julian's quote is also found in Legan's NPR piece. CDC estimates cited are from "With Overdoses Rising, a Push for Syringe Service Programs" by Sandhya Raman, *Roll Call*, September 21, 2022.

**HIV Is Not a Deadly Weapon** (p. 223) Jackson is quoted in *People*'s cover story about twenty-four hours in the AIDS crisis, August 3, 1987. Helms's quote can be found in "Helms Calls for AIDS Quarantine on Positive Tests," *Chicago Tribune*, June 16, 1987. Edwards's quote can be found in the June 26, 1987, issue of the New Orleans *Times-Picayune*. (p. 224) Gary Clements's quote is from the same issue as Edwards's. When this book was completed, CDC figures on HIV criminalization could be found at cdc.gov/hiv/policies/law/states/exposure. As of our final proofread of these notes in November 2025, the page is not available, and the cdc.gov/hiv site has a banner that reads "CDC's website is being modified to comply with President Trump's Executive Orders." (p. 226) Suttle's interview with AIDSVu is titled "Robert Suttle on HIV Decriminalization Advocacy," posted on May 10, 2021, quoted with permission of both AIDSVu and Suttle. We are grateful to the Williams Institute at the UCLA School of Law for their studies on HIV criminalization, the source of our data here. More information can be found at williamsinstitute.law.ucla.edu/issues/hiv-criminalization.

**Timeline: 1987–1991: May 1987** (p. 230) Obama is quoted in "Obama Lifts a Ban on U.S. Entry of HIV-Positive Foreigners" by Frank James at NPR, October 30, 2009. **October 1987** (p. 230) Helms is quoted in "AIDS Booklet Stirs Senate to Halt Funds," *Los Angeles Times*, October 14, 1987. The cited amendment can be found here: congress.gov/amendment/100th-congress/senate-amendment/963%20%20. Kennedy is quoted in "Senator Helms's Callousness Toward AIDS Victims" by Edward I. Koch, *New York Times*, November 7, 1987. (p. 231) Weicker is quoted in "The Senate, Stirred by a Comic Book Showing Safe . . . ," UPI, October 14, 1987. **November 1987** (p. 231) Fraser-Howze is quoted in "Interview: Debra Fraser-Howze" on the nycaidsmemorial.org website. **November 1987** (p. 232) David M. Smith is quoted in "Randy Shilts, Chronicler of AIDS Epidemic, Dies at 42: Journalism: Author of 'And the Band Played On' Is Credited with Awakening Nation to the Health Crisis," *Los Angeles Times*, February 18, 1994. Randy Shilts is quoted in "Randy Shilts, Author, Dies at 42; One of First to Write About AIDS" by William Grimes, *New York Times*, February 18, 1994. **February 1989** (p. 233) The description of Diana's time at the hospital is from "Princess Di Visits Infant AIDS Victims in Harlem," *Jet*, February 20, 1989. **November 1989** (pp. 235–38) The testimonies of the Anger into Direct Action collective are from a public hearing published in the *Yale Journal of Law and Liberation* as "AIDS and Homelessness: Personal Accounts." **July 1990** (p. 239) Examples of ADA protections of PLWHA are taken from "Questions and Answers: The Americans with Disabilities Act and the Rights of Persons with HIV/AIDS to Obtain Occupational Training and State Licensing," a fact sheet created by the US Department of Justice, Civil Rights Division (2009). It can be accessed here: hivlawandpolicy.org/resources/questions-and-answers-americans-disabilities-act-and-rights-persons-hivaids-obtain. **September 1991** (p. 242) The quote from Peter Staley is from his article "In Memory of Jesse Helms, and the Condom on His House," *Poz*, July 8, 2008, poz.com/blog/in-memory-of-je. All *Poz* quotes in this piece reprinted with permission from the magazine/website, which is an essential resource for stories about living with HIV/AIDS.

**As the World Watched: Rock Hudson and Magic Johnson** (p. 246) Quote from the press conference appears in Jonathan Fergenzer's report for UPI, "Actor Rock Hudson, Whose Emaciated Look Shocked the Public . . ." from July 25, 1985. (p. 247) Rivers's comment was made in "Rock Hudson: On Camera and Off" by Jeff Yarbrough, *People*, August 12, 1985. Kearns was quoted in Scott Haller's "Fighting for Life," *People*, September 23, 1985. (p. 247–48) Liz Taylor's quote is from "Liz's AIDS Odyssey" by Nancy Collins, *Vanity Fair*, November 1992. (p. 248) Johnson's statement can be found in many sources, including "Basketball: Magic Johnson Ends His Career Saying He Has AIDS Infection" by Richard W. Stevenson, *New York Times*, November 8, 1991. (p. 249) AP quote from "Day After Magic's Disclosure, People Talk, Reflect and Cry," Associated Press, November 10, 1991. Lakers fan quote is from Stevenson's *New York Times* article cited above. Fauci's quote is from "Magic Johnson's HIV Disclosure Helped to Shatter Stigmas. But 30 Years Later, Disparities in Treatment Remain" by Francine Uenuma, *Time*, November 4, 2021. (p. 250) Johnson's resignation was reported in many places, including "Johnson Slams Bush on AIDS: Basketball Superstar Quits Panel, Criticizes 'Lip Service' Policy" by Mary Jordon, *Washington Post*, September 25, 1992. (pp. 250–51) Video of Broadbent and Johnson can be seen here: youtube.com/watch?v=fcBSXE9FkC8.

**A Little Magic and a Lot of Faith** (pp. 252–55) This essay is reprinted from *Fingernails Across the Chalkboard: Poetry and Prose on HIV/AIDS from the Black Diaspora*, edited by Randall Horton et al. (Third World Press, 2007). Reprinted with the permission of the Third World Press Foundation.

**Pedro Zamora and the New Reality** (p. 257) Zamora's congressional testimony is cited on the National AIDS Memorial website and can be found on YouTube. (p. 258) The *Entertainment Tonight* quote can be found in the article "How *The Real World* Star Pedro Zamora Humanized AIDS (Flashback)" by Stacy Lambe, *ETonline*, June 21, 2018. (p. 259) Zamora quote is from "Pedro Leaves Us Breathless" by Hal Rubenstein, *Poz*, August 1, 1994. (p. 260) Clinton's quote is from "Revisiting 'The Real World' and Remembering Pedro Zamora" by Renée Graham, *Boston Globe*, September 10, 2023. Zamora's first quote is found in many sources, including "Pedro

Zamora" by Oriol R. Gutierrez Jr., *Poz*, October 31, 2011. Chiles is quoted in "Life of 22 Years Ends, but Not Before Many Heard Message on AIDS" by Mireya Navarro, *New York Times*, November 12, 1994. (pp. 260–61) Zamora's second and third quotes are from "Pedro Leaves Us Breathless," cited above. (p. 261) "His one wild and precious life" is a reference to the Mary Oliver poem "The Summer Day." It asks:

> *Doesn't everything die at last, and too soon?*
> *Tell me, what is it you plan to do*
> *With your one wild and precious life?*

We reprint them here with permission from the Mary Oliver Estate. The full poem appears in Mary Oliver's *New and Selected Poems* (Beacon Press, 1992).

**What We Lost** (p. 263) Taylor's words come from his essay "Prodigal Son" in *Loss Within Loss: Artists in the Age of AIDS*, edited by Edmund White (University of Wisconsin Press, 2001). Digital versions of the *Entertainment Weekly* tributes can be found in the archives on their website, although this may not have the same effect as opening up the magazine and seeing face after face, name after name. The tribute from 1994, for example, can be found here: ew.com/article/1994/12/02/faces-aids-1994. (p. 265) The *New Yorker* piece is from the "Goings On About Town" section, December 3, 1990. Reprinted with permission from *The New Yorker*. Carroll's "It was strange timing" quote comes from his interview "Carrolling on Broadway" with Michael Buckley in *Theater Week*, December 16–19, 1990. Michael Jeter is quoted from "Michael Jeter Takes on Hollywood" by Peter Kurth, *Poz*, January 1, 1998. (p. 266) We won't put the links here, but if you search "David Carroll" on YouTube, you too can find these clips.

**Deaths in the Neighborhood** (pp. 268–75) We are deeply indebted to the *Bay Area Reporter* and the GLBT Historical Society for the permission to reprint these obituaries, which come from the January 4, 1990, January 11, 1990, January 18, 1990, and January 25, 1990, issues of the paper. We discovered them through the GLBT Historical Society's invaluable online searchable obituary database, which can be found here: obit.glbthistory.org/olo/index.jsp.

**Blood Sisters** (p. 286) Barbara Vick is quoted in "The Blood Sisters: The Unsung Heroes of the AIDS Crisis" by Amy Chappel, *Diva*, February 8, 2024. (p. 287) Wendy Sue Biegeleisen's quote is from her interview with Steve Wroblewski for the Lambda Archives of San Diego, February 8, 2016. Peggy Heathers is quoted in "The Blood Sisters of San Diego," Women's Museum of California, April 10, 2019. The gay man who said, "Suddenly, the hospitals" and Barbara Vick are quoted in "The Lesbian 'Blood Sisters' Who Cared for Gay Men When Doctors Were Too Scared To" by Kate Lister, *I Paper*, December 13, 2018. (pp. 287–88) Both quotes about what happened in Garden Grove are from "Fear of AIDS Leads Red Cross to Cancel Lesbian Blood Drive" by Kristina Lindgren, *Los Angeles Times*, January 9, 1985.

**Parachute** (pp. 295–98) This poem appeared in Michael Klein and Richard McCann's anthology *Things Shaped in Passing: More "Poets for Life" Writing from the AIDS Pandemic* (Persea Books, 1997). Reprinted with permission from the Estate of Tim Dlugos.

**Tiara** (pp. 301–3) It was very, very hard to choose just one Mark Doty piece for this book, since his poetry and memoir have been such deeply affecting parts of our own education about life during the AIDS epidemic. This poem appears, among other places, in Doty's collection *Fire to Fire: New and Selected Poems* (Harper Perennial, 2008), and is reprinted by permission of HarperCollins.

**What the Living Do** (pp. 304–5) *A note from Gabriel:* In 2020, I attended a conference at the University of Manchester in England: "HIV/AIDS in the Twenty-First Century: Memorialisation, Representation and Temporality," organized by José Saleiro Gomes, Louisa Hann, and Stian Kristensen. Stuart Crowther led an incredibly moving workshop based around a performance of this poem, and the poem has stayed with me ever since. The poem is taken from Howe's collection *What the Living Do* (W. W. Norton & Co, 1998) and is reprinted with permission from W. W. Norton & Co.

**Letter to Roger** (pp. 317–19) This piece first appeared in *Brother to Brother: New Writings by Black Gay Men*, edited by Essex Hemphill (Alyson Books, 1991). It is reprinted with permission from the author.

**Thousands of Angels** (pp. 324–25) This poem first appeared in *Fingernails Across the Chalkboard: Poetry and Prose on HIV/AIDS from the Black Diaspora*, cited above. Reprinted with the permission of the Third World Press Foundation.

**The Names** (p. 326) Photo by Carol M. Highsmith. (p. 328) This grandmother's quote and many of the vignettes mentioned in this chapter come from the book *The Quilt: Stories from the NAMES Project*, by Cindy Ruskin, photographs by Matt Herron (Pocket, 1988). (p. 329) We are indebted to the NAMES Project for the permission to reproduce panels from the Quilt on the following pages, and urge readers to find out more at aidsmemorial.org. (pp. 330–41) We are grateful beyond words to Brian Selznick for creating these illustrations for this book. They are © 2026 by Brian Selznick, printed with permission.

**Aunt Ida pieces a quilt** (pp. 342–45) This poem first appeared in *Brother to Brother: New Writings by Black Gay Men*, cited above.. It is reprinted with permission from the Estate of Melvin Dixon, courtesy of Faith Childs Literary Agency, Inc.

**Refuge in Their Final Days** (p. 346) Angelo's full story can be found in "For Homeless with AIDS, a New Home" by David W. Dunlap, *New York Times*, January 5, 1987. (p. 347) Burks is quoted from "Meet the Woman Who Cared for Hundreds of Abandoned Gay Men Dying of AIDS" by Katherine, on the Mighty Girl website, December 1, 2021. There continues to be uncertainty as to how many men Burks took in, but there is no doubt that she gave refuge to *some* men who had nowhere else to go. Wineland is quoted from NPR's *Morning Edition* on December 5, 2014, in a segment titled "Caring for AIDS Patients, 'When No One Else Would.'" (p. 348) Desrosiers and Rivera are quoted in "New Orleans Priest Founded First Catholic AIDS Hospice" by Peter Finney Jr., *Catholic News Service*, May 3, 2019. (p. 349) Final quote is from "Clara Hale: 'Tell Them How Great They Are'" by Derrick Lane, on the BlackDoctor website, July 5, 2017. It's important to note that the few "refuges" highlighted here are only a small representation of the number of organizations and individuals who stepped up and stepped in to care for people with HIV/AIDS when the federal government wouldn't. Most communities had people who were willing to open doors when others closed; because of space considerations we could feature only a few of them.

**Timeline: 1992–1996: July and August 1992** (pp. 350–51) Hattoy's full speech is posted at towleroad.com/2007/03/bob_hattoys_spe. (pp. 351–53) Glaser's speech can be found at awpc.cattcenter.iastate.edu/2017/03/21/address-at-the-1992-dnc-july-14-1992. To learn more about her, we suggest her memoir, *In the Absence of Angels: A Hollywood Family's Courageous Story* (Penguin, 1991). (pp. 353–57) Fisher's speech can be found at americanrhetoric.com/speeches/maryfisher1992rnc.html, and more can be read in her memoir, *My Name Is Mary: A Memoir* (Scribner, 1995). **January 1993** (p. 358) The 1993 Revised Classification System for HIV Infection and Expanded Surveillance Case Definition for AIDS among Adolescents and Adults can be found here: cdc.gov/mmwr/preview/mmwrhtml/00018871.htm. **May 1993** (p. 359) Kushner's play has become many students' gateway into learning about the AIDS epidemic; besides the print version of the text, the HBO adaptation (directed by Mike Nichols) also makes this work accessible to a wide audience. **June 1993** (p. 360) Johnson's words are reported, among other places, in "Judge Orders the Release of Haitians" by Mary B. W. Tabor, *New York Times*, June 9, 1993. Johnson's description of conditions in Guantanamo are cited in "Detention of HIV-Positive Haitians at Guantanamo—Human Rights and Medical Care" by George J. Annas, *New England Journal of Medicine*, August 19, 1993. (p. 361) Quote from "Judge Orders All Haitians Freed from U.S. Camp" by Mike Clary, *Los Angeles Times*, June 9, 1993. **February 1995** (p. 362) Louganis is quoted from a July 19, 2007, interview he did with *LAYouth*. **December 1996** (p. 364) Quotes from "Turning the Tide" by Philip Elmer-DeWitt, *Time*, December 30, 1996.

**Non, Je Ne Regrette Rien** (pp. 372–74) This poem first appeared in the book *Here to Dare: 10 Gay Black Poets*, edited by Assotto Saint and published by Galiens Press. It is reprinted with permission from the estate of the author.

**Litany** (pp. 375–78) This piece first appeared in *From a Burning House: The AIDS Project Los Angeles Writers Workshop Collection*, edited by Irene Borger (Washington Square Press, 1996). It is reprinted with permission from Gallery Books, a division of Simon & Schuster.

**Timeline: 1997–Present: 1997** (p. 379) Clinton quoted in "Commencement Address at Morgan State University in Baltimore, Maryland," which can be found at presidency.ucsb.edu/documents/commencement-address-morgan-state-university-baltimore-maryland. **1998** (p. 380) Census information is from census.gov/library/publications/1998/demo/p20-508.html. Sulser is quoted from "Money for Hemophiliacs Tied Up in Congress," *CBS News*, January 31, 2002. **1999** (pp. 380–81) Statistics on young people and HIV/AIDS are taken from "Listen, Learn, Live! World AIDS Campaign with Children and Young People," produced by the Joint United Nations Programme on HIV/AIDS (UNAIDS), February 1999. **2002** (p. 381) Figures on HIV/AIDS were taken from "HIV Testing in the United States, 2002" in the CDC's *Advance Data*, no. 363, November 8, 2005. **2003** (pp. 381–82) Bush quoted in "President Delivers 'State of the Union'" in the George W. Bush White House Archives, January 28, 2003. 2023 statistics taken from "Bush Demanded Billions for AIDS in Africa at His 2003 State of the Union. It Paid Off" by Benjamin Ryan, *NBC News*, February 7, 2023. (p. 382) El-Sadr quoted in "George W. Bush's Anti-HIV Program Is Hailed as 'Amazing'— and Still Crucial at 20" by Melody Schreiber, NPR, February 28, 2023. **2007** (p. 384) Brown quoted in "I Am the Berlin Patient: A Personal Reflection," Timothy Ray Brown, in the NIH's National Library of Medicine publication *AIDS Research and Human Retroviruses*, vol. 31, no. 1, January 1, 2015. **2008** (pp. 385–86) "The Swiss Statement" is quoted by *HIV i-Base* at i-base.info/qa/factsheets/the-swiss-statement. **2009** (p. 386) Pelosi is quoted from "Pelosi: Lifting the Ban on Federal Funding for Syringe Exchange Is a Victory for Science and for Public Health," press release December 10, 2009. **2010** (p. 387) Obama is quoted from "National HIV/AIDS Strategy for the United States—July 2010" in the Obama White House Archives. **2012** (p. 387) This survey, "2012 Survey of Americans on HIV/AIDS," was produced by *The Washington Post* and the Kaiser Family Foundation. (p. 388) Loduca is quoted in "FDA Approves Truvada as HIV Preventive" by Victoria Colliver, *SFGate*, July 17, 2012. **2015** (p. 388) Fauci is quoted in "START Trial Finds that Early Treatment Improves Outcomes for People with HIV" by Gus Cairns, *aidsmap*, May 27, 2015. **2017** (p. 388) CDC quotes are from "Those with Undetectable HIV at 'Effectively No Risk' of Transmitting Virus, CDC Says" by Brooke Sopelsa, *NBC News*, September 29, 2017. **2023** (p. 390) In September 2025, this quote from the CDC was up on hiv.gov/hiv-basics/overview/data-and-trends/statistics. The same statistics (still no update since 2022) are up in November 2025, but the heading has been changed from "HIV Surveillance Report" to "US Statistics." **2025** (p. 391) CDC quote is from "National HIV Prevention and Care Objectives: 2025 Update," June 5, 2025, cdc.gov/hiv-data/nhss/national-hiv-prevention-and-care-objectives-2025.html. Headlines in italics are based on "Radical Changes in US Policy Threaten Two Decades' Progress in HIV" by Keith Alcorn, *aidsmap*, March 12, 2025; "Trump's PEPFAR Cuts Upend the Lives of Kenyan Families Battling HIV," *Washington Post*, April 5, 2025; "Withdrawal of HIV Funding Hits Hard in the South" by Heidi Splete, *Medscape*, May 14, 2025; "Risk of 2,000 New HIV Infections a Day After US Aid Freeze, UN says," Reuters, March 24, 2025; "'A Bloodbath': HIV Field Is Reeling After Billions in U.S. Funding Are Axed as USAID's Promises to Support Lifesaving Efforts Are Broken, Putting Millions in Peril" by Ifeoluwa Akinola, *Nigerian Concord News*, March 3, 2025; "US Shutdown of HIV/AIDS Funding 'Could Lead to 500,000 Deaths in South Africa'" by Kat Lay, *Guardian*, February 28, 2025; "'It's Back to Drug Rationing': The End of HIV Was in Sight. Then Came the Cuts" by Kat Lay, *Guardian*, March 18, 2025. (pp. 392–93) Warren is quoted in "Regulators Approve a Twice-Yearly Shot to Prevent H.I.V. Infection" by Apoorva Mandavilli, *New York Times*, June 18, 2025. AIDS activist chants are quoted from "Fired USAid Workers and HIV Activists Hold 'Die-In' to Protest Trump and Musk" by Chris Stein, *Guardian*, February 26, 2025.

**Remembrance** (p. 426) This essay first appeared in *Brother to Brother*, cited above. It is reprinted with permission from the author.

**Happy Anniversary** (pp. 427–28) This essay first appeared in B. Michael Hunter's *Sojourner*, cited above. Reprinted by permission of the author.

**Little Prayer** (p. 429) This poem was first published in Smith's collection *Don't Call Us Dead* (Graywolf Press, 2017). It is reprinted with permission from Graywolf Press.

**Excerpt from Committing to Memory** (pp. 430–31) This poem can be found in Monette's *West of Yesterday, East of Summer: New and Selected Poems* (St. Martin's Press, 1994). Reprinted by permission of both the author's estate and Open Road Integrated Media.

**Excerpt from The Tomb of Sorrow** (pp. 432–33) This poem appeared in, among other collections, *Brother to Brother*, cited above. It is reprinted with permission from New Directions Press, which published *Love Is a Dangerous Word: The Selected Poems of Essex Hemphill* (New Directions, 2025), which also includes the poem.

# Bibliography

The following is a list of books that directly or indirectly informed the creation of this book. We have limited ourselves to works of nonfiction and poetry here. A much longer list would include works of fiction, movies, and TV shows that have inspired and informed us over the years. For citations of magazines, websites, and other nonbook sources, as well as for direct citations of quotations from some of the works below, please see the Notes and Sources section. We do, however, want to highlight two invaluable resources for anyone writing about HIV/AIDS in America: the timeline at hiv.gov/hiv-basics/overview/history/hiv-and-aids-timeline and the ACT UP Oral History Project at actuporalhistory.org.

Works cited or consulted:

Avena, Thomas, ed. *Life Sentences: Writers, Artists, and AIDS.* Mercury House, 1994.

Borger, Irene, ed. *From a Burning House: The AIDS Project Los Angeles Writers Workshop Collection.* Washington Square Press, 1996.

Cahill, Kevin M., ed. *The AIDS Epidemic.* St. Martin's Press, 1983.

Callen, Michael. *Surviving AIDS.* HarperCollins, 1990.

Castiglia, Christopher, and Christopher Reed. *If Memory Serves: Gay Men, AIDS, and the Promise of the Queer Past.* University of Minnesota Press, 2012.

Cheng, Jih-Fei, Alexandra Juhasz, and Nishant Shahani, eds. *AIDS and the Distribution of Crises.* Duke University Press, 2020.

Clark, Philip, and David Groff, eds. *Persistent Voices: Poetry by Writers Lost to AIDS.* Alyson Publications, 2009.

Czerwiec, MK. *Taking Turns: Stories from HIV/AIDS Care Unit 371.* Graphic Mundi, 2021.

Doty, Mark. *Fire to Fire: New and Selected Poems.* HarperCollins, 2008.

Duberman, Martin. *Hold Tight Gently: Michael Callen, Essex Hemphill, and the Battlefield of AIDS.* The New Press, 2014.

Ford, Michael Thomas. *100 Questions & Answers About AIDS: What You Need to Know Now.* Beech Tree, 1993.

Ford, Michael Thomas. *The Voices of AIDS: Twelve Unforgettable People Talk About How AIDS Has Changed Their Lives.* Morrow Junior Books, 1995.

France, David. *How to Survive a Plague: The Inside Story of How Citizens and Science Tamed AIDS.* Alfred A. Knopf, 2016.

Guibert, Hervé. *To the Friend Who Did Not Save My Life.* Semiotext(e), 2020; originally printed by Gallimard, 1990.

Gunn, Thom. *The Man with Night Sweats: Poems.* Farrar, Straus & Giroux, 1992.

Hadas, Rachel. *Unending Dialogue: Voices from an AIDS Poetry Workshop.* Faber & Faber, 1991.

Halkitis, Perry N. *The AIDS Generation: Stories of Survival and Resilience.* Oxford University Press, 2014.

Hein, Karen, Theresa Foy DiGeronimo, and the Editors of Consumer Reports Books. *AIDS: Trading Fears for Facts.* Consumers Union, 1989.

Hemphill, Essex, ed. *Brother to Brother: New Writings by Black Gay Men.* Alyson Books, 1991.

Holleran, Andrew. *Chronicle of a Plague, Revisited: AIDS and Its Aftermath.* Da Capo Press, 2008.

Horton, Randall, M. L. Hunter, and Becky Thompson, eds. *Fingernails Across the Chalkboard: Poetry and Prose on HIV/AIDS from the Black Diaspora.* Third World Press, 2007.

Howe, Marie. *What the Living Do: Poems.* W. W. Norton & Co, 1998.

Howe, Marie, and Michael Klein, eds. *In the Company of My Solitude: American Writing from the AIDS Pandemic.* Persea, 1995.

Hunter, B. Michael, ed. *Sojourner: Black Gay Voices in the Age of AIDS.* Other Countries Press, 1993.

Juhasz, Alexandra, and Theodore Kerr, *We Are Having This Conversation Now: The Times of AIDS Cultural Production.* Duke University Press, 2022.

Klein, Michael, ed. *Poets for Life: Seventy-Six Poets Respond to AIDS.* Persea, 1989.

Klein, Michael, and Richard McCann, eds. *Things Shaped in Passing: More "Poets for Life" Writing from the AIDS Pandemic.* Persea Books, 1997.

Kramer, Larry. *Reports from the Holocaust: The Making of an AIDS Activist.* St. Martin's Press, 1989.

Levithan, Robert. *The New 60: Outliving Yourself and Reinventing a Future.* CreateSpace, 2012.

Luna, G. Cajetan. *Youths Living with HIV: Self-Evident Truths.* Routledge, 1997.

Lyon, Maureen E., and Lawrence J. D'Angelo, eds. *Teenagers, HIV, and AIDS: Insights from Youths Living with the Virus.* Praeger, 2006.

Monette, Paul. *Borrowed Time: An AIDS Memoir.* Harcourt, Inc., 1988.

Monette, Paul. *Last Watch of the Night: Essays Too Personal and Otherwise.* Harcourt Brace & Company, 1994.

Monette, Paul. *West of Yesterday, East of Summer: New and Selected Poems.* St. Martin's Press, 1994.

Nungesser, Lon G. *Epidemic of Courage: Facing AIDS in America.* St. Martin's Press, 1986.

Patton, Cindy. *Fatal Advice: How Safe-Sex Education Went Wrong.* Duke University Press, 1996.

Peck, Dale. *Visions and Revisions: Coming of Age in the Age of AIDS.* Soho Press, 2015.

Peterkin, Allan, and Julie Hann, eds. *Still Here: A Post-Cocktail AIDS Anthology.* Life Rattle Press, 2008.

Petro, Anthony M. *After the Wrath of God: AIDS, Sexuality, & American Religion.* Oxford University Press, 2015.

Preston, John, ed. *Personal Dispatches: Writers Confront AIDS.* St. Martin's Press, 1989.

Richardson, Ann, and Dietmar Bolle. *Wise Before Their Time: People with AIDS and HIV Talk about Their Lives.* Glenmore Press, 2017, first published by Fount, HarperCollins, 1992.

Roscoe, Will, ed. *Living the Spirit: A Gay American Indian Anthology.* St. Martin's Press, 1988.

Ruskin, Cindy. *The Quilt: Stories from The NAMES Project.* Pocket, 1988.

Schulman, Sarah. *Let the Record Show: A Political History of ACT UP New York, 1987–1993.* Farrar, Straus & Giroux, 2021.

Shepard, Benjamin Heim. *White Nights and Ascending Shadows: An Oral History of the San Francisco AIDS Epidemic.* Cassell, 1997.

Shilts, Randy. *And the Band Played On: Politics, People, and the AIDS Epidemic.* St. Martin's Press, 1987.

Smith, Danez. *Don't Call Us Dead: Poems.* Graywolf Press, 2017.

Sycamore, Mattilda Bernstein, ed. *Between Certain Death and a Possible Future: Queer Writing on Growing Up with the AIDS Crisis.* Arsenal Pulp Press, 2021.

Vaucher, Andréa R. *Muses from Chaos and Ash: AIDS, Artists, and Art.* Grove Press, 1993.

White, Edmund, ed. *Loss Within Loss: Artists in the Age of AIDS*. University of Wisconsin Press, 2001.

White, Ryan, and Ann Marie Cunningham. *Ryan White: My Own Story*. Dial Books, 1991.

Wojnarowicz, David. *Close to the Knives: A Memoir of Disintegration*. Vintage, 1991.

# Suggested Reading on the Global AIDS Crisis

Every region of the world has a connection to HIV/AIDS. Infectious diseases don't care about borders: They travel from place to place and body to body. When it comes to the past and present global epidemic, our focus on the United States is just a small snapshot.

The World Health Organization's online resources contain the most accurate information about the circulation of HIV/AIDS in different regions of the world today.

For example:

WHO Information about HIV/AIDS in Africa: afro.who.int/health-topics/hivaids

WHO Information about HIV/AIDS in Europe: who.int/europe/health-topics/hiv-aids

WHO Information about HIV/AIDS in South-East Asia: who.int/southeastasia/health-topics/hiv-aids

Books (all adult nonfiction) about the global impact of HIV/AIDS include:

*To End a Plague: America's Fight to Defeat AIDS in Africa* by Emily Bass

*The Epidemic: A Global History of AIDS* by Jonathan Engel

*Our Kind of People: Thoughts on the HIV/AIDS Epidemic* by Uzodinma Iweala

*28: Stories of AIDS in Africa* by Stephanie Nolen

*Sizwe's Test: A Young Man's Journey Through Africa's AIDS Epidemic* by Jonny Steinberg

*HIV & AIDS: A Very Short Introduction* by Alan Whiteside

While there is little YA nonfiction about global AIDS, here are some recent young adult novels that represent experiences of HIV/AIDS in non-American contexts:

*We Kiss Them with Rain* by Futhi Ntshingila (2018) explores the impact of HIV/AIDS on different generations of women in South Africa. *Where We Go from Here* by Lucas Rocha (2018) depicts a young gay man's experience of HIV/AIDS in contemporary Brazil. *Auma's Long Run* by Eucabeth A. Odhiambo (2017) depicts a young girl's experience of the start of the AIDS crisis in Kenya.

Hopefully this shelf will have become more full by the time you read this, as more stories from around the world are told.

## Acknowledgments

We have worked on this book for over three years now. The list of people who we've discussed it with, who've cheered us on, who've challenged us to do the best job we can, is vast and truly beyond measure.

Thank you to all the people who shared their stories and perspectives with us for the book: Tina Valentin Aguirre, Antonio Boone, Elizabeth Coleman, John D'Amico, Kalee Garland, Milo Miller, Luna Luis Ortiz, Peggy Sue, Kay Poyer, Q, Mallery Jenna Robinson, Sarah Schulman, Floyd Sklaver, Justin Smith, Todd Theringer, Ricky Tucker, Derinthia Williams, and Ed Wolf. Thank you to Mathew Rodriguez for connecting us to the Dandelions.

Thank you to all the other voices whose poems and testimonies we have been grateful to republish as source material. Thanks, too, to those who granted permission for these voices to be heard in this book.

Thank you to the incomparable Gerard Koskovich and all the people who spoke to us at the San Francisco gathering he arranged. Thank you to Isaac Fellman and the GLBT Historical Society Archive in San Francisco, and to the wonderful archivists and librarians at the University of California—San Francisco and the San Francisco Public Library. Thank you to the librarians at the LGBT Community Center National History Archive in New York City and the New York Public Library for facilitating our research.

Thank you to everyone in the USA and around the world who continues to work for HIV/AIDS treatment and prevention to be accessible and affordable for all. Thank you, too, to everyone who is fighting to make sure books like this one remain on the shelves in libraries and classrooms, so the lessons of history can be learned.

Thank you to our early readers, whose insights improved the book: Sayantani DasGupta, Beth Levithan, Alexander Gray, and Charlie Medeiros.

Thank you to Ted Kerr and Sarah Schulman, two writers whose work has been invaluable to our thinking and whose help and wisdom have been enormously appreciated. Thank you to Brian Selznick and David Serlin for artistic and philosophical support. Thank you to Tucker Shaw for your help. Thank you to Kenneth Kidd for support within the scholarly realm, and Hatty Nestor for support in general. Thank you to Michael Ford for being there three decades before us. Thank you to the writers of YA nonfiction we admire, particularly Jason Reynolds, whose *Stamped* (a YA adaptation of Ibram X. Kendi's work) provided a template for how to talk about history to a teen audience. Thank you as well to Deborah Wiles, whose Sixties Trilogy was a structural inspiration for this book.

Thank you to all the various friends and family who have supported us as we've worked on this project. Thanks to everyone who stayed at the Wellfleet house, who were present at the summer of this book's creation (2022) and the summers it was drafted and completed (2023, 2024, 2025). Thank you to everyone in England who helped, especially Joshua Heath, for all that listening. Huge thanks to Beth Levithan for sharing so much wisdom and heart, and to Allen Levithan, whose enthusiasm for both justice and nonfiction is present in these pages.

Immense thanks to Dana Carey, this book's guardian angel. We truly could not have done it without you. Thanks to our editor, Marisa DiNovis, for all your support. Thanks to Nancy Hinkel, Renée Cafiero, Amy Schroeder, and Alix Inchausti for their eagle eyes, and to Christa Angelios and everyone else who helped with permissions. Thank you to Ray Shappell for bringing his care and passion to this book's cover and design, and to everyone whose handwriting was sampled for it. Thank you to everyone in the sales, marketing, library marketing, publicity, manufacturing, and production departments at Random House Children's Books, as well as Barbara Marcus and Mallory Loehr, for turning our labor of love into your labor of love. Thank you to our agent, Bill Clegg, and everyone at The Clegg Agency, as well as all the colleagues who've encouraged us along the way.

Finally, thank you to Bobby Levithan. You inspired this all.

# Resources

If you want to get tested for HIV and sexually transmitted infections, but you're unsure how to begin this process, consider talking to someone you trust: friends, family, your physician, guidance counselors at school or college.

Together TakeMeHome is an organization that offers free at-home HIV testing kits by mail: together.takemehome.org.

If you're interested in learning more about PrEP, check out Healthysexual at healthysexuals.com, an online resource that provides bite-size information about HIV and sexually transmitted infections. Healthysexual offers resources to help you find access to HIV/STI testing and PrEP services.

Here are some other resources that you may find useful—particularly if you're feeling affected by the larger scope of issues we've touched upon throughout this book.

### HIV.gov
hiv.gov/hiv-basics/overview/about-hiv-and-aids/what-are-hiv-and-aids

hiv.gov is one of the most up-to-date and prominent resources for learning more about treating HIV today and preventing HIV transmission.

### The Trevor Project
thetrevorproject.org

The Trevor Project is a suicide prevention and crisis intervention organization that supports LGBTQ+ young people.

### National Association for Children of Addiction

nacoa.org

Substance abuse plays a role in the ongoing transmission of HIV/AIDS. You can learn more about addiction and recovery on the NACoA website, with resources for young people experiencing problems relating to substance abuse in their families.

### RAINN

rainn.org

RAINN (the Rape, Abuse & Incest National Network) is a leading provider of services for people who've experienced sexual violence. RAINN's hotline services for support can be found here: rainn.org/help-and-healing/hotline/

### Advocates for Youth

advocatesforyouth.org

Advocates for Youth is a youth-centered organization dealing with adolescent sexual and reproductive health. The organization's website is overflowing with resources and links to related groups and projects.

None of us are alone. The story of AIDS in America is a story about the power of community, and we hope that this book encourages you to support your community—and to tell your own story.